APHASIOLOGY

Volume 18   Number 5/6/7   May/June/July 2004

33rd Clinical Aphasiology Conference
Editor: Patrick J. Doyle

CONTENTS

33rd Clinical Aphasiology Conference
Orcas Island, Washington, May 27th to May 31st, 2003

Editor
Patrick J. Doyle, Ph.D., Geriatric Research Education & Clinical Center, VA Pittsburgh Healthcare System, & Department of Communication Science & Disorders, University of Pittsburgh, Pittsburgh, PA, USA

Associate Editors
Kirrie J. Ballard, Ph.D., Department of Speech Pathology & Audiology, University of Iowa, Iowa City, IA, USA
Argye Elizabeth Hillis, MD, Department of Neurology, Johns Hopkins University, Baltimore, MD, USA
William Hula, MS, Geriatric Research Education & Clinical Center, VA Pittsburgh Healthcare System, and Department of Communication Science and Disorders, University of Pittsburgh, Pittsburgh, PA, USA
Aquiles Iglesias, Ph.D., Department of Communication Sciences, Temple University, Philadelphia, PA, USA
Mary Kennedy, Ph.D., Department of Communication Disorders, University of Minnesota, Minneapolis, MN, USA
Mikael D. Z. Kimelman, Ph.D., Department of Speech/Language Pathology, Duquesne University, Pittsburgh, PA, USA
Swathi Kiran, Department of Communication Science & Disorders, University of Texas, Austin, TX, USA
Stephen Nadeau, MD, Malcolm Randall DVA Medical Center & Department of Neurology, University of Florida, Gainesville, FL, USA
Katherine Odell, Ph.D., Department of Communication, University of Wisconsin, Madison, WI, USA
Grace Park, Ph.D., National Institute on Deafness and Other Communication Disorders, National Institutes of Health, Bethesda, MD, USA
Anastasia Raymer, Ph.D., Child Study Center, Old Dominion University, Norfolk, VA, USA
Donald Robin, Ph.D., School of Speech, Language, and Hearing Sciences and SDSU-UCSD Joint Doctoral Program in Language and Communication Disorders San Diego State University, San Diego, CA, USA
Susan Shaiman, Ph.D., Department of Communication Science & Disorders, University of Pittsburgh, Pittsburgh, PA, USA
Nina Simmons-Mackie, Ph.D., Department of Communication Science & Disorders, Southeastern Louisiana University, LA, USA
Connie Tompkins, Ph.D., Department of Communication Science & Disorders, University of Pittsburgh, Pittsburgh, PA, USA
Julie Wambaugh, Ph.D., Department of Communication Disorders, University of Utah, and VA Salt Lake City Healthcare System, Salt Lake City, UT, USA

AD-HOC Editorial Consultants

APHASIOLOGY, 2004, *18* (5/6/7), 405

Preface

The papers that appear in this special edition of *Aphasiology* were selected based upon their theoretical importance, clinical relevance, and scientific merit from among the many platform and poster presentations comprising the 33rd Annual Clinical Aphasiology Conference convened in Orcas Island, Washington, USA during the last week of May 2003. Each paper was peer-reviewed by the Editorial Consultants and Associate Editors acknowledged herein consistent with the standards of *Aphasiology* and the rigours of merit review that represent this indexed archival journal.

Patrick J. Doyle, Ph.D.
VA Pittsburgh Healthcare System
Pittsburgh, PA, USA

http://www.tandf.co.uk/journals/pp/02687038.html   DOI:10.1080/02687030444000282

APHASIOLOGY, 2004, *18* (5/6/7), 407–427

Modification of sound production treatment for apraxia of speech: Acquisition and generalisation effects

Julie Wambaugh

University of Utah & VA Salt Lake City Healthcare System, USA

Christina Nessler

VA Salt Lake City Healthcare System, USA

Background: Sound errors are characteristic of acquired apraxia of speech (AOS) and are frequently the focus of treatment. One treatment for AOS, Sound Production Treatment (SPT), has been shown to facilitate improved sound production in trained sounds and untrained exemplars of those sounds (Wambaugh, Kalinyak-Fliszar, West, & Doyle, 1998a). Although the effects of SPT are relatively well understood when the treatment has been applied sequentially to single sounds in words, little is known about its application to multiple sounds. Additionally, the stimulus generalisation effects of SPT have not been well specified.

Aims: This investigation was designed to further investigate the acquisition and stimulus generalisation effects of SPT for AOS. Treatment application was modified from previous investigations to allow for application with multiple sounds and in a different treatment context.

Methods & Procedures: A multiple baseline design across behaviours and contexts was used to assess the effects of treatment with a speaker with chronic AOS and aphasia. Treatment was initially applied within the context of words elicited through repetition. In order to assess stimulus generalisation, the nine consonants of interest were elicited in words through sentence completion. Additionally, the target sounds were elicited in a different word position (i.e., word-final) from that utilised in treatment (i.e., word-initial).

Outcomes & Results: Treatment resulted in increased correct productions of the target sounds in trained contexts. Generalisation to the different stimulus contexts was limited and varied across sounds. Treatment was extended to the sentence completion context and additional treatment gains were observed.

Conclusions: The application of SPT to multiple sounds and to an additional treatment context appears to have promise in the treatment of AOS. Additional replications are required for external validity.

Acquired apraxia of speech (AOS) is characterised by erroneous production of speech sounds, reduced rate of speech, increased time in transitioning between sounds, syllables, and words, and disordered prosody (Croot, 2002; McNeil, Doyle, & Wambaugh, 2000). These core symptoms may be accompanied by behaviours such as articulatory groping, difficulty initiating speech, and motoric perseverations. The sound errors

Address correspondence to: Julie Wambaugh, Research Service 151-A, VA Salt Lake City Healthcare System, 500 Foothill Blvd., Salt Lake City, UT 84148, USA. Email: julie.wambaugh@health.utah.edu

This research was supported, in part, by Rehabilitation Research and Development, Department of Veterans Affairs.

http://www.tandf.co.uk/journals/pp/02687038.html   DOI:10.1080/02687030444000165

observed with AOS take the form of distortions, perceived substitutions (often distorted), omissions, additions (e.g., intrusive schwa), and perseverations (McNeil, Robin, & Schmidt, 1997). Although evidence suggests that AOS sound errors are relatively predictable (McNeil, Odell, Miller, & Hunter, 1995; Mlcoch, Darley, & Noll, 1982; Shuster & Wambaugh, 2003; Wambaugh, Nessler, Bennett, & Mauszycki, 2004), controversy still exists regarding the consistency of AOS errors (Croot, 2002). However, examination of pretreatment baseline data in various treatment investigations clearly reveals that individuals with AOS have consistent difficulty in producing particular sounds that they find problematic (e.g., Knock, Ballard, Robin, & Schmidt, 2000; Raymer, Haley, & Kendall, 2002; Raymer & Thompson, 1991; Wambaugh, in press; Wambaugh et al., 1998a; Wambaugh, Martinez, McNeil, & Rogers, 1999; Wambaugh, West, & Doyle, 1998b)

The majority of investigations that have examined treatments for AOS have focused on approaches to facilitate improved articulation of sounds (Wambaugh, Duffy, McNeil, Rogers, & Robin, 2003). Effects of articulatory-kinematic AOS treatments have generally reported positive results (see McNeil et al., 2000, for a review). Unfortunately, as discussed by Wambaugh (2002), there has been limited replication of findings specific to any given treatment or technique.

One of the few approaches for the treatment of AOS that has received systematic investigation is "Sound Production Treatment" (SPT; Wambaugh et al., 1998a). SPT comprises a combination of repetition, production of minimally contrastive words, integral stimulation, phonetic placement cues, and repeated practice, and was designed to promote improved consonant production. SPT has been demonstrated to have positive results in terms of acquisition of trained sounds and response generalisation to untrained exemplars of trained sounds (Wambaugh, Doyle, Kalinyak, & West, 1996; Wambaugh et al., 1998a; Wambaugh et al., 1999). Response generalisation to untrained sounds has been limited, but maintenance of successfully trained sounds has typically been strong (see Wambaugh, 2001, for a summary of SPT research).

Stimulus generalisation, the occurrence of trained behaviours in untrained contexts, has been examined in two investigations of SPT (Wambaugh et al., 1998a; Wambaugh, in press). Wambaugh et al. (1998a) targeted sounds in single words and measured generalised production of those sounds in phrases with three speakers with AOS and aphasia. Stimulus generalisation results differed across the participants, with consistently positive results for one speaker, inconsistent increases in target sound productions for another speaker, and no generalisation for the remaining speaker. Wambaugh (in press) examined stimulus generalisation effects of SPT by measuring production of trained sounds in unmodelled productions of trained words and in utterances that were longer and phonetically more complex than those used in training. Results were positive for both participants, but varied across stimulus contexts and target sounds.

An understanding of the stimulus generalisation effects of any treatment is critical for obvious reasons. The ecological validity of a behavioural treatment relates to whether or not the desired behaviour has utility for the individual in his/her environment. If the effects of treatment are limited to the training condition, then such effects will necessarily have limited utility. At the current time, there is not a well-developed technology for measuring the impact of therapy on an individual's production of speech in situations that are meaningful for that individual. However, measurement of treatment effects in contexts that systematically vary from those used in training will further our knowledge of the strengths/limitations of that treatment, even if those measurement contexts are somewhat artificial at this point in time.

One should never assume that stimulus generalisation will necessarily occur as a result of any treatment, despite what may be predicted from relevant theory (i.e., scientific measurement is requisite). The authors largely subscribe to the definition of AOS advanced by McNeil et al. (1997) that the speech behaviours observed with AOS result from difficulties in translating an accurate and filled phonologic frame to the previously acquired kinematic parameters required for correct articulation. It is theorised that SPT may act to improve access to or specification of (perhaps a deviation from McNeil et al.) the generalised motor program (GMP; Schmit & Lee, 1999) and/or associated parameters of targeted sounds (see Clark & Robin, 1998, or McNeil et al., 2000, for discussions of motor programs). As indicated previously, when SPT has been applied to a limited number of exemplars of targeted sounds, strong response generalisation to untrained exemplars has consistently occurred. This suggests that production improvements may extend beyond the treatment tasks. That is, the probable improvement in implementation of the GMP or parameterization was not item-specific. Although stimulus generalisation testing, by definition, requires different task demands, improvements that are not item-specific may also be robust enough to generalise to different tasks.

Knock et al. (2000) suggested that principles of motor learning may provide insights into facilitating generalisation with respect to treatment of AOS. They investigated the effects of blocked stimulus presentation versus random stimulus presentation, utilising Phonetic Placement Therapy (Van Riper & Irwin, 1958) with two participants who had severe AOS. Although their findings did not correspond perfectly with the limb motor literature (e.g., blocked and random practice resulted in similar rates of acquisition), the results provided preliminary evidence that random presentation of stimuli may be more effective in promoting retention and transfer of behaviours than blocked presentation for some AOS speakers.

Random practice necessitates training of two or more target sounds concurrently. The majority of investigations of SPT have implemented treatment with only one sound at a time in order to study potential generalisation effects across sounds (Wambaugh, 2001). Concurrent training of multiple sounds offers other possible benefits, such as more efficient use of time. Additionally, multiple sound training may serve to reduce inappropriate, overgeneralised production of trained sounds, which has been reported for SPT as well as other AOS treatments (Knock et al., 2000; Raymer et al., 2002; Wambaugh et al., 1999).

The primary purpose of this investigation was to further examine the stimulus generalisation effects of SPT. Specifically, the study was designed to examine the effects of SPT applied in word-level repetition contexts on sound production in two different stimulus contexts: (1) words elicited in sentence completion tasks, and (2) words in which the target sounds occurred in a different word position from that used in training. SPT was modified to incorporate randomised practice of treatment stimuli in an effort to facilitate generalised responding. Furthermore, the study was designed to extend treatment to the sentence completion context in the event of lack of adequate generalisation effects.

METHOD

Participant

The participant was a male native English speaker with moderate aphasia and moderate-severe AOS. He was 66 years old, premorbidly right handed, and 4 years post-onset of a single left-hemisphere stroke. He had completed 11 years of education, was a retired press operator, and lived at home with his wife. His verbal language production was characterised by non-fluent, agrammatic phrases and short sentences (pretreatment testing data are shown in Table 1). His speech production was consistent with AOS characteristics described by McNeil et al. (1997). Specifically, his speech was consistently slow with syllable segregation and distorted sound errors. His sound errors were relatively predictable in terms of their location and type. In addition to AOS, the participant displayed speech production behaviours consistent with a diagnosis of unilateral upper motor neuron dysarthria, as described by Duffy (1995) (e.g., slow rate, slow AMRs, imprecise articulation [note: all of the preceding are also consistent with a diagnosis of AOS], decreased loudness, occasional harshness, and associated symptoms of drooling, unilateral lower facial and tongue weakness).

The participant had received treatment for consonant production errors in an earlier investigation that had concluded approximately 3 years prior to the initiation of the current study (Wambaugh et al., 1999). Following that study, he received Response Elaboration Training (RET; Kearns, 1997) as well as lexical retrieval treatment and made gains in verbal productivity. However, he continued to have difficulty with sound production. The gains that he had made in production of /p/, /k/, and "sh" in the previous sound training study had not been maintained.

Experimental stimuli

Acquisition and response generalisation stimuli   A total of 72 CV(C) words representing nine consonants served as treatment stimuli: Group 1: /s/, /p/, /v/; Group 2: /k/, "sh", "j"; and Group 3: /m/, /n/, /l/. The words included eight exemplars of each

TABLE 1
Pre-treatment measures

Measures	Scores
Porch Index of Communicative Ability (Porch, 1981)	
Overall average	10.04
Percentile	40th
Western Aphasia Battery (Kertesz, 1982)	
Aphasia Quotient (100 possible)	70
Aphasia classification	Broca's
Apraxia Battery for Adults (Dabul, 1979)	
Severity Score	Moderate to severe
Assessment of Intelligibility of Dysarthric Speech (Yorkston & Beukelman, 1981)	
% of intelligible words	28%
Test of Adolescent/Adult Word Finding (German, 1990)	
Total raw score (107 possible)	64
AOS Characteristics (after McNeil, Robin, & Schmidt, 1997)	
Slow rate in all productions	yes
Inability to increase rate and preserve sound integrity	yes
Phoneme distortions	yes
Distorted perceived sound substitutions	yes
Errors relatively consistent in type and location	yes
Intrusive schwa	rarely
Articulatory groping	yes

consonant with the target in the word-initial position (see Appendix A). The choice of these consonants was determined primarily by the participant's performance during pretreatment testing in which his productions of numerous exemplars of each consonant were evaluated (Wambaugh et al., 1998a). Sounds that were difficult to produce were selected. The groupings of the nine consonants were not determined randomly. The sounds were grouped so that Groups 1 and 2 would be approximately equivalent in terms of composition and difficulty (at least during baseline) for the participant. Both groups included a voiceless stop that had been trained previously with success (i.e., /p/ and /k/). Both included a sibilant: /s/ and "sh". Although "sh" had been trained previously with some success, its production had not been mastered. The choice of the remaining sound in each group, /v/ and "j", was constrained by several factors. Voiced-voiceless cognates were not considered for training because of potential generalisation effects of treatment. Sounds that were used as "replacing" sounds (see below) were excluded, as were sounds that were produced with high levels of accuracy. Thus, the sounds that remained as viable choices were /m, n, l/, /v/ or /f/, and "ch" or "j". Consequently, /v/ and "j" were chosen for Groups 1 and 2, respectively. "j" was chosen instead of "ch" so that it could be more readily differentiated from "sh" and was placed in the same group as "sh" to constrain any potential generalisation to within group. Group 3, /m, n, l/, was recognised as "easier" for this participant on the basis of his pretreatment testing and baseline performance.

The words in each group were selected so that minimal pairs were formed across all three sounds in the group whenever possible (e.g., set-pet-vet). Minimal contrast pairs/triplets were delineated as sets of morphemes that differed by only one sound segment (Edwards, 1992; Shriberg & Kent, 1982), and not necessarily by only one feature (Newman, Creaghead, & Secord, 1985). These words were utilised to assess acquisition effects (i.e., production of trained items in a word repetition probe not occurring during treatment), as well as response generalisation effects (i.e., not all sounds were treated at one time, allowing for assessment of treatment effects to untrained sounds).

For each set of target minimal pair words (e.g., set-pet-vet), an additional minimal pair word was selected for treatment purposes. Treatment (described below) required that the target sounds be practised in contrast to the participant's "replacing" sounds in the context of minimal pair words. The contrast words were chosen on the basis of the participant's typical error productions. For example, the participant usually produced a sound that was perceived as a distorted "th" or a /d/ when attempting to produce most initial fricatives and stops. Therefore, the contrast words for Group 1 (s, p, v) included words beginning with /θ/, /ð/, and /d/ (e.g., sat-pat-vat-*that*) (see Appendix A; treatment contrast column). Real words were chosen as contrast words as frequently as possible.

Stimulus generalisation stimuli.   As indicated previously, stimulus generalisation refers to the use of trained behaviours in untrained contexts. The untrained contexts examined in this investigation were sentence completion contexts and word-final position contexts.

Five words were selected for each sound from the group of 72 words to use to form sentence completion items (e.g., My dog has been very sick for two days. I need to take her to the ... vet; see Appendix B). The sentence completion context was chosen to allow for assessment of trained sounds in words that were produced without a verbal model.

To assess generalisation from word-initial position treatment to word-final position productions, five exemplars for each of the nine consonants were selected. These items were VC and CVC real words that all began with a vowel or the sounds /d/, /t/, or /h/ (see Appendix A; last 3 columns).

Experimental design

A multiple baseline design across behaviours and contexts was utilised. Treatment was applied to one group of sounds while the two other sound groups remained untreated, but were continually probed to assess response generalisation. Following attainment of sound production goals, treatment was terminated with Group 1 sounds and extended to Group 2 sounds, and subsequently to Group 3. Upon completion of training with Group 3, treatment was applied to all sound groups simultaneously to attempt to re-establish productions with Groups 1 and 2.

Because minimal stimulus generalisation was observed as a result of the initial applications of SPT (i.e., treatment of Groups 1, 2, and 3 separately and together), treatment was extended to the stimulus generalisation context. As in the repetition context, sound groups were treated sequentially.

Baseline phase. Production of the targeted sounds was repeatedly examined in word repetition and sentence completion contexts. The 72 words containing the sounds in the word-initial position were presented as a group of items in random order and the participant was instructed to repeat each word. The 45 sentence completion items were also presented as a group in random order as were the 45 word-final position items. The order of presentation of the three groups of stimuli (i.e., word-initial, sentence completion, word-final) was randomised for each probe session.

The participant's productions were transcribed on-line using broad phonetic transcription with audio-recordings used for verification. If the transcription corresponded to the target sound, the production was scored as correct. That is, just the target sound, not the entire word, was required to be produced accurately to achieve a correct score. Probes were conducted seven times in each condition during the baseline phase.

Treatment phase. Treatment was conducted two to three times per week in the participant's home by a certified speech/language pathologist. Probing (as described above) was administered prior to treatment sessions. During the treatment of Groups 1, 2, and 3, probes of the 72 words were conducted prior to each treatment session and stimulus generalisation probes were conducted approximately every two to four sessions. During treatment in the sentence completion context, sentence completion probes were conducted prior to every fourth session and probes of the word-initial items (maintenance—see below) and word-final repetition items were conducted approximately every sixth session. Sentence completion probes were not conducted on a daily basis (as had occurred with treatment of Groups 1, 2, and 3) because the sentence completion training required more time to complete the treatment trials.

Maintenance and follow-up phases. Maintenance of previously trained items was measured during the periods of subsequent training utilising the same probe procedures. During the word repetition training phases, previously trained sound groups were probed on a daily basis. However, during the sentence completion training production of the 72 items in Groups 1, 2, and 3 were measured using a reduced probing schedule. The reduced probing schedule was employed primarily to save time and reduce the probing burden on the participant. However, this reduced schedule also provided a more stringent measure of maintenance. That is, repeated exposures in daily probes may have served to reinforce behaviours. (Note: A reduced schedule of probing was not possible during the word repetition phases because this would have necessitated administering only portions of the group of 72 words.)

Follow-up probes were conducted at 2 and 6 weeks following completion of all treatment.

Treatment

SPT in word repetition context.   SPT was originally designed for application to words or phrases in a repetition context (Wambaugh et al., 1998a). SPT was modified slightly for this investigation in order to try to prevent potential detrimental overgeneralisation (a problem for this participant in a previous study). The modifications included (1) treatment of multiple sounds concurrently, (2) combined use of blocked and randomised practice, and (3) use of minimal contrast practice only upon incorrect responses (to maximise practice time with multiple sounds). The treatment cueing hierarchy (see Appendix C) was applied to each target word, with successive steps being used only upon an incorrect response.

As many trials as possible were conducted in a treatment session. One trial equalled one presentation of each of the 24 words in the group. A total of four to six trials were conducted per treatment session, with the number of trials typically increasing with increasing numbers of sessions within a treatment phase (i.e., increased numbers of trials were possible as the participant became more proficient with the tasks).

The first trial of every session was conducted with *blocked* presentation of the treatment stimuli (e.g., presentation of all eight words of the first sound followed by presentation of all eight words of the second sound, and finally presentation of all eight words of the third sound). Order of the blocked sounds was randomised across sessions. If six of eight items were correct during the blocked trial for all three sounds, then the remaining trials were alternated between blocked and *randomised* presentation (i.e., all exemplars for all three sounds were randomised). Treatment was begun with blocked practice to promote rapid acquisition of correct sound production (Schmidt & Lee, 1999) and to ostensibly provide successful experiences for the participant. However, the employment of randomised practice was considered to be necessary to promote generalisation of the skill (Schmidt & Lee, 1999).

When SPT was applied to all nine sounds simultaneously, the same hierarchy was employed, but all trials were randomised across the nine sounds.

Treatment was scheduled to be applied to each group of sounds until the participant achieved 90% correct responding with all sounds in probes, or until a maximum of 30 sessions were conducted with that group. Across all word repetition training phases (i.e., Group 1, Group 2, Group 3, and all groups), 91 treatment sessions were provided.

SPT in sentence completion context.   A treatment hierarchy was devised that approximated the original hierarchy as closely as possible, while taking into account the different task demands (see Appendix D). Sounds were treated by group, utilising randomised practice. The minimal contrast step was eliminated because of semantic incongruities (i.e., the contrast words were incongruous when inserted into the sentence completion items). Treatment was scheduled to be applied to a sound group until the participant achieved 80% correct responding across three probes for all sounds or until

20 treatment sessions had been conducted. A total of 54 sentence completion training sessions were provided.

RESULTS

SPT in word repetition context

Acquisition and response generalisation data are shown in Figure 1. Each group of sounds is represented on a separate graph, with different symbols used to show each sound within the group. These data represent sound productions during probes, not during treatment. As seen in Figure 1, when treatment was applied to Group 1 (/s,p,v/), the participant rapidly acquired production of /p/ items, and more slowly achieved high levels of correct production of /s/ and /v/. When treatment was applied to Group 2 (/k/, "sh", "j"), increases in correct productions were observed for /k/ and "sh". Productions of /k/ reached 88% correct for four of the five final probes within that phase. Productions of "sh" increased to a high of 88% correct, but then those productions fell to 25–63% correct in the last five probes in that treatment phase. Productions of "j" remained at 0% correct and treatment of "j" was discontinued after 11 sessions due to the participant's frustration with this sound.

Although baseline productions of the sounds in Groups 1 and 2 had been remarkably stable, baseline productions of sounds in Group 3 were variable. During the initial, "true", baseline probes, productions of Group 3 sounds ranged from 0% to 50% for /l/ and 0% to 38% for /m/ and /n/. During training of Group 1, productions of Group 3 sounds remained variable, but similar to those in the true baseline phase. However, during Group 2 training, correct productions of /m/ reached accuracy levels ranging from 63% to 100% (across the last five probes in the phase) without direct training. Upon completion of Group 2 training, two additional probes were conducted to ensure that productions of /n/ and /l/ were not increasing as well. Following application of treatment to Group 3, productions of /n/ and /l/ increased and reached levels of 100% correct, while productions of /m/ remained at high levels (productions of all three sounds ranged from 88% to 100% across the final three probes of the phase).

As indicated above, positive response generalisation was noted when productions of /m/ increased as a result of Group 2 training. This was the only clear occurrence of across sound generalisation.

Maintenance effects were evaluated by continually measuring previously treated sounds during reapplication of SPT to a new sound group. Treated Group 1 items responded differentially: (1) /p/ productions were maintained during Group 2 treatment, and declined during Group 3 treatment, and (2) /s/ and /v/ productions declined through Group 2 and Group 3 treatment, with /v/ eventually returning to baseline levels. /p/ and /s/ productions were extremely variable during Group 3 training, with /p/ productions ranging from 13% to 100% accuracy and /s/ productions ranging from 25% to 100% accuracy. The Group 2 items that had increased in correct productions (i.e., /k/, "sh") also declined (with much variability observed) during withdrawal of treatment, but remained above baseline levels. However, productions of "j" increased to relatively high levels towards the end of Group 3 training. Coinciding with the increase in correct "j" productions was a return to maximum treatment levels for "sh". Reapplication of SPT to all sound groups resulted in reinstatement of previously achieved levels of accuracy for all sounds (note: /p/, /s/, and "sh" had begun to return to treatment levels during the end of Group 3 training).

Stimulus generalisation data for the sentence completion context are shown in Figure 2. Each group of sounds is represented on a separate graph. Vertical arrows indicate when

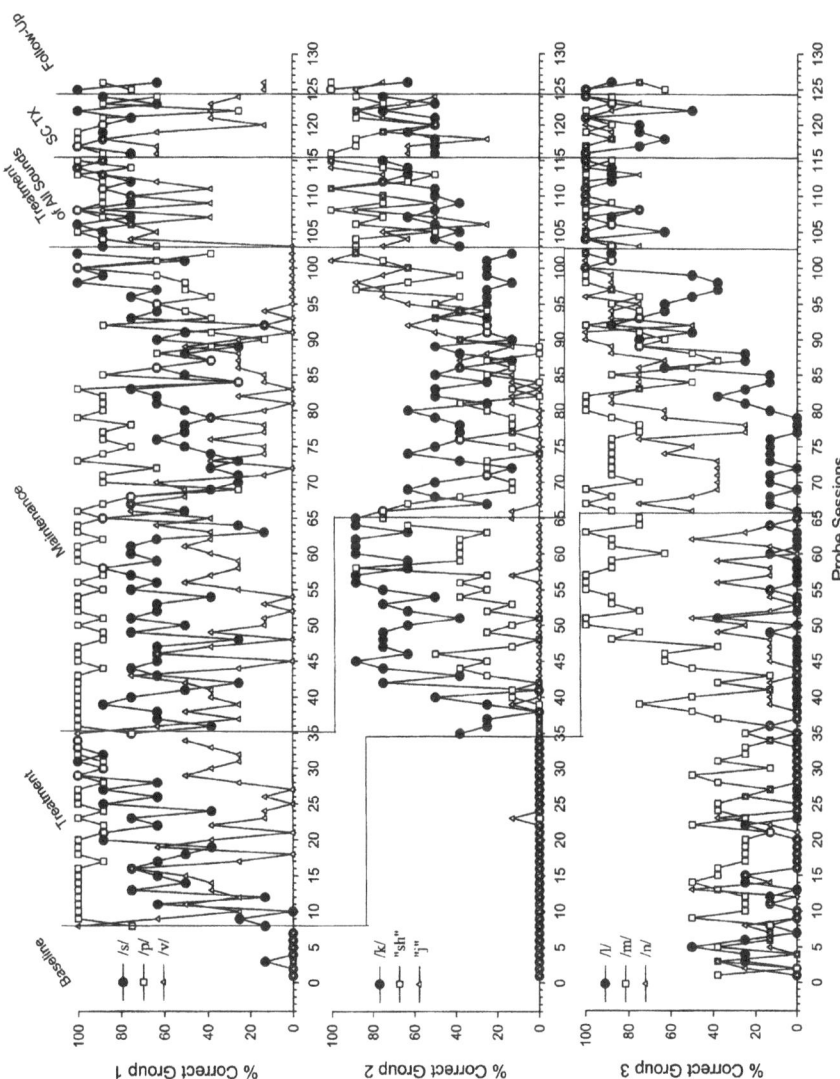

Figure 1. Percent of sounds produced correctly in word repetition probes. Vertical lines indicate different phases of the investigation. SC TX = story completion level training. Treatment discontinued with 'j' after probe #45.

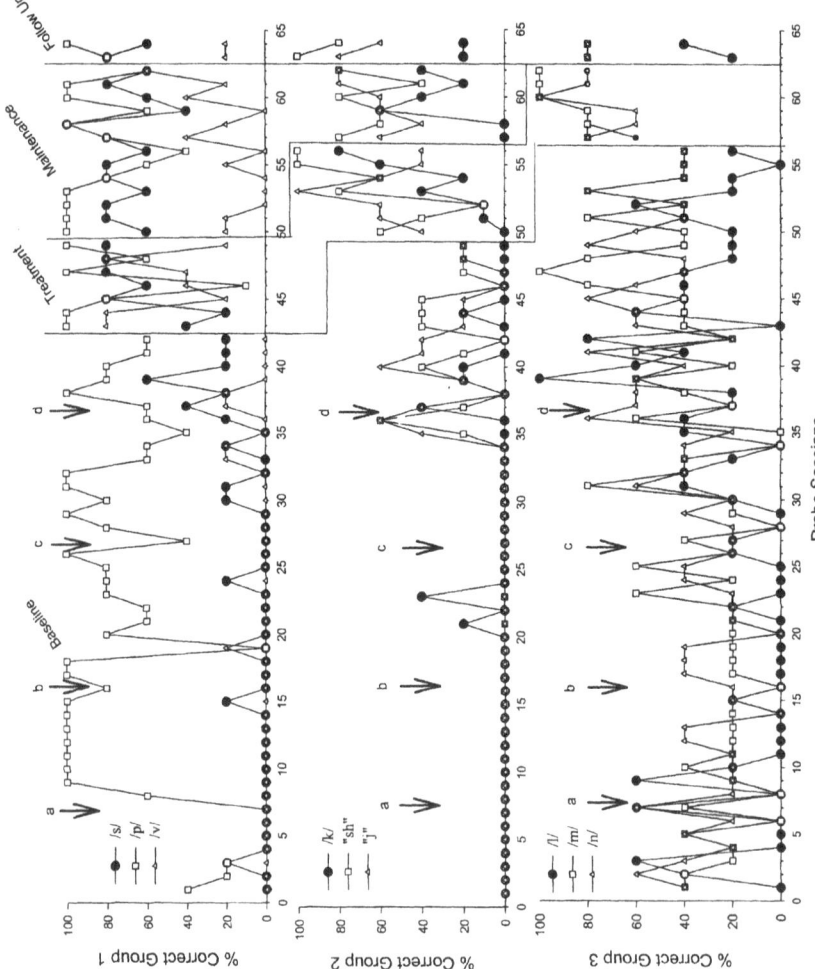

Figure 2 Percent of sounds produced correctly in sentence completion probes. Arrows indicate initiation of treatment. Arrows indicate initiation of treatment at the word repetition level: a = treatment of Group 1; b = treatment of Group 2; c = treatment of Group 3; and d = treatment of all sounds. Vertical lines indicate application of treatment in the story completion context, followed by maintenance, and follow up.

each group of sounds was submitted to SPT in the word repetition context. As seen in Figure 2, word repetition level treatment did not result in changes in sentence completion productions for any of the sounds other than /p/. Productions of /p/ increased rapidly to high levels following application of SPT in the word repetition context. As seen by examining the data following application of treatment to all nine sounds (arrow labelled "d"), increases in correct productions of all remaining sounds (except /m/) coincided with this phase of treatment.

SPT in sentence completion context

Figure 2 also shows correct responses in sentence completion probes conducted during treatment applied in the story completion context. Vertical lines indicate when treatment occurred with each group of sounds. Treatment was applied first to Group 1 sounds and increases were seen in correct responses to /s/ and /v/ items (recall that /p/ responses were at high levels following word repetition treatment). Levels of 80% correct were achieved for /s/ across the final three probes of this phase. Although a high of 80% was reached for /v/, correct productions returned to 20% accuracy in the final probe of the phase.

Treatment was next applied to Group 2 items and relatively consistent increases were seen for "sh" and /k/, with inconsistent increases seen for "j". Specifically, the final three probes of the phase were as follows for these sounds: (1) 60%, 100%, and 100% for "sh"; (2) 20%, 60%, and 80% for /k/; and (3) 60%, 40%, and 40% for "j".

When treatment was applied to Group 3, improvements in accuracy and consistency of production were seen for all three sounds (e.g., 80% to 100% accuracy for all three sounds across the final three probes). Follow-up probes revealed maintenance of high levels of correct production for all sounds, with the exception of /v/, /l/ and /k/.

Figure 1 shows maintenance data for the word repetition items in probes conducted throughout the sentence completion training (labelled "SC Tx."). As seen in the top graph, correct productions of /v/ decreased throughout this phase of training, while productions of the remaining sounds remained above baseline levels (although performance was variable). Productions of word repetition items during follow-up probes remained at relatively high levels, with the exception of /v/.

Changes in the participant's productions of the target sounds in word-final position items are shown in Table 2. Although these items were probed continually throughout the investigation, only data from probes conducted during baseline and at the end of each phase of treatment are shown (note: these data are similar to the data that are not displayed). As seen in the baseline probes, the participant produced several sounds (i.e., /p,k,m,n/) at high levels of accuracy prior to treatment. The accuracy levels of these sounds remained high throughout the investigation. Of the remaining sounds, only /l/ improved in the final position after word-initial training. Of interest is the observation that "sh" and "j" reached 100% and 80% accuracy levels, respectively, following Group 3 training. Also, /s/ reached 80% accuracy after Group 2 training, dropped to 40% accuracy after Group 3 training, and reached 100% accuracy after training of all sounds. All sounds, except /v/, remained at high accuracy levels (i.e., 80–100%) during sentence completion training and at follow-up.

DISCUSSION

As in previous investigations of SPT (Wambaugh et al., 1998a, 1999, 2003), positive acquisition effects were seen for consonants that received treatment. It appears that

TABLE 2
Sound production accuracy in word-final position items

Sounds	Baseline (BL) 1	BL 2	BL 3	BL 4	BL 5	BL 6	BL 7	Final probe following treatment: Group 1	Final probe following treatment: Group 2	Final probe following treatment: Group 3	Final probe following treatment of all Groups	Final probe following sentence completion: Group 1	Final probe following sentence completion: Group 2	Final probe following sentence completion: Group 3
Group 1 Final /s/	**40%**	**40%**	**20%**	**0%**	**40%**	**40%**	**60%**	**60%**	**80%**	**40%**	**100%**	**80%**	**80%**	**80%**
Group 1 Final /p/	100%	100%	80%	100%	100%	80%	100%	100%	100%	100%	100%	100%	100%	100%
Group 1 Final /v/	**0%**	**40%**	**80%**	**0%**	**40%**	**0%**	**0%**	**0%**	**20%**	**60%**	**80%**	**60%**	**60%**	**100%**
Group 2 Final /k/	40%	80%	80%	100%	80%	100%	80%	100%	100%	80%	100%	100%	80%	100%
Group 2 Final 'sh'	**0%**	**0%**	**0%**	**0%**	**0%**	**0%**	**0%**	**0%**	**20%**	**100%**	**100%**	**100%**	**100%**	**100%**
Group 2 Final 'j'	**0%**	**0%**	**0%**	**0%**	**0%**	**0%**	**0%**	**0%**	**0%**	**80%**	**100%**	**80%**	**80%**	**100%**
Group 3 Final /l/	**0%**	**0%**	**0%**	**0%**	**0%**	**0%**	**0%**	**0%**	**0%**	**100%**	**100%**	**100%**	**100%**	**100%**
Group 3 Final /m/	100%	60%	100%	100%	100%	100%	80%	100%	100%	100%	100%	100%	100%	100%
Group 3 Final /n/	100%	100%	100%	100%	100%	80%	100%	100%	100%	100%	100%	100%	100%	100%

Sounds produced poorly in baseline are displayed in bold type.

targeting several sounds simultaneously was not detrimental to acquisition for this participant.

As expected, response generalisation to untrained sounds was minimal. Positive across-sound generalisation was observed only for the sound /m/. The /m/ appeared to be the most likely candidate for positive response generalisation in that it was produced correctly more frequently than any of the other Group 2 and 3 sounds during baseline and the first treatment phase (as well as any of the Group 1 sounds). Like many speakers with AOS, the participant had obvious difficulty with spatial targeting of his articulators. The probe condition may have actually served as a treatment, in that the examiner provided an obvious model of the spatial target for /m/ when she provided a model for repetition. Although verbal models were provided for all target sounds, the visibility of the positioning of the articulators would have been relatively obscured, except for /m/ and /p/. The other bilabial, /p/, did not undergo extended baseline probing, but did improve rapidly with treatment (more so than the other sounds treated in the previous investigation). Another possible factor contributing to the relatively better production of /m/ in baseline and its improvement without treatment is the fact that tongue movement was not required for its production. The participant displayed considerable difficulty in positioning his tongue and consequently /m/ production may have been relatively less difficult than most of the other sounds (/p/ data are consistent with this notion).

It may be argued that /m/ should have been a more difficult sound to produce (and less amenable to change) because of the requirement of "integration and coupling of oral and nasal subsystems" (anonymous reviewer). Obviously, the baseline data indicated that /m/ was an easier sound for this AOS speaker and he had no observed difficulty in coupling the oral and nasal subsystems. The probe words were elicited without a carrier phrase, so that productions were preceded by a presumed resting articulatory state (i.e., the velum would have likely been in non-raised, respiratory status such as required for /m/ production). Consequently, the probe condition did not provide a challenging context for producing nasal sounds. Individual AOS speakers have been observed to have relatively more impairment of one speech subsystem than another (Dworkin & Abkarian, 1996, Marshall, Gandour, & Windsor, 1988). This participant appeared to have relatively intact functioning and coordinated use of the velopharyngeal subsystem. The use of /b/ as a "replacing sound" for /m/ (a possible indication of difficulty in coordination of oral/nasal) did not occur until treatment was initiated for /p/, indicating difficulty with overgeneralisation rather than with velopharyngeal coordination. Thus, it appears likely that the participant found /m/ to be a relatively easier sound to produce, which is also consistent with developmental speech data (Prather, Hedrick, & Kern, 1975; Sander, 1972)

Across-sound generalisation may also have occurred for "j" during Group 3 training. However, improvements in "j" productions had been observed when "j" received direct treatment. These improvements were not reflected in the binary scoring used in graphing because the improved "j" productions remained distorted. It is possible that the participant was able to further refine his "j" productions as overall sound production facility improved.

The changes in /m/ and "j" that occurred independent of treatment may also be interpreted as a loss of some experimental control. However, the fact that changes occurred for the other seven sounds only upon application of treatment speaks against a loss of experimental control. When examining behaviours that may be susceptible to change without intervention, the use of experimental designs that require extensive, repeated probing may be problematic. Repeated exposure alone has been shown to result in improved word finding in aphasia (Fink, Schwartz, Sobel, & Myers, 1997; Nickels, 2002). There are no data currently available that have addressed the issue of repeated exposure on sound production in AOS. In future investigations that may require extended probing of target sound productions in AOS, a design that reduces probing, such as a multiple probe design, may be an appropriate choice. However, the use of a reduced probing schedule would introduce the risk of missing potential generalisation.

Stimulus generalisation effects of SPT applied to repeated words were minimal for the majority of the sounds in terms of changes in production in the sentence completion context. With the exception of /p/, any observed changes were relatively unstable. These findings suggest that production of the target words in the sentence completion context was a more demanding task for this participant than the word repetition task. The sentence completion task required the participant to retrieve the target lexical item without the benefit of a model. Although the lexical item was typically retrieved, its correct articulation was not realised, with incorrect productions being similar to errors observed in the word repetition context. Extension of SPT to the sentence completion context resulted in improved productions for all sounds within this context. However, productions were relatively variable and some decreases in accuracy were seen when treatment was withdrawn and applied to a different sound group. It appears that unless correct productions are well learned, or perhaps overlearned in a repetition context (as with /p/), generalisation should not be expected to an unmodelled production context. It would be difficult to provide training for sound production without employing some form of modelling. However, perhaps treatments such as SPT should incorporate a step at which the AOS speaker could practise production without a model. For example, the SPT hierarchy could be modified to utilise a sentence completion cue as the first step of the hierarchy (i.e., prior to the modelling/repetition step).

Stimulus generalisation effects with respect to generalisation across word positions were positive, but not predictable. For the nine sounds of interest, it appears that the participant had less difficulty with word-final position productions than word-initial (see baseline productions). The re-establishment of production of the problematic sounds did seem to facilitate their production in word-final contexts.

Maintenance effects were also similar to those seen in previous investigations of SPT in that some decreases were observed when training was removed, particularly for sounds that had not reached high, consistent levels of production during training. For this participant, overgeneralization had been a pervasive problem when he received SPT applied to individual sounds (Wambaugh et al., 1999). It appears that, for this participant, training of multiple sounds served to restrict the occurrence of overgeneralisation to some extent. A formal error analysis was not undertaken in this investigation. However, probes in which there was a large decrease in correct productions of sounds that had been produced previously with high levels of accuracy were examined. These probes revealed that the regression errors were generally not due to overgeneralisation of sounds under training. The errors, instead, were similar to those produced in baseline. It appears that the multiple sound training may have facilitated a degree of stimulus discrimination not observed in the previous investigation. Perhaps the relatively temporary decrease in accuracy in previously trained sounds reflected a shifted focus during probes. It would seem to be a natural result of treatment that the sounds undergoing treatment would have received extra attention/effort during probing. If the sounds not undergoing treatment were not produced with relative ease, a decrease in performance would not be surprising. The reinstatement of training on all sounds may have served, in part, to refocus the participant on the previously trained sounds.

The reinstitution of treatment with previously trained groups (in the form of training of all target sounds) re-established high levels of correct production relatively quickly and may be an appropriate consideration in clinical application. Such practice is consistent with motor learning principles which suggest that random practice is important in generalising and maintaining learned behaviours (Schmidt & Lee, 1999). However, it is unlikely that training nine sounds simultaneously would have been a viable choice in establishing correct sound production initially. Specifically, relatively few trials with each sound were possible when practising the nine sounds concurrently. It is likely that training on the sound groups was a necessary precursor to the concurrent training. However, further investigation is required to substantiate this speculation. It is probable that individuals will respond differently to concurrent, multiple sound training, and response variability may be linked to factors such as the chronicity and severity of the speech disruption. Of course, the previous application of SPT several years preceding this investigation may have played a role in this participant's positive response to SPT applied to sound groups.

With the exception of the initial baseline probes for Groups 1 and 2, the participant's productions were variable for most sounds throughout most phases of the investigation. During baseline, the sounds in Groups 1 and 2 were almost never produced correctly, indicating a consistent inability to access the GMPs or parameter specifications required for their production. For sounds that were produced correctly on occasion (i.e., Group 3 sounds in baseline and all sounds following institution of treatment), access remained largely inconsistent. Production of /p/ was the main exception to the observed inconsistency. /p/ productions remained consistently between 88% and 100% for 59 consecutive sessions (with only one deviation to 75%). Of those sessions, 32 occurred during withdrawal of treatment for /p/ and the remaining 27 sessions represented probes that occurred during treatment of /p/. Clearly, /p/ received a great deal of treatment after high levels of accuracy had already been achieved (i.e., numerous opportunities for overlearning were provided). /m/ was the only other sound to receive many treatment sessions after high accuracy levels had been reached. Productions of /m/ remained relatively consistent (i.e., 75% to 100%) after treatment was initiated, with only two exceptions. It is speculated that overlearning may have been required for consistent sound productions for this participant and that insufficient opportunities for overlearning were provided. Furthermore, it appears that even with overlearning, reinforcement of learned sound productions, in the form of additional follow-up training, may be necessary to maintain treatment effects.

This report presents preliminary findings regarding the effects of modifications made to SPT in terms of the organisation and application of treatment. The results were promising in that acquisition and maintenance effects were positive. Treatment effects for the nine word-initial sounds in a repetition context did not generalise to improved production in a sentence completion context. However, treatment effects did appear to generalise to repetition of targeted sounds in word-final position. Application of SPT to a different context (i.e., sentence completion) was successful. However, order effects may have played a significant role in the extension of treatment to the sentence completion context. Additional replications of these findings are necessary, as are further investigations of the stimulus generalisation effects and social validity of this treatment.

REFERENCES

Clark, H. M., & Robin, D. R. (1998). Generalized motor programme and parameterization accuracy in apraxia of speech and conduction aphasia. *Aphasiology, 12,* 699–713.

Croot, K. (2002). Diagnosis of AOS: Definition and criteria. *Seminars in Speech and Language, 23(4),* 267–279.

Dabul, B. (1979). *Apraxia battery for adults.* Tigard, OR: C.C. Publications.

Duffy, J. R. (1995). *Motor speech disorders substrates, differential diagnosis, and management.* St. Louis, MO: Mosby-Year Book, Inc.

Dworkin, J. P., & Abkarian, G. G. (1996). Treatment of phonation in a patient with apraxia and dysarthria secondary to severe closed head injury. *Journal of Medical Speech-Language Pathology, 2,* 105–115.

Edwards, H. T. (1992). *Applied phonetics: The sounds of American English.* San Diego, CA: Singular Publishing.

Fink, R. B., Schwartz, M. F., Sobel, P. R., & Myers, J. L. (1997). Effects of multilevel training on verb retrieval: Is more always better? *Brain and Language, 60,* 41–44.

German, D. J. (1990). *Test of adolescent/adult word finding.* Allen, TX: DLM Publishers.

Kearns, K. P. (1997). Broca's aphasia. In L. L. LaPointe (Ed.), *Aphasia and related neurogenic disorders* (2nd ed., pp. 1–41). New York: Thieme.

Kertesz, A. (1982). *The western aphasia battery.* New York: Grune & Stratton.

Knock, T. R., Ballard, K. J., Robin, D. A., & Schmidt, R. A. (2000). Influence of order of stimulus presentation on speech motor learning: A principled approach to treatment for apraxia of speech. *Aphasiology, 14(5/6),* 653–668.

Marshall, R. C., Gandour, J., & Windsor, J. (1988). Selective impairment of phonation: A case study. *Brain and Language, 35,* 313–339.

McNeil, M. R., Doyle, P. J., & Wambaugh, J. L. (2000). Apraxia of speech: A treatable disorder of motor planning and programming. In L. Gonzalez-Rothi, L. Crosson, & S. Nadeau (Eds.), *Aphasia and language: Theory to practice* (pp. 221–266). New York: The Guilford Press.

McNeil, M. R., Odell, K. H., Miller, S. B., & Hunter, L. (1995). Consistency, variability, and target approximation for successive speech repetitions among apraxic, conduction aphasic, and ataxic dysarthric speakers. *Clinical Aphasiology, 23,* 39–55.

McNeil, M. R., Robin, D. A., & Schmidt, R. A. (1997). Apraxia of speech: Definition, differentiation, and treatment. In M. R. McNeil (Ed.), *Clinical management of sensorimotor speech disorders* (pp. 311–344). New York: Thieme.

Mlcoch, A. G., Darley, F. L., & Noll, J. D. (1982). Articulatory consistency and variability in apraxia of speech. In R. H. Brookshire (Ed.), *Clinical aphasiology conference proceedings* (pp. 235–238). Minneapolis, MN: BRK Publishers.

Newman, P. W., Creaghead, N. A., & Secord, W. (1985). *Assessment and remediation of articulatory and phonological disorders.* Columbus, OH: Charles E. Merrill Publishing Company.

Nickels, L. (2002). Improving word finding: Practice makes (closer to) perfect? *Aphasiology, 16(10/11),* 1047–1060.

Porch, B. (1981). *Porch Index of Communicative Ability [Vol. 2]. Administration, scoring, and interpretation* (3rd ed.). Palo Alto, CA: Pro-Ed, Inc.

Prather, E., Hedrick, D., & Kern, C. (1975). Articulation development in children aged two to four years. *Journal of Speech and Hearing Research, 40,* 179–191.

Raymer, A. M., Haley, M. A., & Kendall, D. L. (2002). Overgeneralization in treatment for severe apraxia of speech: A case study. *Journal of Medical Speech-Language Pathology, 10(4),* 313–317.

Raymer, A. M., & Thompson, C. K. (1991). Effects of verbal plus gestural treatment in a patient with aphasia and severe apraxia of speech. In T. E. Prescott (Ed.), *Clinical aphasiology* (Vol. 20, pp. 285–298). Austin, TX: Pro-Ed.

Sander, E. (1972). When are speech sounds learned? *Journal of Speech and Hearing Disorders, 37,* 55–63.

Schmidt, R. A., & Lee, T. D. (1999). *Motor control and learning a behavioral emphasis.* Champaign, IL: Human Kinetics.

Shriberg, L. D., & Kent, R. D. (1982). *Clinical phonetics.* New York: Macmillan Publishing.

Shuster, L., & Wambaugh, J. L. (2003, May). *Consistency of speech sound errors in apraxia of speech accompanied by aphasia.* Presentation at the Clinical Aphasiology Conference, Orcas Island, Washington.

Van Riper, C., & Irwin, J. (1958). *Voice and articulation.* Englewood Cliffs, NJ: Prentice Hall.

Wambaugh, J. L. (2001). Sound production treatment for apraxia of speech. *ASHA Special Interest Division-2 Newsletter, 11(4),* 9–13.

Wambaugh, J. L. (2002). A summary of treatments for apraxia of speech and review of replicated approaches. *Seminars in Speech and Language, 23*(4), 293–308.

Wambaugh, J. L. (in press). Stimulus generalization effects of sound production treatment for apraxia. *Medical Journal of Speech Language Pathology.*

Wambaugh, J. L., Doyle, P. J., Kalinyak, M. M., & West, J. E. (1996). A minimal contrast treatment for apraxia of speech. *Clinical Aphasiology, 24,* 97–108.

Wambaugh, J., Duffy, J., McNeil, M., Rogers, M., & Robin, D. (2003, November). *Treatment for AOS: A synthesis and evaluation of the evidence.* Paper presented at the meeting of the American Speech-Language-Hearing Association, Chicago, IL.

Wambaugh, J. L., Kalinyak-Fliszar, M. M., West, J. E., & Doyle, P. J. (1998a). Effects of treatment for sound errors in apraxia of speech. *Journal of Speech, Language, and Hearing Research, 41,* 725–743.

Wambaugh, J. L., Martinez, A. L., McNeil, M. R., & Rogers, M. (1999). Sound production treatment for apraxia of speech: Overgeneralization and maintenance effects. *Aphasiology, 9–11,* 821–837.

Wambaugh, J. L., Nessler, C., Bennett, J., & Mauszycki, S. (2004, March). *Apraxia of speech: A perceptual and VOT analysis of stop consonants.* Poster presented at the Conference on Motor Speech, Albuquerque, NM.

Wambaugh, J. L., West, J. E., & Doyle, P. J. (1998b). Treatment for apraxia of speech: Effects of targeting sound groups. *Aphasiology, 12,* 731–743.

Yorkston, K. M., & Beukelman, D. R. (1981). *Assessment of intelligibility of dysarthric speech.* Austin, TX: Pro-Ed.

APPENDIX A
TREATMENT AND PROBE STIMULI

Group 1
treatment contrast:

/s/	/p/	/v/	/ð/, /θ/, & /d/	/s/ (f)	p/ (f)	/v/(f)
sigh	pie	vie	thigh	dice	tap	of
see	pea	vee	thee	toss	ape	dive
sail	pail	veil	thail	ace	deep	have
sat	pat	vat	that	us	up	eve
seal	peel	veal	deal	dose	hip	hive
seer	peer	veer	deer			
Sue	pew	view	due			
set	pet	vet	debt			

Group 2
treatment contrast:

/k/	"sh"	"j"	/ð/, /θ/, /d/ & /t/	/k/(f)	"sh"(f)	"j"(f)
key	she	gee	Thee	tack	ash	age
coo	shoe	Jew	do	oak	dash	dodge
caw	shawl	jaw	thaw	ache	dish	huge
Kate	shade	jade	date	dike	hush	edge
car	share	jar	tar/tear	dock	hash	urge
kale	shale	jail	thail			
cot	shot	jot	tot			
cut	shut	jut	thud			

Group 3
treatment contrast:

/l/	/m/	/n/	/b/, /ð/, & /d/	/l/ (f)	/m/ (f)	/n/ (f)
lit	mitt	knit	bit	tall	am	in
Lee	me	knee	thee	ill	aim	on
low	mow	know	though	ale	time	hen
late	mate	Nate	date	dill	dim	tan
lie	my	nigh	thy	tell	hymn	done
lead	mead	need	bead			
Lou	moo	knew	boo			
light	might	night	bite			

APPENDIX B
STORY COMPLETION ITEMS

(see) Before I can read the newspaper, I need to put on my glasses because I can't _____.

(set) A track and field runner always gets ready when he or she hears the phrase: "On your marks, get _____."

(seal) In order for a passport to be legal, the immigration department has to stamp a _____.

(Sue) My best friend's name is Susan but I call her by the nicknames of Susie or _____.

(sigh) Everybody knows when my father is extremely tired and ready to go to sleep because he tends to yawn and _____.

(pie) Julie usually makes desserts when she has company. Last Saturday, her parents came and she baked a delicious apple _____.

(pail) The little boy wanted to build a sandcastle, so his mom bought him a shovel and a _____.

(pet) We have a goldfish, a hamster, and a dog in my house. I'm responsible for the hamster because she is my _____.

(pat) Every time I get home, my dog wants me to play with him and give him a friendly _____.

(pier) I tied my boat up at the dock or the _____.

("v") The little boy learned today to write words such as violin, van, and vase, which are words that begin with the letter _____.

(veil) A bride bought her wedding gown, shoes, and accessories. But later she realised that she did not buy a _____.

(view) If you live on the mountain and look over the city, you have a beautiful _____.

(vet) My dog has been very sick for the last two days, I need to take her to the _____.

(veal) Instead of making my beef stew with beef, I prefer to use the meat of a calf, which is better known as _____.

(key) I was frustrated because I locked myself out. Fortunately, I remembered that I was carrying an extra _____.

(cut) My hair is too long. I need to go to my hairdresser and get a new hair _____.

(cot) Grandpa came to visit. Mom said to my brother: "Grandpa can sleep in your bed and you can unfold the _____."

(coo) When I went to New York, I visited Central Park. I loved to feed the pigeons and hear them_____.

(car) I've been riding the bus for many years. I finally saved enough money to buy a good_____.

(shoe) The little boy is almost ready to go outside and play. He'll be ready once he ties his left _____.

(shot) The flu can be deadly in older people. That's why older people have been encouraged to have a flu _____.

(shut) The little boy was so tired that when his mom finished reading the story, his eyes were already _____.

(share) At the beginning of the school semester, the teacher did not have enough books for all the children so she said: "We'll have to _____."

(she) We saw a beautiful dog at the pet shop. We wanted to get a "he" so we asked: "Is it a he or a _____?

(jail) A man committed a crime and was caught. He was sentenced to 15 years in _____.

(Jew) Even though my friend is American, he believes in Judaism, so everyone considers him a _____.

(jaw) The boxer threw a punch near his opponent's mouth and broke his _____.

(jar) The little boy was so hungry that he couldn't wait for his lunch and grabbed some cookies from the cookie _____.

("g") The little girl learned in class today that the words girl, game, goat, and guitar begin with the letter _____.

(light) I was reading a book and all of the sudden the room became dark. I told my husband to turn on the _____.

(late) Tim is never on time. He usually gets to school ten to fifteen minutes _____.

(lit) Julie doesn't like to live in a dark house. When she was looking for a home, she made sure that it was well-_____.

(low) Ted wants to apply for medical school but he needs to retake the test because he scored too _____.

(lie) I tried to believe what they said but it was very hard for me because they always _____.

(mitt) Tim was ready to play baseball. He brought a ball and a bat, but then he realised that he forgot to bring his baseball _____.

(me) Julie's mom told her to call home as soon as possible. So when Julie was leaving, mom said: "Don't forget to call _____.

(mate) Ted is always dating but never seems to find the right person. He's still searching for the perfect _____.

(mow) The big kids share the yard work with their dad. The grass is tall and dad asked: "Who is going to _____?"

(moo) I would like to live in a farm. I love to hear the horses neigh, the ducks quack, the pigs oink, and the cows _____.

(knit) I know how to cross-stitch, sew, and crochet, but I don't know how to _____.

(know) The teacher asked a question about what the children were studying in class. A kid raised his hand and said "I _____."

(night) The mom put her son in his bed, covered him with a blanket, gave him a kiss, and said, "Good _____!"

(need) The boy scouts were knocking on every door, asking for donations for families in _____.

(knee) The boy was running and tripped over a rock. He was crying because he scraped his left _____.

APPENDIX C
MODIFIED SOUND PRODUCTION TREATMENT –
WORD LEVEL

1. Clinician produced the target word and requested a repetition;
   A. upon a correct production of the target sound, the clinician requested five additional repetitions* and moved to the next item;
   B. upon an incorrect production of the target sound, the clinician provided feedback and said, ''Now, let's try a different word'' and verbally presented the **contrast word**;
      1) upon a correct production of the contrast word, the clinician said, ''Now, let's go back to the other word'' and moved to Step 2 with the target word;
      2) upon an incorrect production of the contrast word, the clinician provided feedback, and attempted the contrast word with integral stimulation for a maximum of three trials; the clinician then moved to Step 2 with target word.

2. Clinician showed a written letter representing the target sound, produced the target word, and requested a repetition;
   A. upon a correct production of the target sound, the clinician requested five additional repetitions* and moved to the next item;
   B. upon an incorrect production of the target sound, the clinician moved to the next step.

3. Clinician instructed the participant to attempt the target word using integral stimulation (i.e., ''watch me, listen to me, and say it with me'') for a maximum of three trials;
   A. upon a correct production of the target sound, the clinician requested five additional repetitions* and moved to the next item;
   B. upon an incorrect production of the target sound, the clinician moved to the next step.

4. Clinician provided articulatory placement cues, and instructed the participant to attempt the target word using integral stimulation;
   A. upon a correct production of the target sound, the clinician requested five additional repetitions* and moved to the next item;
   B. upon an incorrect production of the target sound, the clinician moved to the next step.

5. Clinician presented next item.

---

* Clinician provided feedback on approximately 60% of the attempts.

APPENDIX D
SENTENCE COMPLETION LEVEL TREATMENT

1. Clinician produced the sentence completion item and requested a completion (e.g., "My dog has been very sick for the last two days. I need to take her to the...". [vet]).

   A. upon a correct production of the target sound, the clinician provided feedback and moved to the next item;

   B. upon an incorrect production of the target sound, the clinician provided feedback and moved to the next step.

   Note: "A" and "B" were included in the following steps.

2. Clinician produced the sentence completion item *including a model* of the correct response. Then, the clinician produced the sentence completion item and requested a completion (i.e., delayed repetition/ modelling) (e.g., "Listen and then you try it... My dog has been very sick for the last two days. I need to take her to the VET. My dog has been very sick for the last two days. I need to take her to the..." [vet].

3. Clinician showed the written letter corresponding to the target sound, produced the sentence completion item, and requested a completion while cueing with the letter (e.g., "Let's try using the first letter of the word. My dog has been very sick for the last two days. I need to take her to the..." [showed the letter V]).

4. Clinician produced the target word alone, then produced the sentence completion item and requested a completion (e.g., "The word is VET. My dog has been very sick for the last two days. I need to take her to the...." [vet]).

5. Clinician produced the target word and requested a repetition of the word. Then, the clinician produced the sentence completion item and requested a completion (e.g., "Say the word after me and then we'll try it with the sentence. Say VET. My dog has been very sick for the past two days. I need to take her to the...." [vet]).

6. Clinician request production of the target word using integral stimulation. Then, the clinician produced the sentence completion item and requested a completion (e.g., "Watch and listen and say the word with me and then we'll try it with the sentence. Say it with me... *VET.* My dog has been very sick for the past two days. I need to take her to the...." [vet]).

7. Clinician produced the sentence completion item and requested completion using integral stimulation with the target word (e.g., "I'll say the sentence and when I get to the word, you try it with me. My dog has been very sick for the past two days. I need to take her to the ... [provided gestural cue to produce word simultaneously]... VET".)

8. Clinician requested production of the target word alone using integral stimulation (e.g., "Say vet with me ... VET").

Integrating the message level into treatment for agrammatism using story retelling

Richard K. Peach and Patrick C. M. Wong

Rush University Medical Center, Chicago, IL, USA

Background: Treatments for agrammatic production generally target sentence forms, inflectional morphology, verb retrieval, thematic roles, or underlying grammatical forms. Reviews of these and related methods suggest that they address Garrett's functional and positional levels of sentence processing. Such reviews also demonstrate that little attention has been given to developing treatments that emphasise the message level of sentence production. Message-level representations appear to have robust potential for influencing sentence-level processes following aphasia, since varying levels of language representation are thought to influence their downstream counterparts.
Aims: The study aimed to determine whether functional and positional-level syntactic training applied in a context requiring structuring of message-level representations would improve expressive syntax in a patient with agrammatism.
Methods & Procedures: A 10-week programme was divided into two 5-week phases requiring story retelling of three fables in each phase with critical oral and written feedback. Story retellings were analysed along three dimensions: grammaticality, complexity, and content. The programme was evaluated using a multiple-baseline across behaviours single-subject design.
Outcomes & Results: Overall, this treatment programme appeared to produce highly beneficial outcomes with regard to improved expressive syntax. Substantial generalisation of treatment effects was observed in post-treatment testing, while long-term maintenance of the gains achieved in treatment was observed.
Conclusions: The story-retelling procedure, with oral and written feedback, stimulated and improved the participant's expressive syntax. Unlike treatment approaches that simply target surface grammar, the story retelling approach appears to be rich with regard to stimulating conceptual syntax as well as lower-level syntactic processes. Functional communication also benefited by treating discourse-level behaviours to improve linguistic processing.

Garrett's model of normal sentence production (1980, 1990) provides a theoretical account of the processes for constructing well-formed sentences and a framework for describing agrammatic errors in language output following aphasia (Berndt, 1998; Garrett, 1984). The model consists of a message level for general conceptual processes, functional, positional, and phonetic levels for sentence processes, and an articulatory level for motor control processes (see Figure 1).

According to Garrett (1990), messages (i.e., the speaker's communicative intent) provide input to the production system; the processes associated with formulation of messages comprise the message level. Message-level representations "are based on the speaker's perceptual and affective state" (Garrett, 1984, p. 173) and provide a con-

Address correspondence to: Richard K. Peach, Rush University Medical Center 1653 West Congress Parkway, Chicago, IL 60612, USA. Email: richard_k_peach@rush.edu

© 2004 by Taylor & Francis.
http://www.tandf.co.uk/journals/pp/02687038.html   DOI: 10.1080/02687030444000147

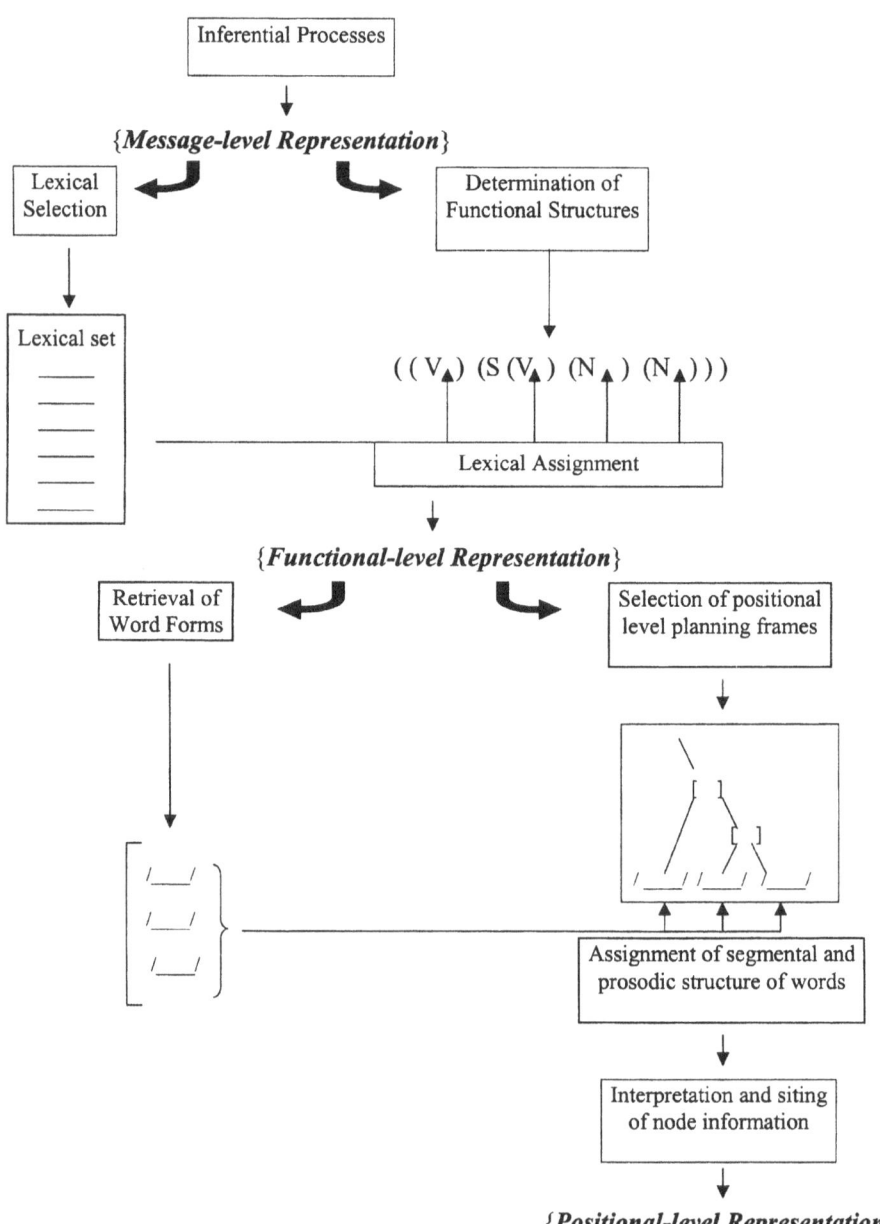

Figure 1. Garrett's model of the internal structure of the sentence level of processing. From D. N. Osherson & H. Lasnik (1990). *An invitation to cognitive science: Language* (p. 164), Cambridge, MA: The MIT Press. Copyright 1990 by the Massachusetts Institute of Technology. Adapted with permission.

ceptual syntax that builds complex expressions. Sentence-level representations are developed at the functional, positional, and phonetic levels using these complex expressions as input. These sentence-level processes provide a control structure for articulation.

The conceptual syntax of the message level is transformed to a more linguistic, logic-oriented representation at the functional level. Lexical items are selected on the basis of meaning relations while such functional structures as predicate for the subject, main verb for the verb phrase, or head noun for the noun phrase are specified. The lexical elements are then assigned to these phrasal roles. A more pronunciation-oriented representation is computed at the positional level. Here, the segmental properties of the lexical items are identified, the surface structure is determined, lexical items are assigned to phrases, and the grammatical formatives are sited. The detailed phonetic character of the elements appearing in these words, subject to regular phonological processes, is then specified at the phonetic level.

As an example of how these processes might unfold, consider the scenario in which a husband wants to tell his wife that he'd prefer to spend a quiet evening at home on New Year's Eve than to go out on the town. This message can be conveyed in a variety of ways that will depend on, among other variables, his perceptions regarding his wife's preferences about this issue, the importance of the outcome vis à vis his own position, and his appreciation of the way previous discussions concerning similar matters were concluded. These nonlinguistic or conceptual influences (message-level representations) determine the linguistic form that the message will take. The words that are retrieved from the mental lexicon and the order in which they are arranged are selected to reflect both the husband's meanings and intentions (e.g., direct/indirect, inquisitive/uninterested, requesting/demanding) and the syntactic conventions of the language (functional-level representations). This information is then used to construct the final form of the sentences that are ultimately produced (positional-level representations). Grammatical encoding then begins at the moment that information available in the message is presented to downstream syntactic processes.

Treatments for agrammatic language production generally target sentence forms and inflectional morphology (e.g., Helm-Estabrooks, Fitzpatrick, & Barresi, 1981), verb retrieval and thematic roles (Byng, 1988; Schwartz, Saffran, Fink, Myers, & Martin, 1994) or underlying grammatical forms (Thompson, 2001). Recent reviews of these and related methods describe them as addressing the functional and positional levels of sentence processing (Chatterjee & Maher, 2000; Mitchum & Berndt, 2001). Such reviews also demonstrate that little attention has been given to developing treatments for agrammatic speakers that include the message level of sentence production.

Treatments targeting one level of language representation are thought to influence downstream representations within this model. Given this, treatments exploiting message-level representations would appear to have robust potential with regard to influencing sentence-level processes following aphasia. According to Garrett (1984), "message level representations are the proximal cause of sentence construction" (p. 173). Chatterjee and Maher (2000) summarise two contrasting positions that attribute agrammatic production to message-level processes. In one account, agrammatic patients make a strategic decision to reduce their output because of the effort that is involved in speaking. In the other account, reduced sentence output is thought to reflect conceptual impoverishment at the message level. Whichever may be the more accurate account is unknown. However, both views provide an impetus for investigating an approach to syntax treatment that specifically attends to the message level.

We wanted to know if syntactic training applied in a context requiring structuring of message-level representations would improve expressive syntax in a patient with agrammatism. To do this, we developed a treatment procedure that purportedly capitalised on message-level representations while emphasising accuracy of syntactic output. In this approach, multiple levels of sentence processing were targeted by the treatment. We modified the story-retelling method described by Chapman and Ulatowska (1992) and Ulatowska and Chapman (1989) for our therapeutic approach. In this approach, patients are asked to retell and elaborate upon fables that are presented auditorily. According to these authors, these tasks place demands on both cognitive processing and linguistic processing.

We believe that the story-retelling procedure provides opportunities for stimulating expressive syntax that are not available using procedures that target functional and/or positional-level processes only. By presenting extended, cognitively complex stimuli for retelling, agrammatic patients are less able to use simple repetition or prescribed roles to produce target sentences. Instead, they are required to extrapolate conceptual information from the fables, use their general knowledge of the world (e.g., the attributes of the characters in the stories, any potential antecedent events, the inferred bases for the reported outcomes) to sequence this information logically, and distil these relationships into novel sentence frames that are syntactically constrained but nonetheless attempt to capture the essential meaning of each story. We believed that a treatment approach targeting functional and positional-level processes to more accurately express crucial conceptual information at the message level would result in improved grammatical encoding overall.

METHOD

Subject

DAB is 42 years old, right-handed, and a former attorney status post left middle cerebral artery infarct. Speech-language evaluation immediately after his stroke resulted in impressions of global aphasia with apraxia. He was subsequently diagnosed with moderate Broca's aphasia approximately 3 years after his stroke. Comprehensive testing prior to entry into this study was undertaken 8 months later (see Table 1).

On the Boston Diagnostic Aphasia Examination (3rd ed.) (BDAE: Goodglass, Kaplan, & Barresi, 2001), DAB performed at the 63rd percentile for the auditory comprehension component and at the 45th percentile for the expressive component. These scores suggested moderately impaired auditory comprehension and markedly impaired expressive language prior to treatment. He demonstrated a complexity index of approximately 1 in narrative discourse, suggesting that his language output was wholly composed of simple sentences. He also achieved an agrammatism index of 45%, suggesting numerous agrammatic deletions. Administration of the Reading Comprehension Battery for Aphasia (2nd ed.) (RCBA-2: LaPointe & Horner, 1998) showed relatively intact reading comprehension but moderately impaired oral reading. Syntactic output assessed by Psycholinguistic Assessments of Language Processing in Aphasia (PALPA: Kay, Lesser, & Coltheart, 1992) showed severely impaired reading and repetition for inflected words. Nevertheless, DAB was a highly functional communicator on Communication Activites of Daily Living (2nd ed.) (CADL-2: Holland, Frattali, & Fromm, 1999). Performance on the Test of Nonverbal Intelligence (3rd ed.) (TONI-3: Brown, Sherbenou, & Johnsen, 1997) was at the 34th percentile.

TABLE 1
Pre- and post-treatment assessment results for DAB

Test	Pre-Treatment	Post-Treatment
BDAE		
Complexity Index (Narrative Discourse)	1.03	1.38
Agrammatism Index	45%	33%
Language Competency Index	54%tile	62%tile
Expressive Component	45%tile	60%tile
Auditory Comprehension Component	63%tile	63%tile
RCBA-2		
Core (Visual)	93%	93%
Extended (Oral)	73%	82%
PALPA		
Inflected Words (Repetition)	40%	80%
Inflected Words (Reading)	13%	67%
CADL-2	8/9	8/9
TONI-3	34%tile	66%tile

BDAE = Boston Diagnostic Aphasia Examination–Third Edition. RCBA-2 = Reading Comprehension Battery for Aphasia–Second Edition. PALPA = Psycholinguistic Assessments of Language Processing in Aphasia. CADL-2 = Communication Activities in Daily Living–Second Edition. TONI-3 = Test of Nonverbal Intelligence–Third Edition.

Stimuli and treatment

Because of DAB's functional skills, it was deemed appropriate to focus treatment at the discourse level with emphasis on grammatical and content accuracy. A 10-week programme consisting of three 1-hour sessions per week was developed to improve syntactic production during discourse. The programme was divided into two 5-week phases.

Treatment stimuli consisted of six fables (see Appendix A). The fables were divided into two sets of three each for the two treatment phases of this study. Each set contained approximately the same number of content units (Set 1 = 279, Set 2 = 275) (McNeil, Doyle, Fossett, & Park, 2001).

During treatment, the clinician presented a complete fable to DAB orally. DAB then retold the story to the clinician while the clinician transcribed his responses. The clinician read each of DAB's utterances to him, one at a time, and asked him after each sentence to listen to the utterance that he had just produced. DAB was then asked to improve on his spoken production in writing. When the patient finished revising his spoken utterance, the clinician immediately provided corrective feedback to the patient regarding errors of grammar and content in the written samples. Feedback consisted of further explanation of the main and inferred details of the story and practice with the appropriate grammatical forms to express these concepts as identified in each of the patient's sentences. DAB reproduced the corrected utterance with and without the corrected transcripts. An example illustrating these procedures is included in Appendix B.

Experimental design

The programme was evaluated using a multiple-baseline across behaviours single-subject design. During each of the three pretreatment baseline sessions, DAB retold two different fables from the larger set of six. In this way, baseline performance levels were obtained over time for all six fables prior to the initiation of treatment. The experimental measures (see below) obtained for each retelling were averaged for each combination of two fables and plotted over the baseline phase. Following the initiation of treatment, progress was probed weekly by having DAB retell all six fables consecutively in random order within a single session without the clinician's feedback. The experimental measures obtained for each retelling were grouped and averaged across the three fables in each treatment set and plotted over the treatment phase of the experiment. DAB was probed weekly in a similar manner after the withdrawal of treatment for each set of fables to evaluate the main-tenance of any treatment effects.

Story retellings were analysed along three dimensions: grammaticality, complexity, and content. Grammaticality was measured by calculating the number of syntactic errors per clause. A complexity index measuring the number of clauses per utterance was computed using the procedures specified in the BDAE (Goodglass et al., 2001). Content was measured by dividing the total number of content units (McNeil et al., 2001) pro-duced by the patient by the total number of content units in each fable.

Reliability

Of the retold stories, 12% (nine fables) were chosen randomly. An independent judge analysed these stories according to the measures discussed above. Correlations for the calculations obtained from the clinician and the judge were .97 for grammaticality, .90 for complexity, and .91 for content.

RESULTS

Figures 2–4 show the grammaticality, complexity, and content of DAB's language production. Figure 2 shows decreasing syntactic errors below baseline levels for both sets of the fables during Phase 1 of the treatment programme. These results demonstrate increased accuracy of grammatical encoding. Since the two sets of fables are related, it is perhaps not surprising that training one set generalised to the other untrained set and that the baselines under the untrained fables showed a decrease in errors as treatment ensued for the trained fables. Thus, it could be that the treatment itself is not the only contributor to the observed improvement in performance (since the baselines for the untreated set were not stable). However, syntactic errors increased at the onset of Phase 2 when the second set of fables was introduced for treatment. Such phase shifts are common in learning and suggest that the treatment itself was, indeed, responsible for these findings. A return to and maintenance of Phase 1 levels of syntactic accuracy for Set 1 fables was observed thereafter, while Set 2 fables also showed improved grammatical encoding. The maintenance phase was characterised by continuation of the levels of syntactic accuracy observed in Phase 2, as well as the return of utterance complexity to Phase 1 levels in the absence of treatment.

Similar patterns of performance were observed regarding the grammatical complexity of the participant's utterances (Figure 3). Utterance complexity increased above baseline levels for both sets of the fables during Phase 1 of the treatment programme but showed a marked decrease for both sets at the onset of Phase 2. Again, this was attributed to learning effects for the two sets of fables. This pattern continued until the termination of Phase 2 after which the complexity of the participant's utterances returned to and were maintained at supra-baseline levels.

DAB's content was strongly associated with the specific fables used during each treatment phase (Figure 4). Baseline results demonstrated that the patient did not increase

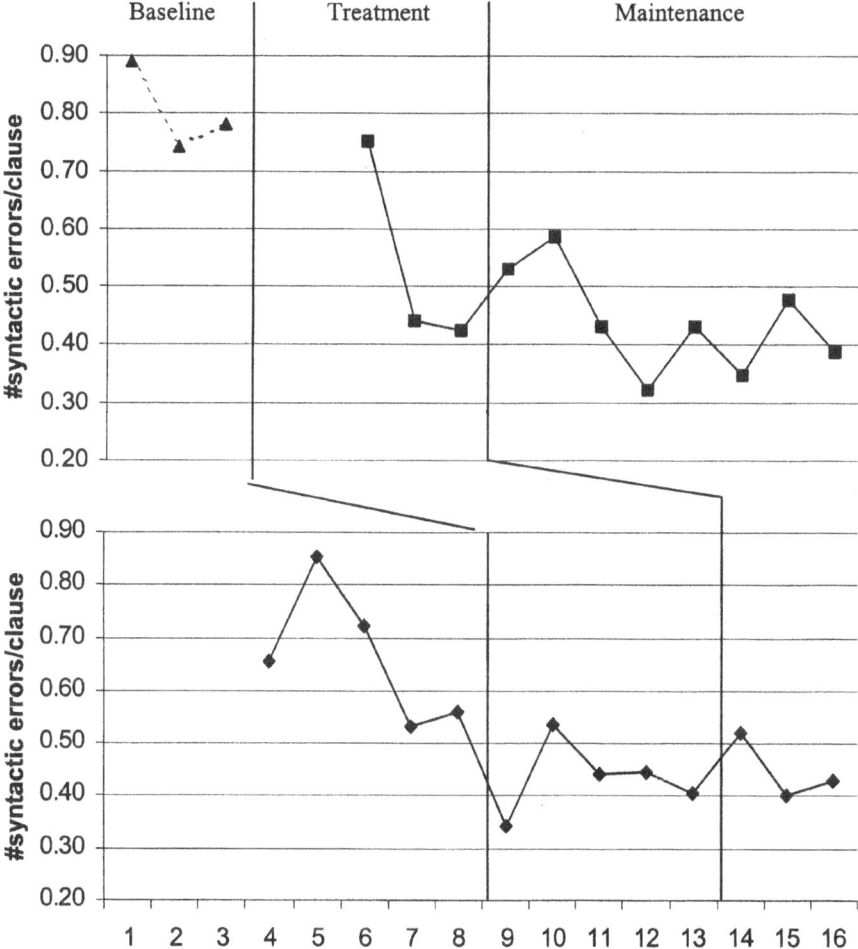

Figure 2.   Grammatical accuracy of language output during baseline, treatment, and maintenance.

the numbers of content units he provided as a function of repeated exposure to the story-retell task. During Phase 1 when the first set of fables was being treated, content units increased substantially for only those stories. During Phase 2 when the second set of fables was being treated, content units for the first set of fables were maintained approximately at the maximum levels attained during treatment, while content units for the second set of fables increased substantially. These results provide additional evidence to suggest that the improvements observed in syntactic accuracy and complexity were not simply a product of repeated exposures to these fables during probing.

Good generalisation of treatment effects was observed on post-treatment testing (see Table 1). Expressive language improved to the 60th percentile. DAB's complexity index increased to 1.38 suggesting an improvement of approximately 10 percentile points. Agrammatic errors also decreased by approximately one third. Substantially increased sensitivity to grammatical markers was suggested by impressive gains on the inflected word subtests of the PALPA.

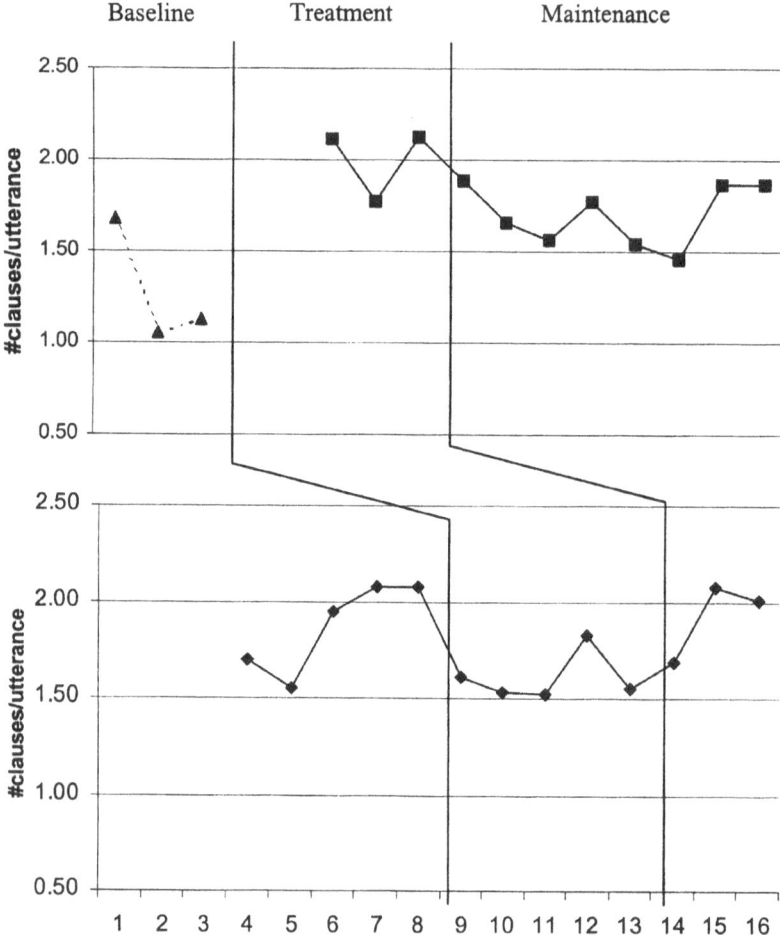

Figure 3.   Sentence complexity for story retellings during baseline, treatment, and maintenance.

The improvements noted in the participant's language following treatment were also observed on long-term follow-up (see Table 2). Improvements in the grammar and complexity of the participant's language output were not only maintained, but further sensitivity to grammatical markers as well as increases in sentence complexity were observed at long-term follow-up.

DISCUSSION

Overall, this treatment programme appeared to produce highly beneficial outcomes with regard to improved expressive syntax. Substantial generalisation of treatment effects was observed in post-treatment testing (see Table 1), while long-term maintenance of the gains achieved in treatment was observed. What mechanisms might be postulated, then, for the improved syntactic production that resulted from emphasising message-level processes with this patient? We return to Garrett's model to explore this issue.

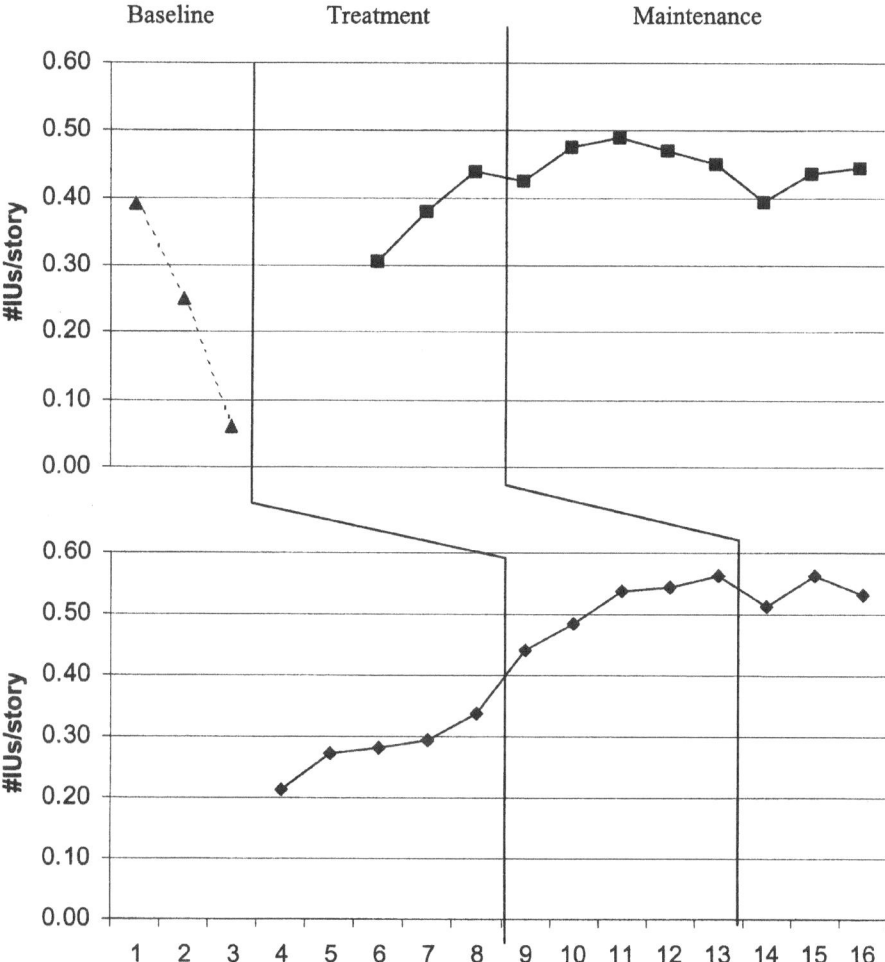

Figure 4. Content measured by total information units for story retellings during baseline, treatment, and maintenance.

The characteristic feature of the agrammatism of Broca's aphasia is failure to produce grammatical morphemes. Agrammatic speakers also appear to have better control of their lexical inventories, as suggested by their relatively superior abilities to comprehend and produce open class vocabulary items. For Garrett, these symptoms suggest impairment in phrasal integration and implicate a mapping deficit from the functional to the positional levels of representation.

Message-level connections are also thought to exist only with the functional level of representation and not with any of the other levels within the model. According to Garrett, "the properties of sentence form that determine meaning are assumed to be fixed at the functional level" (1984, p. 181). As a result, one might conclude that the lack of a direct connection between the message and positional levels would reduce the potential for a message-level approach to influence the impaired positional-level processes of

TABLE 2
Effects of treatment at maintenance phase and at long-term
follow-up relative to baseline performance levels

	Baseline	Maintenance	6-month follow-up
Grammaticality	.80	.43	.37
Complexity	1.29	1.82	2.07
Content	.23	.48	.49

Measures equal mean of probes within each study phase.

agrammatism. However, a lexical approach to grammatical encoding may provide the support for message-level treatment.

The lexical hypothesis suggests that grammatical encoding is lexically driven (Bock & Levelt, 1994; Levelt, 1989). Lemmas activated by conceptual processes at the message level stimulate a variety of syntactic procedures to construct the surface structure. The encoding operations are controlled by the grammatical properties of the lemmas that are retrieved.

For Levelt (1989), lemmas contain declarative knowledge about a word's meaning and grammar. Grammatical encoding procedures are guided by the information that the lemmas make available. That is, the phrasal slots that are required for a given lemma cause dedicated syntactic procedures to set up the appropriate frame. The lemma's syntactic category calls a categorical procedure that provides building instructions for the phrasal category in which the lemma functions as head. So, for example, in the case of a noun lemma, the lemma would call procedure NP.

The categorical procedure transfers control to functional procedures that work in parallel to identify modifying or specifying information such as verb tense, person, or number. This information is attached to the target concepts in the message. In the example, NP calls for the functional procedure DET that generates a determiner. These functional procedures deliver their results to the categorical specialist that called them. The phonological properties of the lemma along with its grammatical parameters are then retrieved by phonological encoding procedures. For Levelt, lemma structure plays a central role in the generation of surface structure.

The story-retelling procedure, with oral and written feedback, stimulated and improved the participant's expressive syntax. Unlike treatment approaches that simply target surface grammar, the story-retelling approach appears to be rich with regard to stimulating conceptual syntax. More than simply a repetition task, retelling of these fables required the participant to integrate the main as well as inferred details of the story, to synthesise them into a cohesive summary, and to activate the grammatical specifications for the reproduced and/or revised phrasal arrangements corresponding to his responses. If agrammatic errors are viewed as a failure of the functional procedures that are involved in the planning of the grammatical features appearing in the surface structure, then the oral and written feedback provided to this participant can be seen as stimulating these mechanisms rather than as a simple and less effective teaching of grammatical rules. It is recognised, however, that the generalisability of the effects obtained with this approach may be limited due to the single case design of this study and the atypical pattern of deficits in this participant (i.e., increased fluency, high level of functional abilities). Nonetheless, it seems plausible that the method could be adapted to additional, more severe patients by reducing the complexity of the stories that are used. Such modifications may then provide opportunities to assess the replicability of the outcomes obtained with this approach in a wider range of agrammatic speakers.

Of course there are additional benefits for functional communication when treating discourse-level behaviours to improve linguistic processing. These include development of communication skills that have greater validity for real-world applications and more effective generalisation of these behaviours to appropriate communication contexts. But functional communication treatments generally ignore language form in favour of more effective language use, which, as in the current case, may fail to address the grammar-specific needs of the agrammatic speaker. Currently, only one well-known procedure, Promoting Aphasics' Communicative Effectiveness or PACE (Davis & Wilcox, 1985) offers the potential to address agrammatism by stimulating message-level representations in a discourse context. But the procedure's reliance on patient-initiated responses to novel stimuli may render it less suitable or effective when compared with story-retelling for re-establishing grammatical encoding routines. The story-retelling procedure with specific grammatical feedback appears to offer an appropriate method to treat agrammatism while reaping the benefits of a discourse-centred treatment.

REFERENCES

Berndt, R. S. (1998). Sentence processing in aphasia. In M. T. Sarno (Ed.), *Acquired aphasia* (3rd ed.) (pp. 229–267). San Diego, CA: Academic Press.

Bock, K., & Levelt, W. (1994). Language production: Grammatical encoding. In M. A. Gernsbacher (Ed.), *Handbook of psycholinguistics* (pp. 945–984). San Diego, CA: Academic Press.

Brown, L., Sherbenou, R., & Johnsen, S. (1997). *Test of nonverbal intelligence* (3rd ed.). Austin, TX: Pro-Ed.

Byng, S. (1988). Sentence processing deficits: Theory and therapy. *Cognitive Neuropsychology, 5*, 629–676.

Chapman, S. B., & Ulatowska, H. K. (1992). Methodology for discourse management in the treatment of aphasia. *Clinics in Communication Disorders, 2*, 64–81.

Chatterjee, A., & Maher, L. (2000). Grammar and agrammatism. In S. E. Nadeau, L. J. G. Rothi, & B. Crosson (Eds.), *Aphasia and language: Theory to practice* (pp. 133–156). New York: The Guilford Press.

Davis, G. A., & Wilcox, M. J. (1985). *Adult aphasia rehabilitation: Applied pragmatics.* San Diego, CA: College-Hill.

Garrett, M. F. (1980). Levels of processing in sentence production. In B. Butterworth (Ed.), *Language production, Volume 1: Speech and talk* (pp. 177–220). London: Academic Press.

Garrett, M. F. (1984). The organization of processing structure for language production: Applications to aphasic speech. In D. Caplan, A. R. Lecours, & A. Smith (Eds.), *Biological perspectives on language* (pp. 172–193). Cambridge, MA: The MIT Press.

Garrett, M. F. (1990). Sentence processing. In D. N. Osherson & H. Lasnik (Eds.), *An invitation to cognitive science: Language* (pp. 133–175). Cambridge, MA: The MIT Press.

Goodglass, H., Kaplan, E., & Barresi, B. (2001). *Boston diagnostic aphasia examination* (3rd ed.). Philadelphia: Lippincott Williams & Wilkins.

Helm-Estabrooks, N., Fitzpatrick, P. M., & Barresi, B. (1981). Response of an agrammatic patient to a syntax stimulation program for aphasia. *Journal of Speech and Hearing Disorders, 46*, 422–427.

Holland, A. L., Frattali, C. M., & Fromm, D. (1999). *Communication activities of daily living* (2nd ed.). Austin, TX: Pro-Ed.

Kay, J., Lesser, R., & Coltheart, M. (1992). *Psycholinguistic assessments of language processing in aphasia.* Hove, UK: Psychology Press.

LaPointe, L., & Horner, J. (1998). *Reading comprehension battery for aphasia* (2nd ed.). Austin, TX: Pro-Ed.

Levelt, W. J. M. (1989). *Speaking: From intention to articulation.* Cambridge, MA: The MIT Press.

McNeil, M. R., Doyle, P. J., Fossett, T. R. D., & Park, G. H. (2001). Reliability and concurrent validity of the information unit scoring metric for the story retelling procedure. *Aphasiology, 15*, 991–1006.

Mitchum, C. C., & Berndt, R. S. (2001). Cognitive neuropsychological approaches to diagnosing and treating language disorders: Production and comprehension of sentences. In R. Chapey (Ed.), *Language intervention strategies in aphasia and related neurogenic communication disorders* (4th ed.) (pp. 551–571). Philadelphia: Lippincott Williams & Wilkins.

Schwartz, M. F., Saffran, E. M., Fink, R. B., Myers, J. L., & Martin, N. (1994). Mapping therapy: A treatment programme for agrammatism. *Aphasiology*, *8*, 19–54.

Thompson, C. K. (2001). Treatment of underlying forms: A linguistic specific approach for sentence production deficits in agrammatic aphasia. In R. Chapey (Ed.), *Language intervention strategies in aphasia and related neurogenic communication disorders* (4th ed.) (pp. 605–628). Philadelphia: Lippincott Williams & Wilkins.

Ulatowska, H. K., & Chapman, S. B. (1989). Discourse considerations for aphasia management. *Seminars in Speech and Language*, *10*, 298–314.

APPENDIX A: STORY STIMULI

Set 1

The Ant and the Dove

An ant went to the bank of a river to quench its thirst, and being carried away by the rush of the stream, was on the point of drowning. A dove sitting on a tree overhanging the water plucked a leaf and let it fall into the stream close to her. The ant climbed onto it and floated in safety to the bank. Shortly afterwards a birdcatcher came and stood under the tree, and laid his lime-twigs for the dove, which sat in the branches. The ant, perceiving his design, stung him in the foot. In pain the birdcatcher threw down the twigs, and the noise made the dove take wing.

The Fox and the Raven

A raven was sitting on a tree holding a piece of cheese in his beak. The fox saw him and decided he wanted the cheese. He stood under the tree and began to praise the raven. He told the raven that he was a very beautiful bird and that he should become a king. The fox said that he would like to hear the raven's voice to be sure that the raven could give orders. Then the raven decided to show off his voice. He opened his beak and the cheese fell out onto the ground. The fox grabbed the cheese and ran away.

The Man and the Serpent

A countryman's son by accident trod upon a serpent's tail, which turned and bit him so that he died. The father in a rage got his axe, and pursuing the serpent, cut off part of its tail. So the serpent in revenge began stinging several of the farmer's cattle and caused him severe loss. Well, the farmer thought it best to make it up with the serpent, and brought food and honey to the mouth of its lair, and said to it: "Let's forget and forgive; perhaps you were right to punish my son, and take vengeance on my cattle, but surely I was right in trying to revenge him; now that we are both satisfied why should not we be friends again?"

"No, no," said the serpent, "take away your gifts; you can never forget the death of your son, nor I the loss of my tail."

Set 2

The Bat, the Birds, and the Beasts

A great conflict was about to come off between the birds and the beasts. When the two armies were collected together the bat hesitated which to join. The birds that passed his perch said: "Come with us"; but he said: "I am a beast." Later on, some beasts who were passing underneath him looked up and said: "Come with us"; but he said: "I am a bird." Luckily at the last moment peace was made, and no battle took place, so the bat came to the birds and wished to join in the rejoicings, but they all turned against him and he had to fly away. He then went to the beasts, but soon had to beat a retreat, or else they would have torn him to pieces. "Ah," said the bat, "I see now, I'm neither."

The Kid and the Wolf

A kid, returning without protection from the pasture, was pursued by a wolf. Seeing he could not escape, he turned round, and said: "I know, friend Wolf, that I must be your prey, but before I die I would ask of you one favour: you will play me a tune to which I may dance." The wolf complied, and while he was piping and the kid was dancing, some hounds hearing the sound ran up and began chasing the wolf. Turning to the kid, he said, "It is just what I deserve; for I, who am only a butcher, should not have turned piper to please you."

The Woman and the Doctor

A certain old woman suffered from a disease of the eyes. She called the doctor. The doctor came every day and rubbed some ointment on her eyes. When the old woman had her eyes closed, the doctor secretly carried her belongings out of her house. When he finished his treatment, he demanded a payment. The old woman refused.

The doctor took her to court. In court, the old woman said that her vision was worse because before the treatments, she saw all of her belongings. But after the treatment, she could not see any of them. That is why she refused to pay.

APPENDIX B: EXAMPLE OF TREATMENT PROCEDURES

1. Clinician reads "The Fox and the Raven" aloud
2. Patient retells story, clinician transcribes the following utterances:
   a. The raven sat on branch and cheese into the beak
   b. The fox see a raven on the branch
   c. Fox said raven you are a king
   d. Fox said to raven want you talk
   e. The raven talk she drop the cheese
   f. After the raven drop the cheese, then the fox pick the cheese up and ran
3. Clinician reads utterance a. aloud and asks patient to correct utterance in writing; patient writes the following:
   A raven sat on the branch and a cheese into the beak.
4. Clinician corrects written sentence, patient attempts to read corrected sentence and then produce it without corrected transcript.
5. Clinician reads utterance b. aloud and asks patient to correct utterance in writing; patient writes the following:
   The fox saw a raven on the branch.
6. Clinician reads utterance c. aloud and asks patient to correct utterance in writing; patient writes the following:
   The fox said to the raven "This which a kings."
7. Clinician partitions first portion of sentence using parentheses and encourages patient to correct remainder of sentence, patient writes:
   "Who is candidate the king."
8. Clinician continues to provide written corrective feedback, patient attempts again, writes:
   "You are a candidate for the king."
9. Patient reads corrected sentence and then produces it without transcript.
10. Clinician continues in this manner with remainder of transcribed utterances.

APHASIOLOGY, 2004, *18* (5/6/7), 443–456

Vowel duration as a cue to postvocalic stop voicing in aphasia and apraxia of speech

Katarina L. Haley

University of North Carolina at Chapel Hill, USA

Background: In American English, vowel duration is, on average, longer preceding post-vocalic voiced stops than preceding postvocalic voiceless stops. Preliminary investigations have reported a preservation of this acoustic contrast for speakers with aphasia and apraxia of speech (AOS) on the basis of mean data. However, clinical interpretation of the available research is difficult due to lack of attention to the range of performance among and within speakers from both normal and disordered populations. Concurrent perceptual analysis is warranted to evaluate functional implications of acoustic variations, but standard approaches using a single listener and presentation may not be sufficiently sensitive to reveal subtle variations.
Aims: (1) To determine whether aphasic and apraxic speakers produce a normal vowel duration differentiation between voiced and voiceless postvocalic stops. (2) To explore whether the produced vowel duration variations are associated with predicted perceptual effects.
Methods & Procedures: Eight speakers with coexisting aphasia and AOS, eight with aphasia and no AOS, and eight normal control speakers produced 24 repetitions of the words "had" and "hat" in a short carrier phrase. For each utterance, the duration of the vowel was measured. Perceptual testing was conducted using three normal listeners and a forced-choice perceptual identification paradigm.
Outcomes & Results: As expected, all normal speakers, and most aphasic and apraxic speakers, displayed a mean vowel duration distinction between the voicing cognates. The magnitude of the distinction did not differ across groups. Instead, there was substantial inter-speaker variability in the magnitude of duration contrast in all three groups. Some aphasic speakers with and without AOS did not distinguish in vowel duration between voicing cognates, and others displayed bimodal, but overlapping, distributions for /d/ and /t/. Results of the perceptual identification experiment indicated that there was good, but not perfect, agreement between variations in vowel duration and voicing perception and that several utterances produced by aphasic and apraxic speakers were perceptually ambiguous.
Conclusions: (1) Although the mean duration for vowels preceding voiced and voiceless stops may be indistinguishable from normal, several abnormal acoustic patterns are found among individual aphasic speakers both with and without AOS. (2) The magnitude of acoustic distinction can vary considerably across normal speakers and this variation must be considered when evaluating disordered speech. (3) Perceptual identification testing facilitates the interpretation of acoustic data, particularly when the two levels of analysis are matched on an utterance-by-utterance basis. (4) Perceptual ambiguity can be demonstrated in disordered speech through perceptual identification testing.

Address correspondence to: Katarina L. Haley, Division of Speech and Hearing Sciences, Department of Allied Health Sciences, Medical School Wing D, CB# 7190, University of North Carolina, Chapel Hill, NC 27599-7190, USA. Email: khaley@med.unc.edu

© 2004 by Taylor & Francis.
http://www.tandf.co.uk/journals/pp/02687038.html   DOI: 10.1080/02687030444000200

Acoustic analysis procedures are becoming increasingly accessible to clinicians. These tools can contribute a wealth of information to the assessment of disordered speech production. However, there is limited knowledge to guide measurement selection and interpretation. In this paper, we consider two factors that are critical to clinical applications of speech acoustics, but have received limited attention in previous research. These include the selection of criteria for normal and impaired acoustic performance and the determination of whether the measured variables have functional implications for speech communication. Whether the purpose is differential diagnosis, intervention planning, or severity estimation, the fundamental focus of clinical speech evaluation is on the performance of individual speakers and on the communicative consequences of production errors. To utilise acoustic measures effectively, clinicians need to know how each patient's acoustic profile compares to the range of both normal and disordered speech and whether the observed variations make a perceptual difference to listeners. The purpose of the present investigation was to provide preliminary information about these factors and how they may be addressed in future research involving speakers with aphasia and apraxia of speech (AOS).

Our experience in working with persons who have these disorders is that there is a range of qualitative and quantitative performance both within and across diagnostic groups, and that group means often do not correspond with the performance of individual speakers. Previous work in our laboratory has provided preliminary results about different performance profiles for persons with aphasia with and without AOS. In two separate investigations, we examined the achievement of spectral contrast for front vowels and sibilant fricatives produced by aphasic speakers with and without AOS and by normal controls (Haley, Ohde, & Wertz, 2000, 2001). Both apraxic and aphasic speaker groups produced the anticipated phonetic distinctions and their mean spectral content did not differ from the normal group. Yet the performance of individual apraxic and aphasic speakers was not normal. Some speakers displayed partially overlapping spectra for adjacent places of articulation, whereas others failed to distinguish between targets altogether. Such patterns were not seen in the normal speakers, indicating that they were likely associated with impaired speech production. The source may include any combination of linguistic, motor programming, or motor execution factors. Yet, if robust, their presence in aphasic speakers both with and without AOS must be acknowledged in clinical characterisation and theoretical accounts of these disorders.

A primary purpose of the present investigation was to replicate and extend our findings on spectral properties to a phonetic contrast based on a temporal acoustic differentiation. The targeted contrast was the variation in vowel duration seen prior to voiced and voiceless postvocalic stops. When speakers of American English produce single words and sentences, they use a longer duration for vowels that precede voiced stops than for vowels that precede voiceless stops (Chen, 1970). Similarly, studies of both natural and synthetic speech have demonstrated that vowel duration serves as a cue to the perception of postvocalic stop voicing (Hogan & Rozsypal, 1980; Raphael, 1972).

A handful of investigations have examined the production of this acoustic contrast in aphasia and AOS, and in all investigations the focus has been on the overall existence or magnitude of the contrast, with minimal attention to the range of individual speaker performance. The most consistent finding is that there is a mean vowel duration distinction between postvocalic voicing cognates for speaker with these disorders (Baum, Blumstein, Naeser, & Palumbo, 1990; Caligiuri & Till, 1983; Duffy & Gawle, 1984). Thus, neither aphasia nor AOS appears to result in a consistent loss of a phonologic rule for postvocalic stop voicing. However, it cannot be inferred that individual speakers in the two groups do not make phonemic errors, or that all speakers achieve this duration distinction. Duffy and Gawle (1984) and Tuller (1984) reported a tendency for vowel duration distributions for voiced and voiceless postvocalic stops to overlap for individual aphasic and apraxic speakers, but not for normal control speakers. If this temporal acoustic distinction is affected similarly to the spectral distinctions examined in our previous research (Haley et al., 2000, 2001), we would expect varying degrees of overlap, primarily for aphasic speakers with AOS, but also for some aphasic speakers without AOS.

In regard to the magnitude of the distinction, the duration difference between vowels that precede voiced stops and vowels that precede voiceless stops is often expressed as a ratio. Rogers (1997) compared the voiced-to-voiceless vowel duration ratios produced by three speakers with coexisting aphasia and AOS, four speakers with aphasia and no AOS, four speakers with dysarthria, and six normal speakers. Mean ratios were 1.3 for the normal, dysarthric, and aphasic groups and 1.4 for the apraxic-aphasic group, indicating that all speaker groups, on the average, produced longer vowel duration preceding voiced stops than preceding voiceless stops. The mean differences in ratios across groups prompted Rogers to characterise the results as a potential vowel-lengthening exaggeration effect in speakers with AOS, and to hypothesise that the exaggeration effect may facilitate the differentiation of AOS from aphasia and from dysarthria. This suggestion has obvious implications for differential diagnosis, but its empirical basis did not consider potential overlap across populations in the range of performance. Inspection of individual speaker data reported in other investigations indicates that the magnitude of vowel duration differences may vary substantially across aphasic speakers (Baum et al., 1990; Duffy & Gawle, 1984), thereby challenging the notion of a diagnostic marker.

Wertz and Rosenbek (1992) cautioned that speech deviations detected by instrumentation have no communicative importance, unless listeners hear them. In our previous investigations, the selected quantification of spectral content corresponded well with phonetic transcription of place of articulation for the fricative consonants (Haley et al., 2000) but not for the vowels (Haley et al., 2001), leading us to conclude that acoustic variations other than those examined must have contributed to the vowel perception. Duffy and Gawle (1984) reached a similar conclusion regarding the relationship between vowel duration variations and postvocalic voicing perception in speech produced by persons with aphasia and AOS. In light of these observations and the fact that several acoustic properties are known to affect the perception of postvocalic stop voicing (Hillenbrand, Ingrisano, Smith, & Flege, 1984), the interpretation of observed duration variations should benefit from concurrent perceptual analysis.

One problem with perceptual analysis is that the tools clinicians and researchers typically use may not be sufficiently sensitive to detect variations of interest. Buckingham and Yule (1987) noted that listeners have limited ability to detect the unusual and sub-linguistic acoustic variations that are often present in disordered speech, because their language knowledge orients them away from these variations and towards properties that are phonemically important in their language. To the extent that acoustically ambiguous or deviant utterances are classified perceptually as either correct productions or segmental substitutions, variable perceptions may be expected across listeners and presentations. A summary of this perceptual variability may better reflect how a production is perceived than a single judgement of phonetic accuracy made by a single listener.

The present investigation addressed both the acoustic performance patterns of individual speakers and the auditory-perceptual effects of the analysed utterances. The dual aims were to determine if aphasic and apraxic speakers produce a normal vowel duration distinction between voiced and voiceless postvocalic stops and to explore the relationship between this acoustic measure and listeners' voicing perception. The approach was a combination of quantitative and qualitative analyses, with a focus on individual performance patterns.

METHOD

Speakers

Speech samples were recorded from 8 normal speakers and 16 individuals with a clinical diagnosis of aphasia secondary to a cerebrovascular accident (CVA). Participants were native speakers of American English and reported no previous speech or language difficulties. All aphasic speakers were at least 3 months post-onset of the CVA, as confirmed by a review of the medical records. Please refer to Table 1 for a summary of speaker characteristics.

Eight aphasic speakers were diagnosed with coexisting apraxia of speech (A-AOS) and eight were diagnosed with aphasia uncomplicated by apraxia of speech (APH). No speaker was included who carried a suspected or confirmed diagnosis of dementia or moderate dysarthria.

Presence and absence of AOS and dysarthria were based on the consensus of three speech-language pathologists specialising in the assessment and management of adults with acquired neurogenic communication disorders. Traditional criteria for AOS were used (Wertz, LaPointe, & Rosenbek, 1984). Specifically, to receive a diagnosis of AOS the speaker had to present with the following speech characteristics: (1) effortful speech with attempts to self-correct, (2) frequent articulatory errors, such as substitutions, distortions, omissions, additions, and repetitions, (3) articulatory variability across repeated productions of the same utterance, and (4) abnormal prosody. The three clinicians listened jointly to an audio-recording of a standard motor speech evaluation (Wertz et al., 1984). They then independently rated the severity of AOS and dysarthria on an 8-point rating scale from 0 (no impairment) to 7 (severe impairment). Inter-observer agreement within one scale level for at least two of the clinicians was 100%. Following the independent rating, the clinicians discussed their impressions and reached consensus about AOS and dysarthria severity. Eight speakers were diagnosed with mild to moderate AOS and six of these were judged to have mild coexisting dysarthria.

The Aphasia Quotient subtests of the Western Aphasia Battery (WAB: Kertesz, 1982) were given to estimate the severity of aphasia and classify the aphasia type. The mean aphasia quotients (AQ) were similar in the two aphasia groups; 75.0 for the A-AOS group and 77.4 for the APH group. A single word intelligibility test (Kent, Weismer, Kent, & Rosenbek, 1989) was administered to estimate the magnitude of speech impairment. Each speaker produced 70 monosyllabic words. These words were presented to normal listeners, who transcribed them orthographically. An intelligibility score was computed as the percentage of words that listeners identified accurately. The administration and scoring of the intelligibility test for these speakers have been reported in detail previously (Haley, Wertz, & Ohde, 1998). Mean intelligibility was 95% in the normal group, 75% in the A-AOS group, and 86% in the APH group. These results indicate that a satisfactory matching was achieved in overall language severity and that both groups presented with impaired speech production. However, the degree of speech production impairment was greater in the apraxic group, and this difference should be kept in mind when interpreting the results (see McNeil, Robin, & Schmidt, 1997, for a discussion of conceptual problems

TABLE 1
Demographics and test results

Speaker	Age	Gender	MPO	Aphasia	AQ	AOS	Dys.	Intell.
NOR1	50	F	NA	NA	99.8	0	0	97.5
NOR2	71	F	NA	NA	99.9	0	0	97.0
NOR3	56	M	NA	NA	99.8	0	0	96.5
NOR4	52	M	NA	NA	99.4	0	0	93.9
NOR5	59	M	NA	NA	97.0	0	0	88.5
NOR6	70	M	NA	NA	100.0	0	0	96.0
NOR7	72	M	NA	NA	98.8	0	0	97.7
NOR8	63	F	NA	NA	100.0	0	0	92.3
MEAN	*61.6*				*99.3*	*0*	*0*	*94.9*
A-AOS1	57	M	45	Broca	59.5	5	2	39.4
A-AOS2	64	M	11	Broca	73.9	4	1	85.1
A-AOS3	45	F	30	Broca	72.3	4	0	90.2
A-AOS4	47	M	63	Broca	67.5	1	0	92.4
A-AOS5	57	M	23	Anomic	80.6	4	2	70.9
A-AOS6	63	M	180	Anomic	94.8	2	1	66.4
A-AOS7	74	F	13	Anomic	79.5	2	2	89.4
A-AOS8	56	F	44	Conduction*	71.9	4	2	63.9
MEAN	*57.9*		*51.1*		*75.0*	*3*	*1*	*74.7*
APH1	59	M	78	Wernicke	68.2	0	0	89.3
APH2	61	M	13	Wernicke	54.0	0	0	88.6
APH3	28	M	91	Wernicke	70.9	0	0	88.2
APH4	74	F	13	Conduction	64.3	0	0	61.0
APH5	81	M	27	Anomic	87.8	0	0	88.1
APH6	37	M	8	NC	85.8	0	0	88.8
APH7	67	M	9	NC	90.4	0	0	91.3
APH8	48	M	22	NC	97.8	0	0	93.8
MEAN	*56.9*		*32.6*		*77.4*	*0*	*0*	*86.1*

Demographics and test results for speakers in the normal (NOR), aphasia and apraxia of speech (A-AOS), and aphasia only (APH) groups.

MPO = Months postonset; Aphasia; Syndrome classification on the Western Aphasia Battery (Kertesz, 1982); NC = Not classifiable; AQ = WAB Aphasia Quotient; AOS = AOS severity rating (0–7); Dys = Dysarthria severity rating (0–7); Intell = Single word intelligibility in percent (Haley et al., 1998; Kent et al., 1989).

*Classification according to the WAB cutoff scores. The clinicians agreed, based on traditional criteria (Wertz et al., 1984), that her speech difficulties were most characteristic of AOS.

associated with the use of aphasic comparison groups with minimal or no speech production errors).

Speech samples

Speech samples were recorded in a sound treated IAC booth, using a Tascam 22 reel-to-reel recorder and a head-mounted microphone (AKG-C410) with a constant mouth-to-microphone distance. The speaker was seated in a chair facing the experimenter. The experimenter displayed a 3″ × 5″ index card with a target phrase printed on it, read the card, and asked the speaker to repeat the utterance. The target words "had" and "hat" were elicited 24 times each in the context of the carrier phrase "The word _____".
Occasionally, speakers responded with more than one repetition of the target phrase.

These repetitions were accepted as valid production attempts. All utterances were digitised and stored on a Pentium II PC with a 22 kHz sampling rate and a 10 kHz low pass filter setting. They were edited so that only the final target word in each phrase was retained for acoustic and perceptual analysis. A perceptual screening across three listeners ensured that subsequent acoustic and perceptual analyses were appropriate for the examined contrast. A total of 25 utterances (2% of the sample) were excluded from further analysis due to perceived substitution of place or manner of articulation. None of the listeners perceived any voicing errors for any of the normal speakers. Several voicing substitutions were perceived among the aphasic and apraxic speakers, but these utterances were not excluded from analysis. The resulting speech sample consisted of 1137 utterances.

Vowel duration measures

Waveform and wide-band (300 Hz) spectrographic analyses were obtained through CSpeech (Milenkovic, 1996). The analyses were displayed simultaneously on the computer screen and referred to for duration measures. Aspiration typical for /h/ was visible for all productions, although sometimes voicing was noted during this portion of the utterance. The duration of the vowel nucleus was measured from the end of the aspiration noise in /h/ to the onset of closure for /d/ or /t/. On the spectrographic display, the vowel segment was defined operationally as the duration between the initial and final vertical striations that were visible through the first and second formant regions.

Intra-observer agreement was estimated by repeating measurements for 20% of the vowel segments 6 months after the original measures. Analyses were distributed equally across all speakers in the three speaker groups and across both voicing contexts. Point-to-point agreement was 98% within 10 ms and 84% within 5 ms.

Perceptual identification

Three graduate students in speech-language pathology participated as listeners in a forced choice perceptual identification test. They were all female native speakers of American English, ranged in age from 22 to 35, and passed a hearing screening at 20 dB for the octave frequencies between 500 Hz and 8000 Hz.

The entire set of productions produced by each APH and A-AOS speaker was presented in five separate random orders, yielding five presentations to each listener. Speakers were presented one at a time, and the order of speakers was randomised separately for each listener. The listening task was conducted in a sound treated IAC booth, with utterances presented over headphones at a comfortable listening level. A response box with two buttons labelled "had" and "hat" was positioned in front of the listener. The listeners were asked to press the button corresponding to the perceived utterance and to guess if they were not sure. Each listener was tested separately in two 1-hour sessions.

RESULTS

Vowel duration

The duration of vowel segments across individual utterances and speakers are displayed in Figure 1. For all groups and all speakers, the mean duration of the vowel nucleus was longer in the context of a voiced postvocalic stop than in the context of a voiceless postvocalic stop.

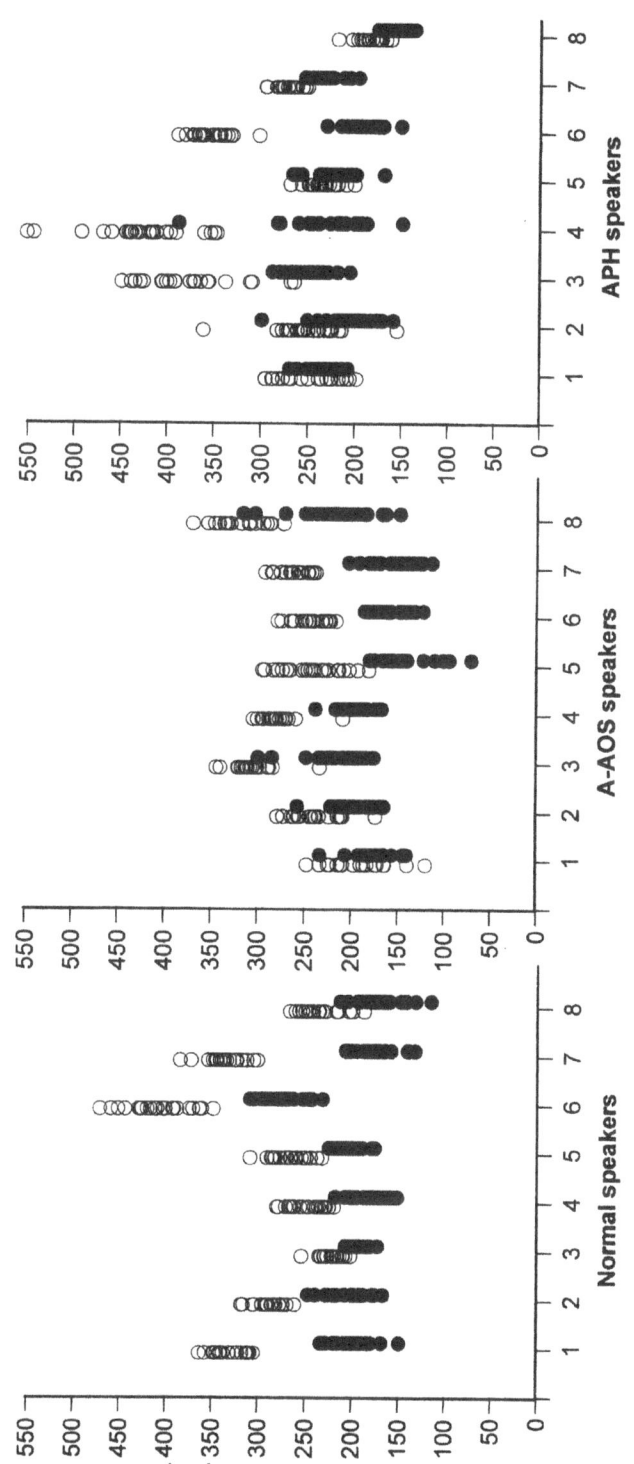

Figure 1. Vowel duration across repeated utterances for speakers in the normal, A-AOS, and APH groups. Open circles represent voiced targets (had) and closed circles represent voiceless targets (hat).

449

To examine the group effects for the acoustic data, we used a hierarchical linear model approach (Snijders & Bosker, 1999), which does not assume equal variance across conditions. A mixed model, treating the speakers as random effects, was fitted to the data using SAS PROC MIXED. Several possible covariance structures were tested with different constraints on the between- and within-speaker variability. We chose a final model that provided the best fit based on the differences in the goodness-of-fit statistic (ΔG^2), which has a chi-square distribution. In a model constraining the covariance structure to have equal variances for "had" and "hat", the goodness of fit statistic was significantly larger than in a model where the variance was allowed to vary across voicing contexts, $\Delta G^2(1) = 9555$, $p < .001$. Therefore, we selected a model with a within-subject covariance structure that permitted unequal variances for the duration of the vowel nucleus in "had" and "hat", with "had" displaying the greatest variability. As can be seen in Figure 1 and Table 2, whereas the vowel duration remained relatively stable across speakers for "hat", there was substantial inter-speaker variability for "had" in both the

TABLE 2
Mean vowel duration (ms) and voiced-to-voiceless
vowel duration ratio across speakers and
speaker groups

Speaker	had	hat	Ratio
NOR1	329.0 (17.3)	199.9 (20.0)	1.65
NOR2	292.0 (15.8)	207.8 (22.2)	1.40
NOR3	222.4 (11.3)	192.0 (9.7)	1.16
NOR4	248.9 (18.0)	181.4 (17.2)	1.37
NOR5	268.4 (18.7)	205.2 (12.5)	1.31
NOR6	407.3 (32.6)	277.3 (21.4)	1.47
NOR7	335.2 (19.6)	179.0 (21.5)	1.87
NOR8	231.5 (22.0)	166.8 (23.0)	1.39
Mean	*291.8 (62.6)*	*201.2 (33.8)*	*1.45*
A-AOS1	191.5 (31.9)	173.6 (21.7)	1.10
A-AOS2	242.6 (25.9)	196.2 (21.4)	1.24
A-AOS3	305.8 (21.0)	214.0 (30.8)	1.43
A-AOS4	279.6 (18.4)	194.1 (17.4)	1.44
A-AOS5	243.5 (31.3)	145.8 (29.2)	1.67
A-AOS6	243.6 (17.6)	162.2 (17.6)	1.50
A-AOS7	263.2 (14.6)	155.2 (22.0)	1.70
A-AOS8	321.8 (26.2)	219.0 (40.3)	1.47
Mean	*261.4 (41.1)*	*182.5 (27.3)*	*1.44*
APH1	248.2 (32.9)	230.1 (15.0)	1.08
APH2	251.6 (34.5)	206.3 (29.4)	1.22
APH3	378.2 (50.0)	251.3 (19.1)	1.50
APH4	428.5 (52.2)	232.9 (46.9)	1.84
APH5	237.6 (15.1)	223.5 (21.7)	1.06
APH6	353.3 (18.7)	193.0 (16.3)	1.83
APH7	270.4 (12.8)	233.4 (13.4)	1.16
APH8	184.1 (13.4)	153.2 (11.5)	1.20
Mean	*294.0 (83.2)*	*215.5 (30.8)*	*1.36*

Standard deviations for each speaker's duration measures are reported in parentheses. Group means are listed in *italics* and the associated standard deviations reflect inter-speaker variations.

normal and the aphasic groups. Allowing the covariance structure to have unequal variance across speaker groups did not improve the fit significantly, $\Delta G^2(4) = 3.6, p > .05$. Therefore, we concluded that duration variability did not differ significantly across speaker groups. Using the selected model, we found no significant group difference in vowel duration for either the voiced, $F(2, 21) = 0.63, p = .54$, or the voiceless, $F(2, 21) = 2.31, p = .12$, context. As expected, all three speaker groups displayed a statistically significant vowel duration differentiation between voiced and voiceless stop targets, $F(1, 30) = 32.02, p < .0001$.

Analysis of the performance of individual speakers was based on visual inspection of Figure 1. As can be seen, distributions for voicing cognates overlapped slightly for two normal speakers (NOR3 and NOR8). However, the degree of overlap in these two normal speakers was limited, and the distributions were clearly bimodal. Dramatically different patterns were observed for several aphasic and apraxic speakers. Whereas some speakers displayed a distribution overlap that was almost complete (A-AOS1, APH1, APH5), others displayed minimal or no overlap (A-AOS5, A-AOS6, A-AOS7, APH6), and the majority presented with partially overlapping distributions.

A vowel duration ratio was computed for each speaker by dividing the mean duration in the context of postvocalic voiced targets with the mean duration in the context of postvocalic voiceless targets (see Table 2). An analysis of variance was performed across speaker groups. The omnibus effect was not significant, $F(2, 23) = 0.31, p < .74$, indicating that the magnitude of the duration ratios did not differ across groups. More importantly, ratios varied substantially across speakers, ranging from 1.2 to 1.9 in the normal group, from 1.1 to 1.7 in the A-AOS group, and from 1.1 to 1.8 in the aphasic group.

Perceptual identification

The results of the identification test yielded different profiles for individual speakers. In the interest of brevity, Figure 2 presents results for only eight of the A-AOS and aphasic speakers. The remaining eight speakers produced patterns comparable to those illustrated. In general, there was good correspondence between acoustic and perceptual levels of analysis. This was true not only for accurate productions, but also for production errors. For example, speaker APH1 presented with completely overlapping duration distributions for the voicing cognates. Perceptually, numerous substitutions were recorded and shorter vowel duration was consistently associated with "hat" perceptions, whereas longer vowel duration was associated with "had" perceptions.

However, several other aphasic and apraxic speakers' utterances were perceptually ambiguous with regard to the postvocalic voicing, and this was evidenced by variable voicing responses across repeated presentations both within and among listeners. As illustrated in Figure 1, vowel duration for speaker A-AOS1 was similar for voiced and voiceless stops. Figure 2 shows that the majority of the productions were perceived as "hat". Only the "had" targets with the longest vowel duration were perceived as "had", and a number of "had" targets with intermediate vowel duration were perceived at chance level. Speaker A-AOS2 produced bimodal, but overlapping, vowel duration distributions for the voicing cognates. Perceptually, several productions, particularly those with intermediate duration values, were identified at near chance levels. A similar tendency for greater perceptual ambiguity to be associated with intermediate vowel durations was noted for speakers A-AOS3, A-AOS5, A-AOS6, APH2, and APH3. For some speakers, there was disagreement between the acoustic and perceptual levels of

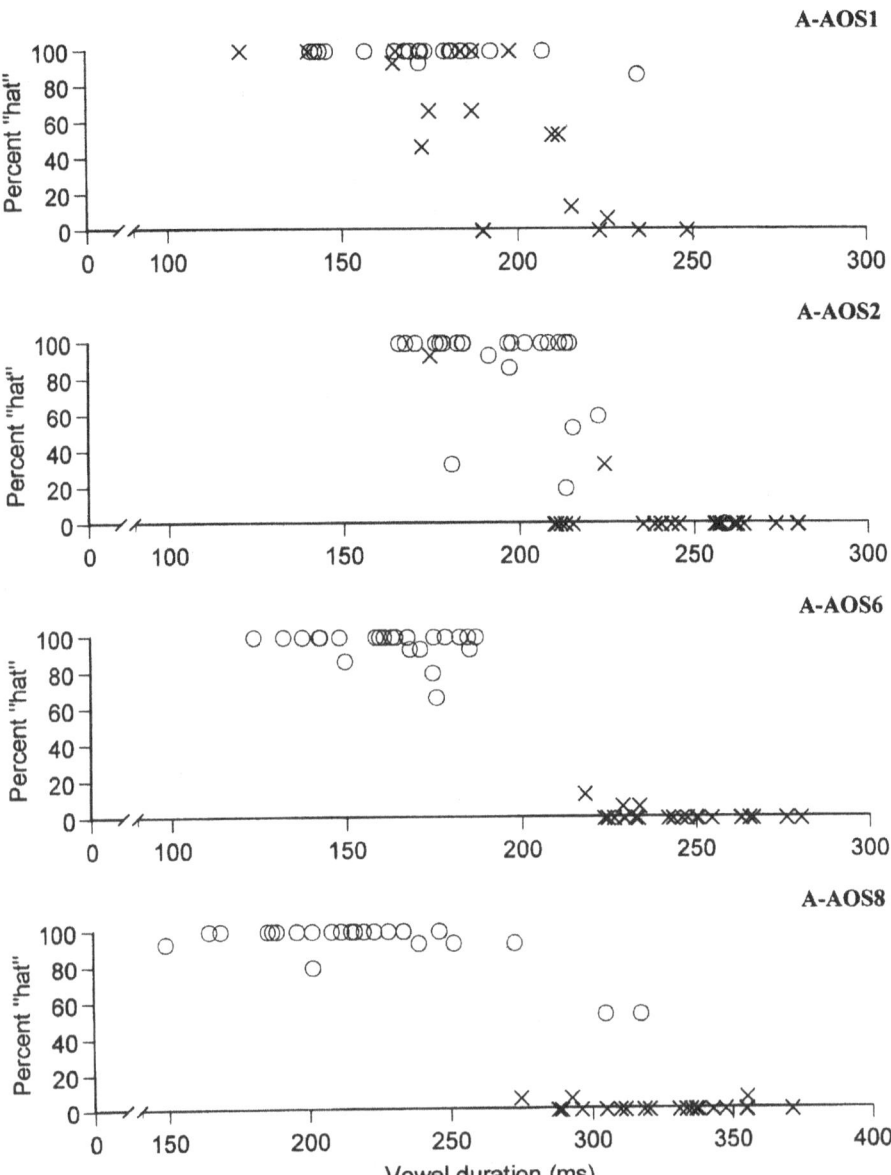

Figure 2 (above and opposite). Percent ''hat'' responses as a function of vowel duration for four A-AOS speakers and four aphasic speakers. Circles represent target words with voiceless postvocalic stops (hat) and Xs represent target words with voiced postvocalic stops (had). Note that the scale on the abscissa varies across speakers to accommodate variations in absolute duration and magnitude of duration contrast.

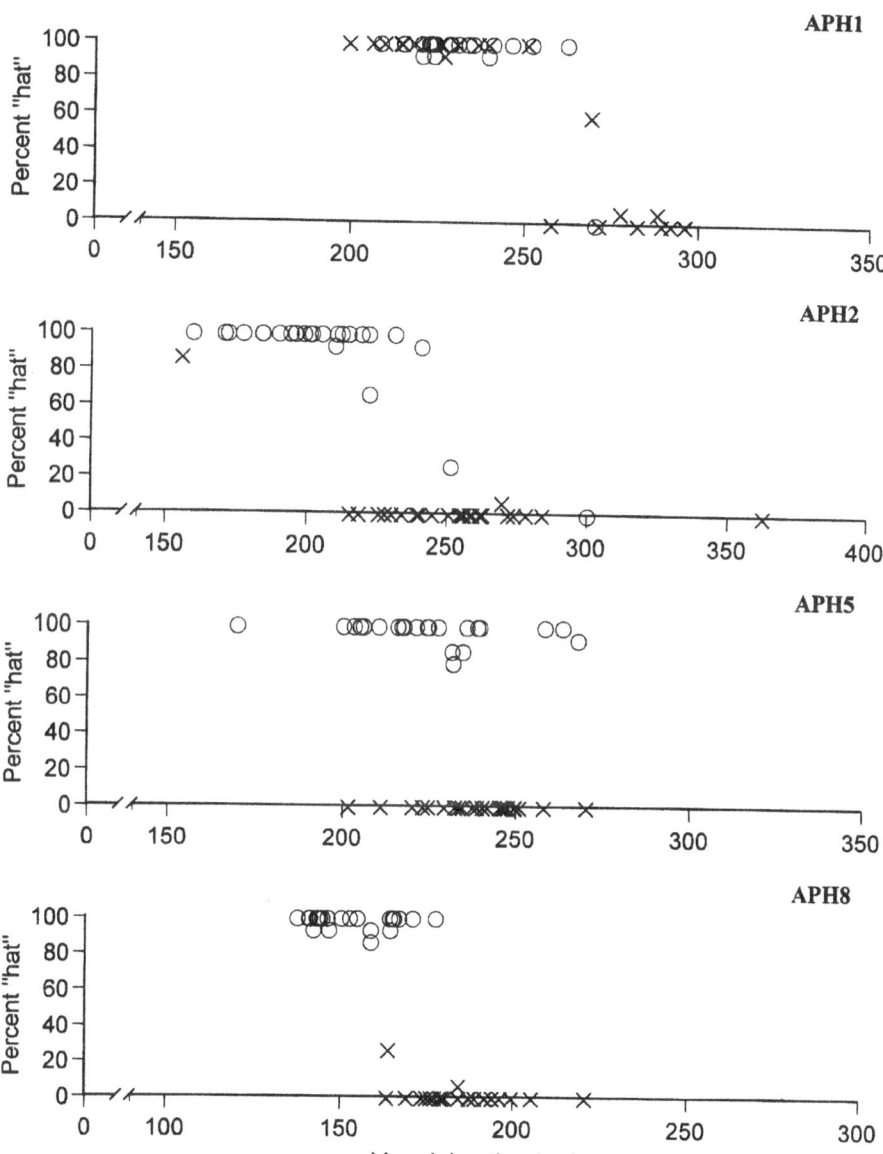

analysis. The most extreme example is speaker APH5. Despite complete overlap in voiced and voiceless vowel duration distributions, listeners identified the target word with 100% accuracy for almost all utterances.

DISCUSSION

The results of the vowel duration analysis are consistent with our previous observations using spectral measures (Haley et al., 2000, 2001). Despite a statistically significant duration difference between voiced and voiceless postvocalic stop contexts, many speakers displayed an inconsistent differentiation and some failed to distinguish between the two voicing cognates altogether. Several examples of abnormal acoustic performance were seen among the aphasic and apraxic speakers.

On the assumption that AOS severity ratings and single word intelligibility scores quantify some aspect of impairment magnitude, there was not a strong correspondence between speech severity and achievement of phonetic contrast. However, most speakers who displayed limited perceptual and acoustic ambiguity had intelligibility scores above 89%. Similarly, speaker A-AOS1 presented with the lowest intelligibility score, the highest AOS severity rating, and the acoustically and perceptually most abnormal profile. Most of his utterances were perceived as "hat" and the vowel duration distributions overlapped almost completely for voiced and voiceless stops. Interestingly, this speaker's production of fricative consonants yielded a similar collapse of phonetic distinctiveness (Haley et al., 2000). Future studies should examine the correlation between severity and achievement of phonetic contrast in a larger and more varied speaker sample. Of related interest is whether shifts from one distinction pattern to another occur during recovery. For example, motor learning accounts of coordinated movement acquisition predict both an increase in inter-trial variability as new movement patterns are explored and a decrease in such fluctuations as movements later stabilise (Schmidt & Lee, 1999). For some speakers, a transition from complete to partial acoustic overlap may reflect an increase in movement fluctuations as more phonetic targets are approximated, whereas a transition from partial to minimal overlap may suggest stabilisation of the underlying speech movements.

A comparison of voiced to voiceless vowel duration ratios showed that the magnitude of the distinction did not differ across groups and that it varied substantially among individual speakers. Thus, the results do not support Rogers' (1997) hypothesis regarding a vowel lengthening exaggeration in AOS, at least not for the target words and phrase position used in the present investigation. Additionally, the classification of a property as a diagnostic marker implies that persons with a given diagnosis differ consistently from persons without that disorder with respect to the given property. Thus, it is not sufficient to demonstrate a high probability of population differences in the mean. For the marker to assist with differential diagnosis, the observed property must have a value outside the typical range of normal and within the range of the disorder, so each individual can be appropriately diagnosed. The conditions for the potential marker must also be determined. Over the years, it has been shown that a large number of factors influence vowel duration and that these factors interact with each other in rather complex ways (Crystal & House, 1988; Klatt, 1973; Smith, 2002; Umeda, 1975; Weismer & Ingrisano, 1979). Certain combinations of segmental, supra-segmental, linguistic, and pragmatic conditions are likely to yield a greater magnitude of vowel duration differences for postvocalic voiced and voiceless stops than other combinations. Similar interactions may be expected between these conditions and properties associated with disorders such as aphasia and

AOS. Thus, the magnitude observations in the present investigation, and in Rogers (1997), may have been different with another phrase position, vowel target, elicitation format, and/or stress pattern.

The observation of substantial inter-speaker variability in the normal group was important, because it demonstrates the need to collect normative data on the range of individual speaker performance. Some of the variability may have been associated with natural differences in speaking rate. Although we attempted to achieve consistency in the rate of stimulus presentation and in the experimenter's speaking rate, we did not attempt to control the rate of speech production formally. It is possible, at least among the normal speakers, that those who produced a relatively smaller magnitude difference may have used a relatively faster speaking rate. However, it is unlikely that all, or even most, of the inter-speaker variation can be explained by rate variations. In a recent investigation, Smith (2002) examined the effects of experimental variations in speaking rate on several durational measures for 15 normal speakers. Although 13 of the speakers reduced the duration difference for vowels preceding postvocalic voiced and voiceless stops when they increased their speaking rate from normal to fast, the magnitude of this difference was small in comparison to the naturally occurring inter-speaker variations. Based on these observations, Smith called for increased attention in research to the range of performance across normal speakers.

The results of the perceptual identification experiment have several clinical implications. First, the generally good agreement between acoustic and perceptual levels of analysis indicates that measures of vowel duration provide meaningful information about the accuracy of postvocalic voicing in speakers with aphasia and AOS. Vowel duration is relatively easy to quantify and may therefore be useful in clinical assessment and intervention outcome measures that address or include postvocalic voicing production. Second, many utterances produced by speakers with aphasia and AOS were perceptually ambiguous and could not be clearly classified as either voiced or voiceless. The effects of this ambiguity were seen upon repeated presentations of the utterances to a group of listeners. Clinical assessment of phonetic accuracy may consider replacing standard perceptual screening or phonetic transcription procedures with a similar test approach when subtle acoustic or sub-phonemic variations are expected. Third, occasional incongruity between acoustic and perceptual levels of analysis suggests that acoustic properties other than vowel duration must have contributed to the perception of postvocalic stop voicing. A systematic investigation of what other acoustic properties may have been involved was beyond the scope of this study. However, preliminary analyses of one potential cue helped to resolve most discrepancies, including the surprisingly intact voicing perception for APH5 and the minimal acoustic overlap for NOR3 and NOR8. Specifically, the overlap in vowel duration for these speakers was balanced by non-overlapping variation in the presence or absence of voicing during stop closure. Examination of the extent to which such trade-off among acoustic properties occurs in normal and impaired speech production would be valuable.

Finally, the observation of acoustically and perceptually ambiguous utterances in both aphasic groups is difficult to explain within traditional dichotomies of apraxic/aphasic and phonetic/phonemic speech errors (Haley et al., 2000, 2001). It remains to be determined whether the overlap is best explained relative to the neural substrate affected for individual speakers, to the interaction among dimensions or levels of speech motor control and language processing, or to methodological limitations.

REFERENCES

Baum, S., Blumstein, S., Naeser, M., & Palumbo, C. (1990). Temporal dimensions of consonant and vowel production: An acoustic and CT scan analysis of aphasic speech. *Brain and Language, 39*, 33–56.

Buckingham, H. W., & Yule, G. (1987). Phonemic false evaluation: Theoretical and clinical aspects. *Clinical Linguistics and Phonetics, 1*, 113–125.

Caligiuri, M., & Till, J. (1983). Acoustical analysis of vowel duration in apraxia of speech: A case study. *Folia Phoniatrica, 35*, 226–234.

Chen, M. (1970). Vowel length variation as a function of the voicing of the consonant environment. *Phonetica, 22*, 129–159.

Crystal, T. H., & House, A. S. (1988). A note on the variability of timing control. *Journal of Speech and Hearing Research, 31*, 497–502.

Duffy, J. R., & Gawle, C. A. (1984). Apraxic speakers' vowel duration in consonant-vowel-consonant syllables. In J. C. Rosenbek, M. R. McNeil, & A. E. Aronson (Eds.), *Apraxia of speech: Physiology, acoustics, linguistics, management* (pp. 167–196). San Diego, CA: College-Hill.

Haley, K. L., Ohde, R. N., & Wertz, R. T. (2000). Precision of fricative production in aphasia and apraxia of speech: A perceptual and acoustic study. *Aphasiology, 14*, 619–634.

Haley, K. L., Ohde, R. N., & Wertz, R. O. (2001). Vowel quality in aphasia and apraxia of speech: Phonetic transcription and formant analyses. *Aphasiology, 15*, 1107–1123.

Haley, K. L., Wertz, R. T., & Ohde, R. N. (1998). Single word intelligibility in aphasia and apraxia of speech. *Aphasiology, 12*, 715–730.

Hillenbrand, J., Ingrisano, D. R., Smith, B. L., & Flege, J. E. (1984). Perception of the voiced-voiceless contrast in syllable-final stops. *Journal of the Acoustical Society of America, 76*, 18–26.

Hogan, J. T., & Rozsypal, A. J. (1980). Evaluation of vowel duration as a cue for the voicing distinction in the following word-final consonant. *Journal of the Acoustical Society of America, 67*, 1764–1771.

Kent, R. D., Weismer, G., Kent, J. F., & Rosenbek, J. C. (1989). Toward phonetic intelligibility testing in dysarthria. *Journal of Speech and Hearing Disorders, 54*, 482–499.

Kertesz, A. (1982). *Western Aphasia Battery.* New York: Grune & Stratton.

Klatt, D. H. (1973). Interaction between two factors that influence vowel duration. *Journal of the Acoustical Society of America, 54*, 1102–1104.

McNeil, M., Robin, D., & Schmidt, R. (1997). Apraxia of speech: Definition, differentiation, and treatment. In M. McNeil (Ed.), *Clinical management of sensorimotor speech disorders* (pp. 311–344). New York: Thieme.

Milenkovic, P. (1996). CSpeech [computer program], Department of Electrical and Computer Engineering, University of Wisconsin-Madison.

Raphael, L. J. (1972). Preceding vowel duration as a cue to the perception of the voicing characteristic of word-final consonants in American English. *Journal of the Acoustical Society of America, 51*, 1296–1303.

Rogers, M. A. (1997). The vowel lengthening exaggeration effect in speakers with apraxia of speech: Compensation, artifact, or primary deficit? *Aphasiology, 11*, 433–445.

Schmidt, R. A., & Lee, T. D. (1999). *Motor control and learning: A behavioral emphasis.* Champaign, IL: Human Kinetics

Smith, B. L. (2002). Effects of speaking rate on temporal patterns of English. *Phonetica, 59*, 232–244.

Snijders, T. A. B., & Bosker, R., J. (1999). *Multilevel analysis: An introduction to basic and advanced multilevel modelling.* London: Sage Publications.

Tuller, B. (1984). On categorizing aphasic speech errors. *Neuropsychologia, 22*, 547–557.

Umeda, N. (1975). Vowel duration in American English. *Journal of the Acoustical Society of America, 58*, 434–445.

Weismer, G., & Ingrisano, D. (1979) Phrase-level timing patterns in English: Effects of emphasic stress location and speaking rate. *Journal of Speech and Hearing Research, 22*, 516–533.

Wertz, R. T., LaPointe, L. L., & Rosenbek, J. C. (1984). *Apraxia of speech in adults: The disorder and its management.* San Diego, CA: Singular.

Wertz, R. T., & Rosenbek, J. C. (1992). Where the ear fits: A perceptual evaluation of motor speech disorders. *Seminars in Speech and Language, 13*, 39–54.

APHASIOLOGY, 2004, *18* (5/6/7), 457–471

Treatment of word retrieval deficits with contextual priming

Nadine Martin

Temple University, and Moss Rehabilitation Research Institute, Philadelphia, USA

Ruth Fink

Moss Rehabilitation Research Institute, Philadelphia, USA

Matti Laine

Åbo Akademi University, Åbo, Finland

Background: Repetition priming is often a component of treatments for word-finding disorders. It can facilitate or interfere with naming success depending on a number of factors. Here we investigate the effectiveness of massed priming coupled with semantic or phonological context as a treatment for naming impairments arising from semantic and phonological deficits.

Aims: We aimed to determine whether (1) this procedure, used previously in a short-term facilitation study, would effectively improve word retrieval in a treatment study, and (2) the pattern of facilitation or interference observed in the facilitation study would carry over to the treatment programme.

Methods & Procedures: We used a single subject multiple baseline design. There were two participants: LP with a phonological encoding deficit and AS with both semantic and phonological deficits. Treatment involved identifying and repeating the names of words that were related semantically or phonologically, or unrelated. Pre and post measures of naming were used to assess overall effectiveness of the treatment. Acquisition, maintenance, and generalisation were measured with baseline tests at the start of each session. Correct responses and errors on within-training naming probes were used to measure sensitivity to priming in a particular context.

Outcomes & Results: LP benefited from this procedure regardless of the training context. AS showed interference in the semantic context during training and only modest short-term gains. These outcomes were predicted by their performance on an earlier facilitation study.

Conclusions: Contextual repetition priming has different effects on naming and these differences appear to be related to the context of training (semantic or phonological) and the primary source of an individual's naming impairment (semantic or phonological). This procedure is most effective when semantic processing of words is relatively spared.

Address correspondence to: Nadine Martin, Department of Communication Sciences, Temple University, Weiss Hall, 1701 N. 13th Street, Philadelphia, PA 19122, USA. Email: nmartin@temple.edu

This study was supported by a grant from the National Institutes of Deafness and Communication Disorders (DC19024) awarded to Temple University (PI: Nadine Martin). We thank Kelly Bowes and Farah Hussain for their help with data collection. Many thanks go to LP and AS for their participation in this study.

http://www.tandf.co.uk/journals/pp/02687038.html   DOI: 10.1080/02687030444000129

Priming access to words is a technique that is incorporated into many therapy approaches for word retrieval impairments (e.g., Patterson, Purell, & Morton, 1983). Priming can involve simple exposure to a stimulus (e.g., a spoken or written word) that is related to or identical to the target word, or it can involve an additional response from the individual undergoing treatment (e.g., repeating the prime or identifying a picture to match the prime). In the present study, we explored the effectiveness of contextual priming, a relatively recent approach to treatment of word retrieval that combines massed repetition of picture names with context effects by training pictures in small sets that are related in some way semantically or phonologically.

Laine and Martin (1996) first investigated the effectiveness of contextual priming in a single case study, IL, whose naming was affected by a breakdown in the links between semantic and lexical-phonological representations. In this short-term facilitation study, they found that whereas semantic context facilitated IL's naming, phonological context interfered with it. In a second study, Martin and Laine (2000) identified another individual, JL, who displayed a different pattern of sensitivity to context. JL was diagnosed with Wernicke's aphasia and had deficits in both semantic and phonological processing. In contrast to IL, he benefited from training with a phonological context but not with semantic context. Martin, Fink, Laine, and Ayala (2004) investigated immediate and short-term effects of contextual repetition priming on naming abilities of 11 aphasic individuals. In all but one of the participants, they found that contextual priming had an immediate interference effect on naming (increased errors on naming probes during training in at least one context), but was facilitative for all participants in the short term (significantly better naming on a post-test 5 minutes after treatment). This pattern of interference followed by facilitation is consistent with predictions of an interactive activation model of word retrieval (e.g., Dell & O'Seaghdha, 1992), the theoretical framework that guides our work. According to this model, massed priming of a set of related target words would create a highly active set of lexical neighbours during training, because the interactive activation that occurs as each word is primed spreads to representations of each word in the set. Thus, the probabilities of substitution errors involving words within the training set will be high at this time. After priming is stopped, for a short period the words should each be more accessible for production due to residual activation of their representations, but the probability of intrusion from one of the words in the training set will be less.

Martin et al. (2004) also found evidence that individuals respond differentially to contextual priming depending on the nature of their naming disorder (i.e., semantic or phonological). This finding corroborates evidence for differential sensitivity to context that was observed in the case studies described above (IL: Laine & Martin, 1996; JB: Martin & Laine, 2000).

The studies reviewed so far have examined the short-term effects of contextual priming. Two other studies have used contextual priming in a treatment protocol. Renvall, Laine, Laakso, and Martin (2003) applied the technique to treatment of YK, an individual whose word retrieval was impaired and who demonstrated good semantic processing, but impaired phonological processing. The most important finding from this study concerned generalisation of naming improvements to untrained items. Training was carried out with semantic, phonological, and unrelated contexts. Facilitation was observed in all contexts, but generalisation to untrained items was evident in the semantic context only. These effects were present at a 1.5-month follow-up assessment. Renvall et al. noted that these results suggested that context effects are, by themselves, short-lived, and that repetition priming is the most significant contributor to facilitation. This question remains unresolved however, as we have also identified participants who do not show facilitation over the short term in all context conditions (Martin et al., 2004).

A second study using contextual priming was conducted by Cornelissen, Laine, Tarkiainen, Järvensivu, Martin, and Salmelin (2003). They combined repetition priming with semantic context to rehabilitate the naming abilities of three chronic left-hemisphere-damaged aphasic individuals. Both behavioural and magnetoencephalographic measurements were obtained before and after treatment. All three participants' naming of the trained items improved, and in all participants a single source area, located in the left inferior parietal lobe close to the lesioned area, displayed statistically significant training-induced changes beginning 300–600 ms after picture presentation. Cornelissen et al. attributed these training effects to improved phonological encoding and storage of the trained items through the engagement of a left hemispheric word learning system, an interpretation that is consistent with functional imaging studies that link the left inferior parietal lobe activity to the phonological storage component of the verbal working memory (e.g., Paulesu, Frith, & Frackowiak, 1993).

In this paper, we report the results of a long-term treatment programme for word retrieval using contextual priming. We examined whether this procedure would effectively improve word retrieval and whether the pattern of facilitation or interference observed following a one-session contextual priming treatment would carry over to an extended treatment protocol using contextual priming. The two participants in this study, LP and AS, had completed the facilitation study described above (Martin et al., 2004). Based on their performances in that study, we hypothesised that AS and LP would demonstrate different patterns of sensitivity to context; that is, AS would show interference in both semantic and phonological contexts, and LP would show no significant interference in any context.

METHOD

Participants

Our two participants, LP and AS, demonstrated moderate naming deficits following left middle cerebral artery infarctions. A series of background tests revealed different profiles of semantic and phonological impairments underlying their naming difficulty (see Table 1 for selected background information). LP, a 41-year-old female, demonstrated relatively intact semantic abilities but poor phonological encoding. AS, a 66-year-old male, demonstrated moderate deficits in both semantic and phonological processing, but with a primary difficulty in accessing the word form from semantics. The differences in semantic/phonological profiles of these two individuals are especially apparent in their rates of semantic and phonological errors in naming (AS: high rates of semantic errors; LP: high rates of phonological errors) and repetition (AS: relatively intact; LP: impaired).

Both participants were native English speakers. They each passed a hearing screening and neither reported or exhibited any visual difficulties. Neither participant was involved in a treatment programme while participating in this study. Also, they were not enrolled in therapy between the end of treatment and follow-up measures.

Design

We used a single subject multiple baseline design (McReynolds & Kearns, 1983). Before treatment, subjects were administered a 652-item naming test with pictures from 15 categories drawn from three context conditions (semantic, e.g., animals, professions;

TABLE 1
Selected participant information

	AS	LP
Demographics		
Age	66 years/10 months	41 years/9 months
Gender	Male	Female
Time post-onset	5 years/11 months	1 year/9 months
Aetiology	LMCA	LMCA
Aphasia subtype	Broca's	Conduction
WAB[1] AQ	68.8	79.7
Output measures		
PNT[2] (Oral Picture Naming)		
% Correct	65	55
% Phonological Errors	11	37
% Semantic Errors	16	2
PRT[3] (Oral Repetition)	91	73
Input measures		
PPVT[4] (Standard Score)	90	89
PCB[5] (% Correct)		
Lexical Comprehension	100	100
Synonymy Triplets	87	93
Concrete/Abstract Synonymy[6] (% Correct)		
Concrete	92	100
Abstract	58	83

[1] Western Aphasia Battery (WAB: Kertesz, 1982).
[2] Philadelphia Naming Test (PNT: Roach, Schwartz, Martin, Grewal, & Brecher, 1996).
[3] Philadelphia Repetition Test (PRT: Dell, Schwartz, Martin, Saffran, & Gagnon, 1997).
[4] Peabody Picture Vocabulary Test (PPVT: Dunn & Dunn, 1981).
[5] Philadelphia Comprehension Battery (PCB: Saffran, Schwartz, Linebarger, Martin, & Bochetto, 1988).
[6] Concrete/Abstract Synonymy (Martin & Saffran, 1997).

phonologic, e.g., words beginning with /k/, /s/, etc.; unrelated). Difficult-to-name items from each of nine categories were used to create three 60-item baseline naming tests to be used in three treatment modules. Each module consisted of one category from each relatedness context (e.g., Module 1: animals, K-words, unrelated words). Each corresponding baseline test consisted of 20 items from each relatedness context. Prior to each treatment module, a corresponding baseline naming test was administered until a stable baseline was obtained. From the set of 20 items, 5 items that were difficult to name over repeated presentations were chosen for training and 5 items matched in frequency, length, and difficulty were chosen as control items. Easy-to-name items were not used in training but were probed daily in the 60-item baseline and maintenance measure.[1]

Procedure

The treatment approach combined intensive repetition priming with systematic manipulation of linguistic relationships (semantic, phonologic, and unrelated) among pictures in a treatment set. Each of three treatment sessions per week included: a 60-item baseline test, 20 words from each of three context conditions; a 10-item pretest with words from the

---

[1] Stimulus words used as experimental and control items for each subject are available upon request.

context undergoing training (5 trained and 5 untrained); multiple priming trials followed by naming probes; and a 10-item post-test. A priming trial consisted of three steps: spoken word-to-picture matching; repetition; and naming (see Appendix for details of treatment procedures). The purpose of the pre- and post-tests within a training session was to observe any evidence of short-term facilitation effects on items being trained and their matched controls. Treatment of each context within a treatment module continued until 80% of the trained items were named correctly on the repeated baseline measure over two consecutive sessions. Following criterion or a maximum of nine treatment sessions, treatment began on another relatedness condition. The 5 items previously trained were then tested for maintenance as part of the 60-item baseline/generalisation probe. When training was completed for all three contexts, we initiated two replications of the treatment (Treatment Modules 2 and 3) using different categories within each context.

Upon completion of the three Treatment Modules participants were administered the 652-item naming test to compare performance on trained and untrained items before and after therapy. In addition, each 60-item baseline test was administered sequentially following the completion of all three treatment modules.

Scoring

We scored final attempts at naming. A response was scored as correct if it was the target name or an acceptable alternative name based on the responses of five normal control subjects. Participants were allowed 20 seconds to produce a name. Correct responses had to be phonologically accurate.

Data analyses

We used McNemar tests of change to examine naming improvement on the 652-item naming test. We graphed correct responses on the baseline tests administered at the beginning of each session to track acquisition, maintenance, and generalisation. We also measured context sensitivity from responses to naming probes during training. To do this, we compared rates of correct responses and contextual errors on probes in related contexts with the same in unrelated contexts using chi square analyses. These comparisons yielded measures of immediate interference or facilitation effects of contextual priming on naming.

RESULTS

Results are shown in Figures 1–6 and Table 2. These graphs plot the correct responses on trained and matched control items probed at the beginning of each training session (as part of the 60-item baseline–maintenance measures).

Acquisition/maintenance

As Figures 1–6 show, performance on trained and untrained items remained low until treatment was initiated in each phase. For both participants, correct responses on trained items increased when training began, although the effects were stronger for LP. Acquisition effects for LP (Figures 1–3) were strong in all contexts, occurred in fewer sessions and were maintained at or near criterion. These gains were maintained at follow-up testing.

Participant AS (Figures 4–6) never reached criterion in semantic contexts and while his performance in phonological and unrelated contexts improved, it was variable and not

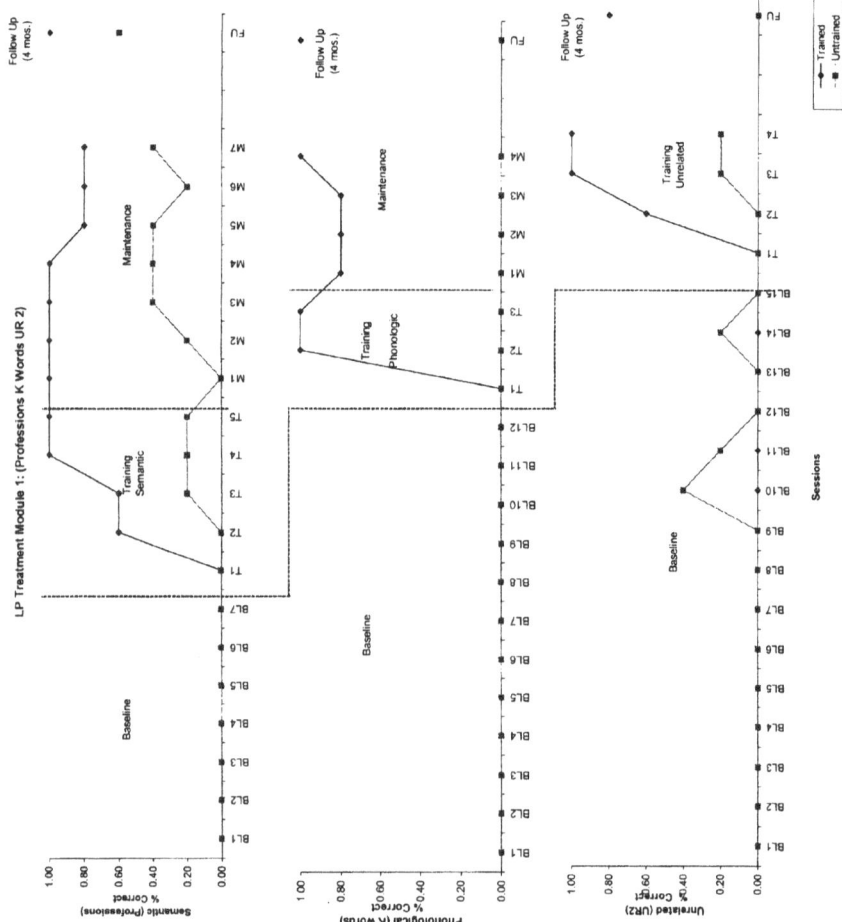

Figure 1. LP: Module 1 (professions, K-words, unrelated–UR2) baseline, acquisition, and maintenance.

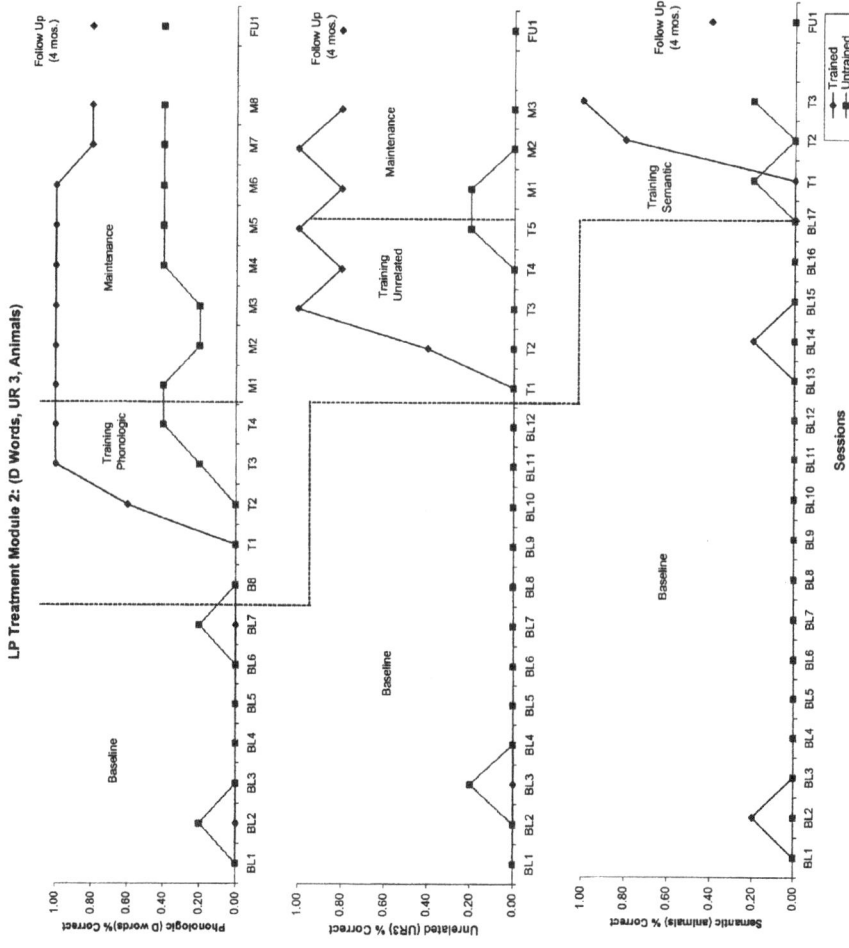

Figure 2. Module 2 (D-words, unrelated—UR3, animals) baseline, acquisition, and maintenance.

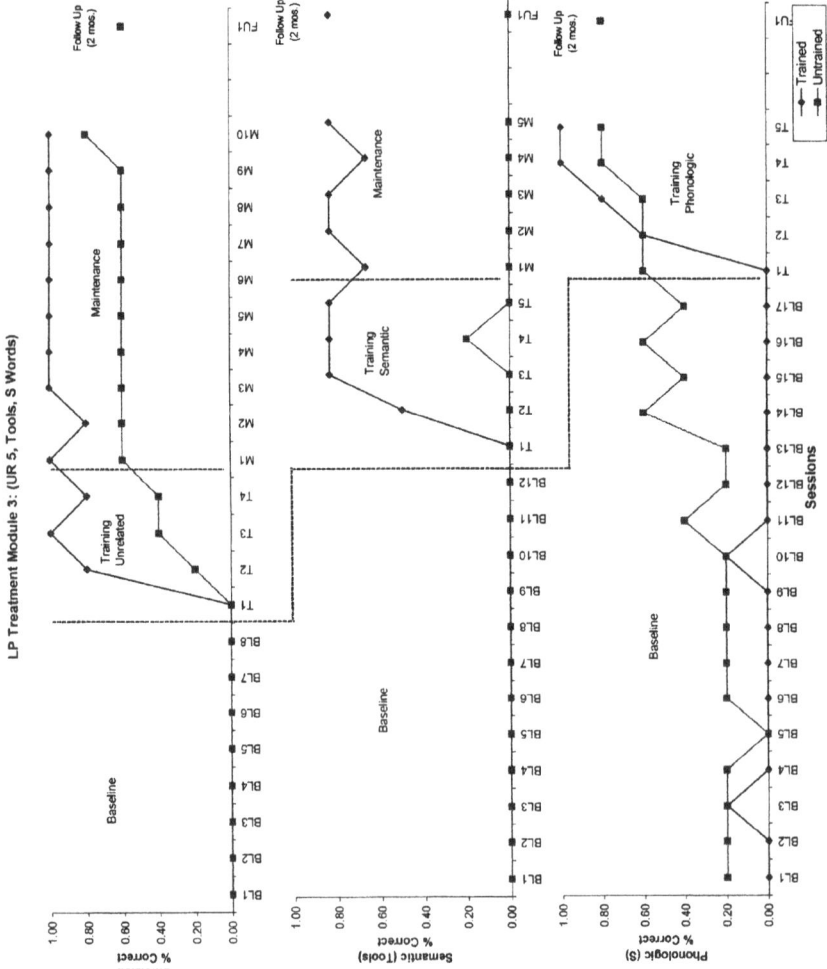

Figure 3. LP: Module 3 (unrelated–UR5, tools, S-words) baseline, acquisition, and maintenance.

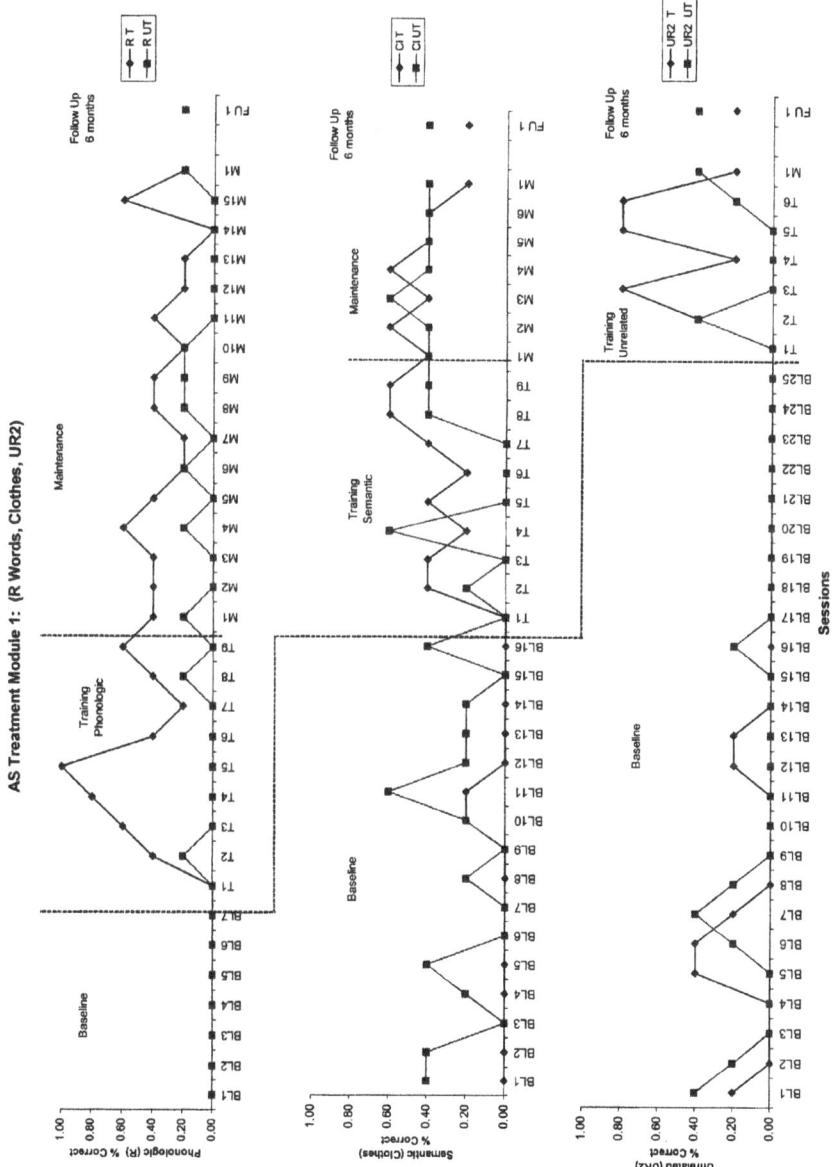

Figure 4. AS: MOdule 1 (R-words, unrelated-UR 2, clothes) baseline, acquisition, and maintenance.

465

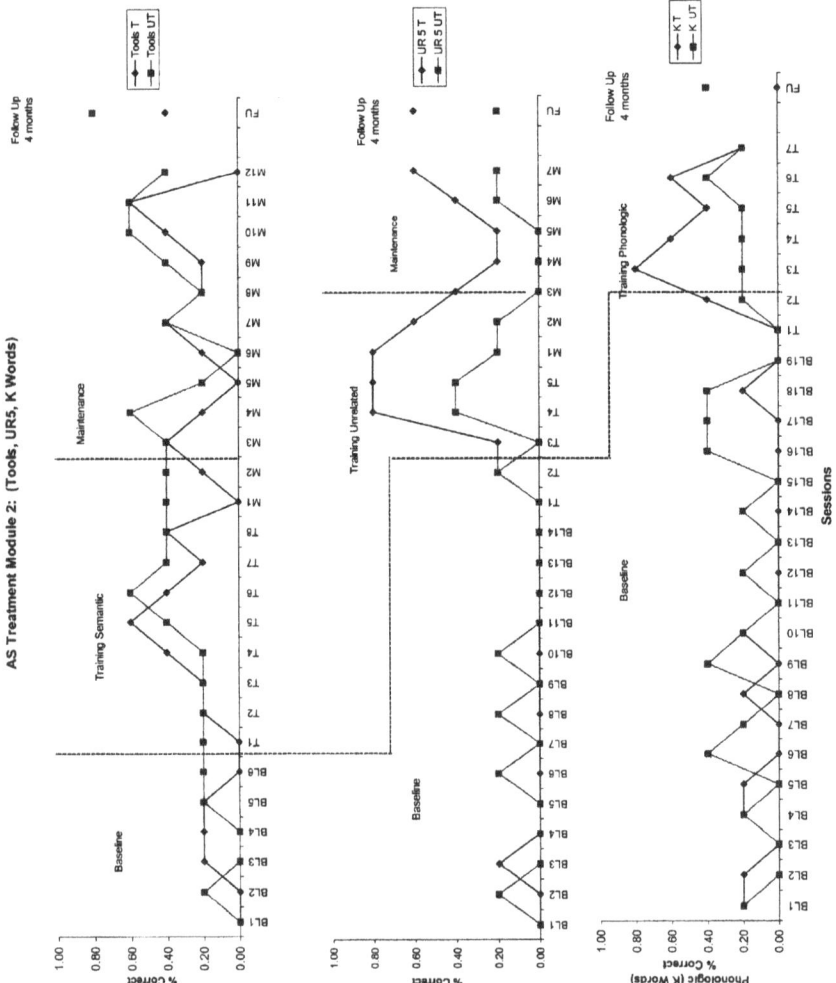

Figure 5. AS: Module 2 (tools, unrelated–UR 5, K-words) baseline, acquisition, and maintenance.

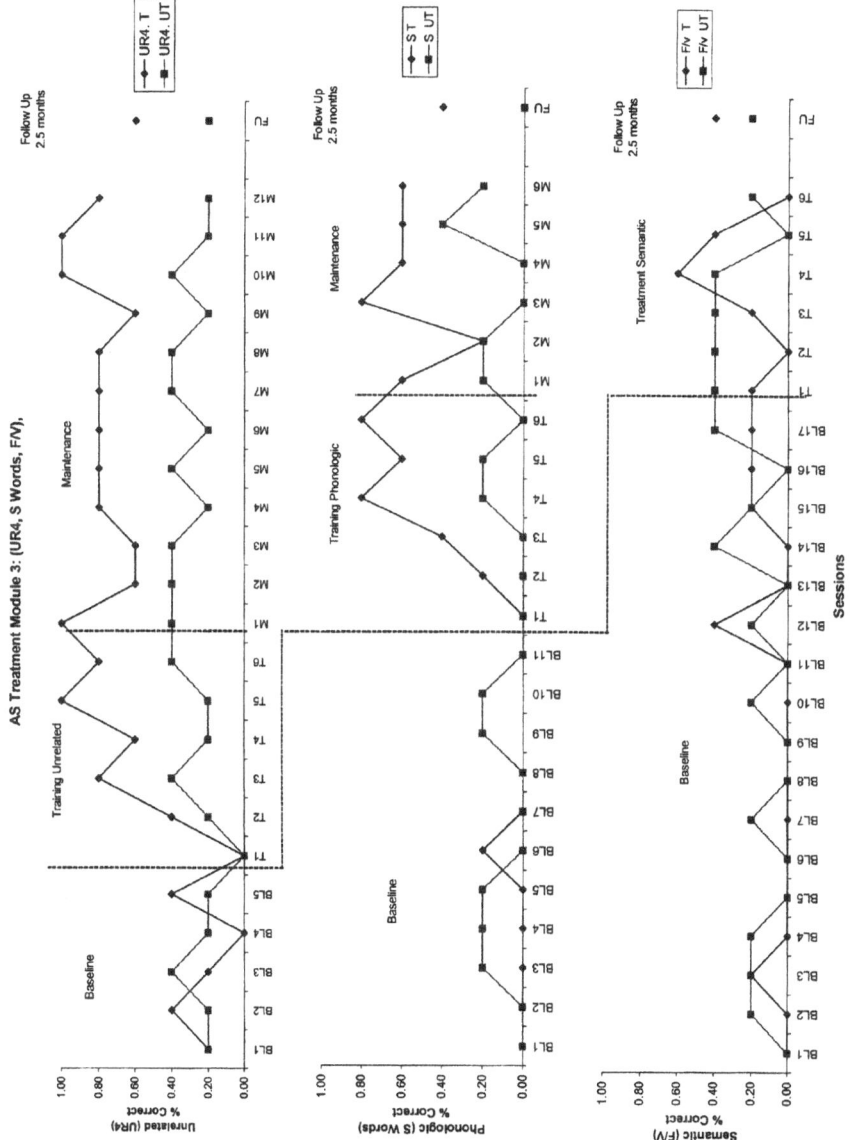

Figure 6. AS: Module 3 (unrelated–UR 4, S-words, fruits and vegetables) baseline, acquisition, and maintenance.

consistently maintained immediately following training or at follow-up testing. As can be seen in Figure 6, for example, AS shows both learning and maintenance of items in the unrelated condition when tested at 2.5 months following treatment (Module 3). For items from Module 2 (Figure 5) tested at 4 months following treatment, performance in the unrelated context was maintained at above baseline levels. Gains made in Module 1(Figure 4) were not maintained at follow-up testing (6 months after this module was trained).

Generalisation

For the most part, acquisition was limited to trained items. Although we see small gains in untrained items when treatment is initiated (see LP, Figure 1: semantic and unrelated contexts; Figure 2: phonological; Figure 3: unrelated and phonological contexts), there is no consistent pattern related to context of training.

McNemar tests of change, used to evaluate pre- and post-performance on the 652-item naming test (see Table 2), revealed significant improvement in picture naming for both participants overall. For LP this improvement was observed in all context conditions, but for AS these gains were found only in the unrelated and semantic contexts. Furthermore, and contrary to the acquisition data, for both participants, we see significant changes in naming both trained and untrained items.

An important issue is whether simple exposure played a role in improvement of naming. We found some evidence of this in our results. Not only did we observe improved performance on the untrained control items, but also on the remaining untrained items that were probed only in the 60-item baseline measure—LP: $\chi^2(1) = 72.99$, $p < .0001$; AS: $\chi^2(1) = 54.98$, $p < .0001$. Additionally, for those untrained items that were never exposed in any of the daily probe measures but were tested within the 652-item naming test before and after the entire experiment, a significant increase in correct responses was observed for AS, $\chi^2(1) = 13.82$, $p < .001$, but not for LP, $\chi^2(1) =$

TABLE 2
Performance on 652-item pre- and post-treatment naming test

Pre and post measure	LP			AS		
	Pre	Post	χ^2	Pre	Post	χ^2
	(% correct)			(% correct)		
All items (n = 652)	0.39	0.57	p < .0001	0.41	0.46	p < .05
Trained-semantic (n = 15)	0	0.67	p < .01	0	0.33	p < .05
Trained-phonological (n = 15)	0	0.75	p < .001	0	0.27	p < .10 NS
Trained-unrelated (n = 15)	0	0.60	p < .01	0	0.33	p < .05
Trained items (n = 45)	0	0.69	p < .0001	0	0.31	p < .001
Untrained control items (n = 45)	0.02	0.24	p < .01	0	0.20	p < .01

0.8421, NS. Thus, while simple exposure does appear to have some role in facilitating word retrieval, it is clear that gains made on treated items are noticeably greater than on untreated matched controls (see Table 2).

Context sensitivity

To further assess differences in context sensitivity, we looked at two types of responses in the naming probe trials during training: (1) contextual errors (substitution of the names of other pictures in the training set) and (2) correct responses. Rates of these responses in semantic and phonological contexts were compared to rates in unrelated contexts using chi square. AS produced many contextual errors, with more occurring in semantic contexts (96 of 455 attempts to name) than in unrelated contexts (20 of 300 attempts to name), $\chi^2(1) = 27.86$, $p = .0001$, or in phonological contexts (35 of 425 attempts to name), $\chi^2(1) = 27.69$, $p = .0001$. Additionally, compared to the unrelated context, he produced significantly fewer correct responses in the semantic, $\chi^2(1) = 24.88$, $p = .0001$, and phonologic, $\chi^2(1) = 20.36$, $p = .0001$, contexts. In contrast, LP produced fewer attempts to name on probes overall (semantic: 217; phonological: 194; unrelated: 214) and showed no evidence of sensitivity to context, producing only one contextual error (in the semantic context) and roughly equivalent rates of correct responses across conditions (semantic: 179; phonological: 166; unrelated: 180).

GENERAL DISCUSSION

These two case studies indicate that contextual priming affects naming in different ways that may be related to the type of naming deficit. Additionally, we found that the patterns of context sensitivity observed in this study for each participant were consistent with those observed in the facilitation study (Martin et al., 2004). Overall, the effects of the priming procedure on AS's naming were selective and not robust. We observed immediate interference effects during training, particularly in the semantic context, as predicted. At the same time, gains were observed in the semantic and unrelated condition in the 652-item post-training test. This pattern of interference during training followed by improved naming some time after training is consistent with findings reported by Martin et al. (2004).

LP benefited greatly from this kind of training. For her, repetition priming improved naming in the short term in the semantic training context as well as in phonological and unrelated contexts. These gains were maintained for up to 4 months following treatment. Furthermore, LP did not show any interfering effects during the training.

Generalisation

Renvall et al. (2003) observed generalisation using contextual priming, but in the semantic condition only. In the present study, evidence of generalisation was inconsistent. AS showed some generalisation in semantic contexts and LP showed some in all contexts, but not consistently. Some evidence of generalisation comes from the pattern of non-contextual errors produced in response to within-training naming probes. Non-contextual errors are whole word substitutions that are related to the target but are not in the training set. Laine and Martin (1996) interpreted these errors as results of activation spreading from the target words in the training set to other related lexical "neighbours", priming their activation. In interactive activation models of word retrieval (e.g., Dell & O'Seaghdha, 1992), spreading activation is the medium of priming. Both subjects showed some evidence of this "generalisation priming". LP produced phonologically related non-contextual errors in phonological contexts more than other contexts, and AS produced semantically related non-contextual errors in semantic contexts more than in other contexts. Thus, the contextual priming procedure promoted some activity that is associated with generalisation in treatment.

The role of semantic ability in the effectiveness of repetition priming treatments

Lexical-semantic processing impairments impede learning of new verbal information via repetition priming (Martin & Saffran, 1999) and therefore would likely impact effectiveness of such treatments for language impairments. The data from the two participants in this study confirm that the benefits of repetition priming on naming are dependent, at least in part, on the integrity of lexical-semantic processing. LP, who demonstrated good lexical-semantic processing, showed robust and long-lasting benefits from the repetition priming. AS, with impaired lexical-semantic processing, showed only short-term improvement from the contextual priming treatment. Other participants with significant semantic deficits who are currently enrolled in this treatment programme are also making only short-term gains with no lasting improvement.

One account of lack of facilitation by contextual priming in cases of lexical-semantic processing impairment is that this procedure stimulates access to lexical and semantic representations (e.g., word-to-picture matching) on the basis of phonological input, thus priming the mapping from lexical to semantic representations. It does not necessarily prime the output mapping from semantics to lexical and phonological representations. Therefore, in the case of damaged connections between lexical and semantic representations (e.g., anomic aphasia or transcortical sensory aphasia), repetition priming treatments could bypass this connection to semantics altogether. The mapping that needs to be primed in word retrieval disorders is the output connection between semantics and the lexicon (and from there to phonological representations). Treatments that train semantic features of words are presumably stimulating this pathway, as are self-generated semantic cues, and these approaches have met with some success (Boyle & Coelho, 1995; Marshall, Freed, & Karow, 2001). Massed priming of the output semantic-lexical-phonological pathway could be accomplished with a task that promotes naming of the target rather than just repetition. It would be of interest to know if alternative priming approach that stimulates this pathway would have more of an impact on naming than repetition priming. We are currently exploring this possibility.

REFERENCES

Boyle, M., & Coelho, C. A. (1995). Application of semantic feature analysis as a treatment for aphasic dysnomia. *American Journal of Speech-Language Pathology, 4*, 94–98.

Cornelissen, K., Laine, M., Tarkiainen, A., Järvensivu, T., Martin, N., & Salmelin, R. (2003). Adult brain plasticity elicited by anomia treatment. *Journal of Cognitive Neuroscience, 15*, 444–461.

Dell, G. S., Schwartz, M. F., Martin, N., Saffran, E. M., & Gagnon, D. A. (1997). Lexical access in aphasic and non-aphasic speakers. *Psychological Review, 104*, 801–838.

Dell, G. S., & O'Seaghdha, P. G. (1992). Stages in lexical access in language production. *Cognition, 42*, 287–314.

Dunn, L., & Dunn, L. (1981). *Peabody Picture Vocabulary Test - Revised.* Circle Pines, MN: American Guidance Service.

Kertesz, A. (1982). *Western Aphasia Battery.* New York: The Psychological Corporation, Harcourt Brace Jovanovich, Inc.

Laine, M., & Martin, N. (1996). Lexical retrieval deficit in picture naming: Implications for word production models. *Brain & Language, 53*, 283–314.

Marshall, R. C., Freed, D. B., & Karow, C. M. (2001). Learning the subordinate category names by aphasic subjects: A comparison of deep and surface-level training methods. *Aphasiology, 15*, 585–598.

Martin, N., Fink, R., Laine, M., & Ayala, J. (2004). *Immediate and short-term effects of contextual priming of word retrieval.* Manuscript submitted for publication.

Martin, N., & Laine, M. (2000). Effects of contextual priming on word retrieval in anomia. *Aphasiology, 14*, 53–70.

Martin, N., & Saffran, E. M. (1997). Language and auditory-verbal short-term memory impairments: Evidence for common underlying processes. *Cognitive Neuropsychology, 14*, 641–682.

Martin, N., & Saffran, E. M. (1999). Effects of word processing and short-term memory deficits on verbal learning: Evidence from aphasia. *International Journal of Psychology, 34*(5/6), 330–346.

McReynolds, L. V., & Kearns, K. P. (1983). *Single-subject experimental designs in communication disorders.* Baltimore: University Park Press.

Patterson, K. E., Purell, C., & Morton, J. (1983). Facilitation of word retrieval in aphasia. In C. Code & D. J. Müller (Eds.), *Aphasia therapy* (pp.76–87). London: Edward Arnold.

Paulesu E., Frith C. D., & Frackowiak R. S. J. (1993). The neural correlates of the verbal component of working memory. *Nature, 362*, 342–345.

Renvall, K., Laine, M., Laakso, M., & Martin, N. (2003). Anomia rehabilitation with contextual priming: A case study. *Aphasiology, 17*, 305–308.

Roach, A., Schwartz, M. F., Martin, N., Grewal, R., & Brecher, A. (1996). The Philadelphia Naming Test: Scoring and rationale. *Clinical Aphasiology, 24*, 121–134.

Saffran, E. M., Schwartz, M. F., Linebarger, M., Martin, N., & Bochetto, P. (1988). *Philadelphia Comprehension Battery* [unpublished test battery].

APPENDIX

Training procedure: Priming trials and test probes

Following the 10-item pre-test, the five pictures designated for training are displayed in front of the participant. A priming trial consisted of three steps: spoken word-to-picture matching; repetition, and naming, as follows:

1. *Spoken word-to-picture matching*: The examiner names a picture and asks the participant to <u>point to</u> the picture in the array of pictures ("Show me ____ ").
2. *Repetition of the name*: The examiner says the name of the picture and asks the participant to <u>repeat</u> it ("Say ___ ").
3. *Independent naming (delayed repetition)*: The examiner asks the participant to <u>name</u> the picture ("What is this?").
4. Steps 1–3 are carried out for each of the five pictures, selected randomly by the examiner.
5. Steps 1–4 are repeated four times.
6. *Within-training test probe*: Following the above described training cycle, the participant is asked to name a randomly presented picture.
7. This entire procedure (steps 1–6, the training and within-training probes) is repeated twice more within each session.

Post-test. Following a 5-minute break the 10-item pre-test is re-administered.

APHASIOLOGY, 2004, *18* (5/6/7), 473–492

A biological model of aphasia rehabilitation: Pharmacological perspectives

Steven L. Small

The University of Chicago, IL, USA

Background: Aphasia is a multi-modality disturbance of speech, language, and memory caused by neurological injury, particularly stroke.
Aims: This review article views aphasia as fundamentally a disease of the brain, and aims to survey biological treatments for aphasia that address amelioration of brain injury.
Main Contribution: The review examines the effects of different drugs on both direct and indirect mechanisms of neural circuit reorganisation, gauged through effects on multi-modal measures of speech, language, and memory. Based on this review, therapists might choose to analyse and change the pharmacological state of their patients with aphasia.
Conclusions: We conclude that (a) both biological and behavioural therapies affect brain repair and reorganisation; (b) pharmacotherapy is not yet proven, but has promise, but only when accompanied by concomitant behavioural therapy; (c) the most important biological interventions that can be accomplished at present are to withdraw certain drugs that impede aphasia recovery and to administer anti-depressants to all patients with major or minor post-stroke depression.

Aphasia is a multi-modality disturbance of speech, language, and memory caused by neurological injury, particularly stroke. The main premise of this article is that aphasia is fundamentally a disease of the brain, and thus treatment for aphasia must focus on repair of brain injury. As will become clear later, this does not mean in any way that traditional therapies for aphasia are inappropriate or unhelpful. The point will be that they are both appropriate and helpful to the extent that they work towards repair and reorganisation of the brain, which many of them do.

There are many possible purposes for aphasia therapy, perhaps most importantly, the quality of life of the person with aphasia. There are many ways to achieve this goal without changing communication or neurobiology. If we as clinicians are going to help our patients remediate aphasia, rather than compensate for it, outcome measures that require actual language use are necessary. Although this is not in conflict with most views in clinical aphasiology research, it is in conflict with many contemporary efforts in medical cost containment. In this paper, we advocate a medical model in which aphasia recovery directly reflects repair of neural circuits for language and associated cognitive functions, such as memory and attention. Although it is possible to measure directly the neural circuits underlying language performance, these are only relevant insofar as they

Address correspondence to: Steven L. Small, Department of Neurology, The University of Chicago, 5841 S. Maryland Avenue, MC-2030, Chicago, IL 60637, USA. Email: small@uchicago.edu

This research was supported by the National Institute of Deafness and other Communication Disorders, National Institutes of Health, under grant NIH DC R01-3378. Their support is gratefully acknowledged.

http://www.tandf.co.uk/journals/pp/02687038.html   DOI: 10.1080/02687030444000156

coexist with language recovery. Thus, our view on the importance of biology is based on the critical assumption that intervening in the biology will have direct effects on language recovery. Remediation of aphasia is the underlying principle of the biological model advocated here.

A BIOLOGICAL MODEL

Research in animal models suggests that the cerebral cortex undergoes plasticity for months following stroke, and that these adaptive changes occur both in the intact tissue surrounding the lesion, and in areas remote from the site of injury (Jenkins & Merzenich, 1987; Nudo & Friel, 1999; Nudo, Wise, SiFuentes, & Milliken, 1996; Xerri, Merzenich, Peterson, & Jenkins, 1998). Many pharmacological and cellular approaches to neuro-remediation have been proposed—e.g., dextro-amphetamine (Goldstein, 2000a; Stroemer, Kent, & Hulsebosch, 1998), neurotrophins (Kent et al., 1999; Zhang et al., 1999), cell transplantation (Kondziolka et al., 2000). However, it is important to note that the biological organism develops skill though interaction with the environment. For example, studies of pharmacological intervention for stroke rehabilitation have consistently shown that successful drug therapy is always accompanied by behavioural practice (Small, 1994, 2001). Furthermore, when computational neural network models are experimentally damaged, by removing "neurons" or adding noise, restoring them to perform their original functions is not possible solely by replacing the lost "tissue", but requires additional training (Gernsbacher & St. John, 1998; McCloskey & Cohen, 1989).

In the (prevalent) educational perspective for rehabilitation, therapy is understood as "re-education" (Féré, 1886; Lecours, Lhermitte, & Bryans, 1983), with a goal of teaching lost knowledge or skills. Patients and families are typically given low expectations, since the relearning of lost skills can be quite meagre and can take tremendous effort over a long time, limiting the patience of both the patient and the insurance company. In the biological model, the assumption is that a damaged brain is producing the impairment, and that neural circuit repair or reorganisation can produce a cure for the disease. The biological model emphasises both behavioural and biological interventions to effect the necessary neural changes. Biological remediation can take two different forms neurobiologically, although the outcome, i.e., restoring function, remains the same. Whereas in direct restoration, the original (damaged) neural circuits are reinstated, in indirect restoration, adjacent or related neural circuits perform the original functions (Friel & Nudo, 1998). In both cases, a combination of behavioural training and biological intervention can be used to effect the desired (direct or indirect) circuit changes.

In this article we focus on one type of biological intervention, namely pharmaco-therapy. We will not address several more radical approaches that are still in their infancy. For example, it might be possible in the future to directly alter the aphasic brain to increase synaptic connectivity among existing brain regions or between existing brain regions and new tissue that has been artificially implanted. There is increasing therapeutic interest in the direct repair of damaged brain tissue, through a combination of tissue or cell transplantation (Johansson, 2000; Kondziolka, Wechsler, & Achim, 2002; Kondziolka, Wechsler, Gebel, DeCesare, Elder, & Meltzer, 2003; Macklis, 1993; Snyder, Yoon, Flax, & Macklis, 1997) and administration of growth factors (Castren, Zafra, Thoenen, & Lindholm, 1992; Olson et al., 1994; Rocamora, Welker, Pascual, & Soriano, 1996). Genetic manipulations have been proposed as a possible way to achieve both of these interventions (Zlokovic & Apuzzo, 1997). All of these methods entail the same basic requirement that biological interventions be accompanied by behavioural practice.

In this article we will focus solely on pharmacotherapy, and examine its effects on both direct and indirect mechanisms of neural circuit reorganisation, gauged through effects on multi-modal measures of speech, language, and memory.

INTRODUCTION TO PHARMACOTHERAPY

For over a century, clinicians have sought to use pharmacological agents to remediate aphasia or to aid compensation, and this work has generally been unsuccessful (Small, 1994). However, in several limited areas, the use of drug treatment as an adjunct to traditional (behavioural) speech therapy has shown some promise. Furthermore, the future for pharmacological and other biological treatments is bright, with new research in neurotrophins and cell transplants holding tremendous promise (Small, 2000).

Although aphasia is a brain disorder, and its remediation will ultimately depend on brain repair, the language and memory disturbances that characterise aphasia depend on highly complex neural circuits (Neville & Bavelier, 1998; Small & Burton, 2001) that develop through a lifetime of learning (Helmuth, 2003). Thus, the necessary brain repair cannot be completely achieved by direct biological intervention, but will require accompanying "re-education". Thus, although we advocate a biological perspective, reflecting a goal of brain remediation, such remediation is unlikely to occur solely through biological interventions. In fact, many lines of evidence suggest that any bio-logical intervention will require a matched behavioural intervention to "re-educate" appropriate neural circuits and influence plausible mechanisms of reorganisation or remodelling.

There is strong evidence that behavioural interventions can influence the anatomical and physiological structure of the brain. In the motor system, a relative increase in the use of one muscle group compared to another can lead to motor cortical changes reflecting this use (Merzenich, Nelson, Stryker, Cynader, Schoppmann, & Zook, 1984). In animals given experimental cortical lesions and then trained on motor tasks, cortical reorgani-sation occurs adjacent to the damaged region (Jenkins & Merzenich, 1987). This provides tantalising data for neurobiological approaches to rehabilitation in humans, including treatment of cognitive disorders and aphasia.

Data such as these suggest an approach to aphasia treatment that focuses on biology rather than education, whether the intervention used is specifically biological (e.g., neuro-pharmacological) or behavioural (e.g., stimulation-based, neurolinguistic). If certain types of aphasia therapies, whether linguistic, neuropsychological, stimulation-based, pharmacological, or surgical, can alter brain anatomy and physiology, and if particular patterns of such altered states can be shown to be associated with better outcome, then there is a precise and scientific method of designing, monitoring, and evaluating treat-ment. This would alter significantly both the goals of aphasia therapy, and the respon-sibility of therapists (Small, 2000).

ANIMAL MODELS OF APHASIA PHARMACOTHERAPY

Of course there are no animal models of aphasia pharmacotherapy *per se*, yet there are animal studies aimed at treating the subacute and chronic sequelae of stroke, particularly motor function. In addition, there are basic studies of the effects of certain types of agents on the neurophysiology of certain animal model systems. It is important to note that there is an enormous literature on mechanisms of recovery and repair after brain injury, and a large number of articles addressing the potential of diverse pharmacological agents to affect this recovery (for a review, see Goldstein, 1998b, or Freund, Sabel, & Witte, 1997).

For the present purposes, we have selected a small number of articles that are particularly relevant to an interpretation of human studies in stroke recovery (especially aphasia recovery). This necessarily excludes discussion of some animal model systems (e.g., fluid percussion injury as a model of traumatic brain injury) and some pharmacological systems (e.g., glutamate antagonism in early acute injury).

The most important agents used in aphasia pharmacotherapy are the catecholamines, particularly dopamine and norepinephrine. Since the catecholamines do not cross the blood-brain barrier, they must either be administered directly into the brain or spinal fluid, or other agents must be administered that act as catecholamine agonists or increase catecholamine concentrations. Dextro-amphetamine is the most widely studied experimental drug of this latter sort, acting non-specifically to increase the concentrations of all the catecholamines at synaptic junctions.

The concentrations of catecholamines in the rat and cat brainstem (Brown, Carlson, Ljungren, Seisjö, & Snider, 1974; Cohen, Woltz, & Jacobson, 1975) and the subcortex of the rat (Robinson, Shoemaker, & Schlumpf, 1980) are decreased following cerebral cortical infarction. After the acute phase (40 days), there remain decreases in ipsilateral norepinephrine concentrations in the cortex and brainstem, and decreases in ipsilateral brainstem (but not cortical) dopamine concentrations (Robinson, Shoemaker, Schlumpf, Valk, & Bloom, 1975). More specifically, lesions to the dorsal noradrenergic bundle have an effect on recovery of animals with contralateral sensory-motor cortical injuries, but have no effect on animals with sham cortical injuries (Goldstein & Bullman, 1997). The general conclusion of this research on central norepinephrine (NE) suggests that efforts to deplete NE, to block α-adrenergic receptors, or to decrease NE release impede recovery, whereas drugs that increase NE release or block reuptake facilitate recovery (Goldstein, 1999).

These basic data have led to a number of therapy studies in animal models (Goldstein, 2000a). In the early studies of this type, a single dose of *dextro*-amphetamine (*d*-amphetamine), which augments post-synaptic catecholamines including both norepinephrine and dopamine, led to accelerated recovery in a beam-walking task in rats with unilateral motor cortex ablation (Feeney, Gonzalez, & Law, 1982; Goldstein, Miller, Cress, Tyson, & Davis, 1988). By contrast, a single dose of haloperidol, a dopamine antagonist, blocked the amphetamine effect. When given alone, haloperidol delayed spontaneous recovery, whereas phenoxybenzamine, an α-adrenergic antagonist, reproduced the deficits in recovered animals. Paradoxically, treatment with intraventricular norepinephrine, but not dopamine, reproduced the beneficial effect of *d*-amphetamine (Boyeson & Feeney, 1984). Analogous results have been obtained with *d*-amphetamine therapy of motor system injury in the cat (Feeney & Hovda, 1983; Hovda & Feeney, 1984).

These motor system results generalise to the visual system (Feeney & Hovda, 1985). Bilateral ablation of the primary visual cortex of the cat causes impairment of visual depth perception. When given both visual experience and dextro-amphetamine, such cats demonstrate marked improvement in function. The effect is not seen when the dextro-amphetamine is unaccompanied by visual experience or when the visual experience is accompanied by saline instead of active drug.

Animal models thus suggest that endogenous and exogenous catecholamines, particularly norepinephrine, acting through α receptors, play an important role in recovery from stroke. A number of neurophysiological mechanisms are postulated as underlying the beneficial effects of catecholamine enhancement. None of these is proven. One study showed that growth-associated protein expression (GAP-43) increases in neocortical regions medial and lateral to infarction early (weeks 1–2) and that synaptic density (synaptophysin) increases later (2–10 weeks) in a pattern correlated with behavioural recovery (both temporally and spatially) (Stroemer, Kent, & Hulsebosch, 1995). These authors showed subsequently that such neurite growth and synaptogenesis in the neocortex increases with the addition of dextro-amphetamine, possibly due to protein upregulation via functional activation of pathways able to remodel in response to active behavioural performance (Stroemer et al., 1998).

These data also suggest that the effect of catecholamine augmentation therapy depends on concomitant experience. Thus motor recovery following stroke, while facilitated by pharmacotherapy, depends on the presence of motor practice, just as visual recovery depends on visual experience.

One monoamine that is not a catecholamine—5-hydroxy-triptophan (5-HT or serotonin)—is also important in stroke recovery because it is the main target of the antidepressant medications. Several studies have investigated both tricyclic antidepressants and the newer "selective" serotonin reuptake inhibitors (SSRI) in their effects on stroke recovery in animal models (Boyeson, 1996; Boyeson & Harmon, 1993; Boyeson, Harmon, & Jones, 1994). One study, aiming to assess the issue of transmitter selectivity, also evaluated the role of 5-HT itself in mediating this process. Of particular interest were the results that neither the SSRI fluoxetine nor direct administration of 5-HT was effective in improving motor function in a rat model (Boyeson et al., 1994). The results with the tricyclics, with much less specific effects on monoamine uptake, were not as clear, particularly since desipramine (Boyeson & Harmon, 1993) and amitryptyline (Boyeson et al., 1994) seemed to have opposite effects.

Another class of agents that have been used in neurological injury to improve memory function and to increase neuroplasticity is the group of drugs that increase cerebral acetylcholine (ACh). These agents have been particularly relevant to the treatment of Alzheimer's disease, where there is a cholinergic model that relates atrophy in the nucleus basalis of Meynert (nbM; the source of all cerebral ACh) to the pathophysiology of AD (Whitehouse, Price, Clark, Coyle, & DeLong, 1981). Acetylcholine is thought to be involved in a number of aspects of cognition, including perception, selective attention, associative learning, and memory (Yu & Dayan, 2002). Early data on this mechanism came from evaluations of scopolamine, an ACh blocker, which inhibits certain types of learning (Petersen, 1977). Although scopolamine has been shown to have some beneficial effects in (early) recovery from animal models of traumatic injury (Lyeth et al., 1992), possibly by reducing cholinergic neuronal activation (Saija et al., 1988), the window for such advantage is very short (15 minutes) (Hamm, O'Dell, Pike, & Lyeth, 1993), and later on it appears that the effects of scopolamine are to impair learning and memory (Dixon, Hamm, Taft, & Hayes, 1994).

Some additional data relate to the role of ACh in stimulating neural plasticity, with simultaneous stimulation of the basal forebrain and behavioural training leading to improved learning (Bakin & Weinberger, 1996; Kilgard & Merzenich, 1998). One view is that with their diffuse projections from the basal forebrain, ACh neurons serve a modulatory function in marking important stimuli (Kilgard & Merzenich, 1998). In any event, there is agreement that ACh input from nbM plays an important role in the cortical response to experience (Baskerville, Schweitzer, & Herron, 1997).

A third agent that has received attention in animal studies is γ-amino butyric acid (GABA). GABA is particularly interesting since it is uniformly inhibitory, and accounts for about 25% of all cortical neurons and about 20% of all cortical synapses (Hendry, Schwark, Jones, & Yan, 1987). Further, inhibition may play a fundamental role in cortical neuroplasticity (Jacobs & Donoghue, 1991). Intracortical infusion of GABA exacerbates the hemiparesis produced by a small motor cortex lesion in rats (Schallert, Jones, Weaver, Shapiro, Crippens, & Fulton, 1992). The short-term administration of diazepam (a benzodiazepine and indirect GABA agonist) permanently impedes sensory cortical recovery from the anteromedial neocortical injury. Furthermore, administration of phenobarbital, which may have some agonist effects on GABA receptors, also impedes recovery from brain injury (Hernandez & Holling, 1994; Montanez, Kline, Gasser, & Hernandez, 2000).

PHARMACOTHERAPY OF APHASIA

There is an interesting history of pharmacotherapy studies (Bergman & Green, 1951; Linn, 1947; Sarno, Sarno, & Diller, 1972; West & Stockel, 1965) that were generally unsuccessful, often because of poor rationales based on inadequate medical knowledge of the time (for a review of these studies, see Small, 1994 or 2001). Modern studies of pharmacological treatment of aphasia have focused on neurotransmitter systems, particularly catecholaminergic systems. A number of studies have been conducted, not all well designed (see Small, 1994, for some critical analysis), aiming to assess several different agents. This section reviews the existing literature on drug therapy of aphasia. Only three agents have been studied in a controlled manner for treatment of aphasia: bromocriptine (dopamine agonist), dextro-amphetamine (sympathomimetic), and piracetam ("nootropic" agent). However, none of these agents has been adequately shown to help aphasia recovery to the degree that would be necessary to recommend its general use (Greener, Enderby, & Whurr, 2001; Small, 1994). Thus, while these drugs remain promising candidates for helping aphasia recovery, none has yet been proven to do so.

Bromocriptine and dopamine agonists

Several studies have examined the role of dopamine in aphasia treatment. One case report prompted this, suggesting that the dopamine agonist bromocriptine helped restore speech fluency in a patient with transcortical motor aphasia (Albert, Bachman, Morgan, & Helm-Estabrooks, 1988). Fluency improved when the patient was taking bromocriptine and evaporated following cessation of the drug. A multiple baseline single subject experimental design failed to find a similar benefit from bromocriptine in an analogous clinical situation (MacLennan, Nicholas, Morley, & Brookshire, 1991). A second multiple baseline trial of bromocriptine involved two patients with "left frontoparietal infarcts" and "nonfluent aphasia" who showed improvement in fluency (Gupta & Mlcoch, 1992).

Several larger studies have been conducted. A prospective open-label trial of seven patients with non-fluent aphasia showed some improvement in moderately affected patients during dose-escalation and remission during dose-withdrawal (Sabe, Leiguarda, & Starkstein, 1992). In a double-blind dose-escalation study of 11 patients with non-fluent aphasia with high-dose bromocriptine and behavioural therapy, patients improved statistically on several of the tested measures, but more than half dropped out due to side effects (Bragoni, Altieri, Di Piero, Padovani, Mostardini, & Lenzi, 2000). Only one bromocriptine study fulfils the Cochrane group evidence-based medicine standards (CEBM, 2003; Mulrow & Cook, 1998; Sackett, Richardson, Rosenberg, & Haynes, 2000) for utility in medical decision making regarding aphasia therapy (Greener et al., 2001). That investigation was a double-blind, placebo-controlled crossover study in non-fluent aphasia, which showed that, compared with placebo treatment, bromocriptine did not significantly improve the patient's speech fluency, language content, overall degree of aphasia severity, or nonverbal cognitive abilities (Gupta, Mlcoch, Scolaro, & Moritz, 1995).

Dextro-amphetamine and sympathomimetics

Dextro-amphetamine is perhaps the most widely studied biological treatment for the chronic effects of stroke, including aphasia (Walker-Batson, 2000), yet both its clinical efficacy and mode of action remain unclear (Goldstein, 2000a). Nonetheless, the strong evidence from animal model systems, and some suggestive evidence from human studies, still make this a promising drug for treatment of aphasia. There is very suggestive evidence that dextro-amphetamine (Clark & Mankikar, 1979; Crisostomo, Duncan, Propst, Dawson, & Davis, 1988; Goldstein, 2003; Walker-Batson, Smith, Curtis, Unwin, & Greenlee, 1995) and possibly methylphenidate (Grade, Redford, Chrostowski, Toussaint, & Blackwell, 1998) can help with the speed and/or degree of recovery in motor function after stroke.

In aphasia, an early study used methylphenidate, another sympathomimetic, in a double-blind placebo-controlled study (Darley, Keith, & Sasanuma, 1977). Statistical analysis of the data revealed no difference in language performance between any of the conditions for the patients as a group. In a more recent study of six patients (Walker-Batson, Devous, Curtis, Unwin, & Greenlee, 1991), dextro-amphetamine administered with therapy seemed to lead to improvement over their expected levels (Porch, 1967). Although this is a rare study incorporating a series of patients in a group design, its use of the "expected" outcomes, rather than a control group, diminishes its importance.

Both dextro-amphetamine and methylphenidate can act as anti-depressants, and given the high prevalence of post-stroke depression (Gustafson, Nilsson, Mattsson, Astrom, & Bucht, 1995; Robinson, 1998; van de Weg, Kuik, & Lankhorst, 1999), particularly in patients with aphasia (Robinson, Kubos, Starr, Rao, & Price, 1984; Starkstein, Bryer, Berthier, Cohen, Price, & Robinson, 1991), this could play an important role in therapeutic effectiveness. Two studies have specifically suggested a benefit of methylphenidate in post-stroke depression (Grade et al., 1998; Lazarus et al., 1992).

Of importance, and in concordance with the animal model studies (Feeney et al., 1982; Feeney & Hovda, 1985; Goldstein et al., 1988), the studies showing beneficial effects of sympathomimetics (on motor or language) (Crisostomo et al., 1988; Grade et al., 1998; Walker-Batson et al., 1991, 1995), share the common feature of evaluating dextro-amphetamine as an adjunct to behavioural or physical therapy, rather than alone. This is consistent with the view espoused at the outset about the role of behaviour in modifying neural circuits, and the notion that without training, even extensively reorganised or remodeLled neural circuits are not likely to improve performance.

Cholinergics and anticholinergics

Despite the significant neurophysiological data on the role of cholinergic projections in modulating neural plasticity and the neuropsychological data on its role in learning and memory, there have been relatively few attempts to modulate this system for the treatment of aphasia. There is one case report of cholinergic treatment of post-traumatic amnesia, which showed improvement in verbal recall but not verbal recognition, visual memory, or conceptual reasoning (Goldberg, Gerstman, Mattis, Hughes, Sirio, & Bilder, 1982). Another study involved three patients with anomia, one of whom had a lesion in the basal forebrain (although the other two did not), who were administered physostigmine and seemed to have benefit in confrontation naming but not on other cognitive measures (Jacobs et al., 1996). A subsequent study was initiated based on the postulate that patients with damage to the left temporal lobe, with concomitant fluent aphasia, might be best suited for such therapy since there might be a relative lateralisation of cholinergic projections (Bracco, Tiezzi, Ginanneschi, Campanella, & Amaducci, 1984) and since methylscopolamine, an anticholinergic, can impair phonological and lexical processing in normal adults (Aarsland, Larsen, Reinvang, & Aasland, 1994). This double blind, placebo-controlled study of four patients compared the cholinergic agent bifemelane to placebo and saw definite improvements in the treatment pair as opposed to the placebo pair (Tanaka, Miyazaki, & Albert, 1997).

Several therapeutic attempts have focused on donepezil, the reversible acetyl-cholinesterase inhibitor with a selective central action that is used to improve language and cognitive deficits in AD. One single case study involved a patient with a small subcortical lacunar infarction. Dopamine agonist therapy was ineffective, but donepezil led to a significant improvement in fluency (Hughes, Jacobs, & Heilman, 2000). Other single cases have also reported benefit (Pashek & Bachman, 2003; Tsz-Ming & Kaufer, 2001), but these cases reflect a diverse group of subjects. In an open label trial of 10 chronic aphasic patients (mixed type and stroke aetiology), receiving medication for 16 weeks, all improved on a number of language measures (Berthier, Hinojosa, Martin Mdel, & Fernandez, 2003).

Piracetam

Piracetam is a derivative of GABA, but instead of GABA agonist or antagonist activity, acts as a "nootropic agent" on the central nervous system, facilitating cholinergic and excitatory amine neurotransmission (Giurgea, Greindl, & Preat, 1983; Vernon & Sorkin, 1991). It is said that this agent improves learning and memory, but it is not clear which of its multitudinous biological effects (e.g., neuroprotective, circulatory) are responsible for the purported cognitive benefit.

This drug is particularly interesting because of all the pharmacological agents that have ever been evaluated for use in aphasia therapy, it is the only one for which the Cochrane report feels that there is some reasonable evidence. In their report, they evaluated only randomised controlled trials. Unfortunately this report, which aimed to be objective, was written by the author of the only trial that was positively evaluated in the report. Furthermore, for this drug and no other did the Cochrane report consider both published and unpublished data. Finally, the report accepted trials for this drug that included a post hoc analysis of questionable validity and a study with considerable dropout; conditions that generally lead this highly conservative group to disqualify studies.

But what are the actual data on piracetam? One large multi-centre trial ($n = 927$) aimed to treat all stroke patients within 12 hours and used a variety of outcome measures, including aphasia. This study showed no effect on the primary outcome measure of neurological status (Barthel Index and Orgogozo scale) at 4 weeks (De Deyn, Reuck, Deberdt, Vlietinck, & Orgogozo, 1997). A post-hoc analysis of an "early treatment subgroup" (defined prospectively as within 6 hours, but retrospectively as within 7 hours), showed some benefit of piracetam. This was particularly true in the moderate to severe subgroup (De Deyn et al., 1997; Orgogozo, 1999). Of these patients, about a third ($n = 373$) were aphasic, and aphasia recovery at 12 weeks was better in the piracetam group than the control group, particularly for the early treatment subgroup (Huber, 1999; Orgogozo, 1999).

In post-acute and chronic aphasia, one randomised controlled trial showed significant improvement on a multivariate analysis of Aachen Aphasia subtest scores relative to baseline in favour of piracetam ($p = .02$) at 12 weeks. This effect was no longer present at 24 weeks (Enderby, Broeckx, Hospers, Schildermans, & Deberdt, 1994). A later double-blind, placebo-controlled study in chronic aphasia showed improvement on a single subtest of the AAT (written language) (Huber, Willmes, Poeck, Van Vleymen, & Deberdt, 1997). Integrating functional neurological measures into a treatment trial, another study showed an increase of activation in several left hemisphere language regions over the course of the treatment period, more in the treatment group than the placebo group. The piracetam group improved on six language measures; the placebo group on three (Kessler, Thiel, Karbe, & Heiss, 2000).

The benefits of piracetam, if there are such benefits, appear to be in the early treatment (Huber, 1999). Although this might turn out to be beneficial, it is important to realise that virtually all pharmacotherapy efforts have been focused on subacute and chronic patients. Early treatment of stroke is of tremendous importance (Grotta, 1987), and many approaches are either in clinical use—e.g., thrombolytics (Hacke et al., 1995; The NINDS rt-PA Stroke Study Group, 1995)—or in intensive investigation (Connors, 2002; De Keyser, Sulter, & Luiten, 1999; Lutsep & Clark, 2001). If an acute stroke therapy is proposed as "aphasia therapy", it should be evaluated by comparison with these other approaches, not by comparison with therapies aimed at the subacute or chronic phase.

Depression

Post-stroke depression is incredibly prevalent, with estimates ranging from 30% to 60% (Starkstein & Robinson, 1989; van de Weg et al., 1999). Post-stroke depression is highly underdiagnosed (Robinson, 1998), since not all post-stroke depression fits into the classic DSM-IV (Task Force on DSM-IV, 1994) category of major depression, which requires depressed mood or loss of interest, at least five of nine DSM-IV criteria, and a duration of at least 2 weeks. Such patients are more likely to have minor depression (Task Force on DSM-IV, 1994), including depressed mood or loss of interest or pleasure, but fewer than five symptoms of major depression.

A crucial issue that must be addressed as part of aphasia rehabilitation is depression, since it can adversely affect language recovery. Following stroke, it has been demonstrated that patients with depression have more cognitive impairment than patients with comparable lesions but no depression (Downhill & Robinson, 1994). Furthermore, in stroke patients matched for severity and lesion localisation, patients with depression had worse recovery than their non-depressed counterparts in functional status and cognitive performance (Morris, Raphael, & Robinson, 1992).

Some data suggest that depression is more common in patients with left hemisphere stroke than right (Starkstein et al., 1991), which would be of major importance for aphasia rehabilitation, but these data are somewhat controversial (Singh, Herrmann, & Black, 1998). Nevertheless, treatment of depression should be considered a fundamental part of any aphasia rehabilitation programme.

Of the agents available for treatment of depression, some are not recommended after stroke. In particular, drugs with α-1 adrenergic antagonist properties (trazadone, amitriptyline) have been shown to slow motor recovery in animal models (Boyeson & Harmon, 1993; Boyeson et al., 1994). Other agents have been associated with more rapid recovery (desipramine) (Boyeson & Harmon, 1993) or with no effect on motor recovery (fluoxetine) (Boyeson et al., 1994).

TABLE 1

Summary of aphasia pharmacotherapy studies (three non-aphasia studies on dextro-amphetamine also included)

Drug	Reference	Subjects	# Subjects	Duration of aphasia	Cause of lesion	Dose	Time of dose	Duration of drug therapy	Therapy	Study design	Results
Amobarbital	(Linn, 1947)	Aphasia, mutism	2	Minimal (but unknown)	Tumour, stroke	4cc 5% soln	Challenge (immediately before testing)	Once	None	Two cases	+
Amobarbita 1	(Bergman & Green, 1951)	Aphasia	27	Unknown	Multiple etiologies	0.25–0.5 g	Challenge (immediately before testing)	Once	None	Multiple cases	−
Meprobamate	(West & Stockel, 1965)	Aphasia	29	19 > 6 months; 10 < 6 months	Stroke	Not stated	Daily	2 years	Routine controlled SLP	AB or BA × 4	−
Hyperbaric O$_2$	(Sarno, Sarno, & Diller, 1972)	Aphasia, Right hemiplegia	16	3–108 months	Stroke	100% O$_2$ at 2 atm	Daily	2 days	None	AB or BA	−
Bromocriptine	(Albert, Bachman, Morgan, & Helm-Estabrooks, 1988)	Transcortica 1 motor aphasia	1	3.5 years	Stroke	15 mg → 30 mg	Daily	43 days	None	One case test-retest	+
Bromocriptine	(MacLennan, Nicholas, Morley, & Brookshire, 1991)	Transcortica 1 motor aphasia	1	4 years	Stroke	4 mg → 20 mg	Daily	7 weeks	None	One case	−
Bromocriptine	(Gupta & Mlcoch, 1992)	Nonfluent aphasia	2	> 18 months	Stroke	3 mg → 30 mg	Daily	3 months	None	Open label	+ (dose dependent)
Bromocriptine	(Sabe, Leiguarda, & Starkstein, 1992)	Nonfluent aphasia	7	1–3 yrs	Stroke	3.75 mg → 60 mg	TID	14 weeks	Routine SLP	Open label	+ moderate − severe
d-amphetamine	(Walker-Batson, 2000)	Hemiplegia	10	16–30 days	Ischemic Cerebral Stroke	10 mg	45 minutes before therapy (q 4 days)	6 weeks	Intensive PT	P, R, DB, PC	+

Drug	Citation	Diagnosis	N	Time	Etiology	Dose	Timing	Duration	Therapy	Design	Outcome
d-amphetamine	(Clark & Mankikar, 1979)	Elderly "rehab failures"	88	Rehab failures	28 stroke; 8 PD; others non-neuro)	5 mg → 20 mg	BID	21 days	Not stated	Open label	+
d-amphetamine	(Crisostomo, Duncan, Propst, Dawson, & Davis, 1988)	Hemiparesis	8	< 10 days	Stroke	10 mg	Within 45 min of therapy	Once	PT	P, R, DB, PC	+
d-amphetamine	(Walker-Batson, Smith, Curtis, Unwin, & Greenlee, 1995)	Aphasia	6	10–30 days post	Stroke	10–15 mg	30 minutes before therapy (q4 days)	6 weeks	Routine controlled SLP	Open label	+
Methylphenidate	(Grade, Redford, Chrostowski, Toussaint, & Blackwell, 1998)	Stroke	21	Acute rehab	Stroke	5 mg → 30 mg	8 AM/noon		With PT	P, R, DB, PC	+ depression ± function
Methylphenidate	(Darley, Keith, & Sasanuma, 1977)	Aphasia	14	> 21 days post	12 Stroke; 2 TBI	20 mg	2.5 hrs post lunch, 45 min before eval	3 doses	None	P R, DB, PC	–
Chlordiazepoxide						20 mg					–
d-amphetamine	(Walker-Batson, Devous, Curtis, Unwin, & Greenlee, 1991)	Broca Aphasia and Right Hemiparesis	1	21 days post stroke	Stroke	10 mg	45 minutes before a 75 minute session (q4 days)	6 weeks	Routine SLP	Single case	+
Bifemelane	(Tanaka, Miyazaki, & Albert, 1997)	Fluent aphasia	4	6–8 weeks post stroke	Stroke	300 mg daily	Daily	1 month	Routine controlled SLP	P, R, DB, PC	+
Donepezil	(Berthier, Hinojosa, Martin Mdel, & Fernandez, 2003)	Aphasia	10	10 months to 7 years	Stroke	5 mg → 10 mg	Daily	16 weeks	Routine controlled SLP	Open label	+

(Continued)

TABLE 1
(Continued)

Drug	Reference	Subjects	# Subjects	Duration of aphasia	Cause of lesion	Dose	Time of dose	Duration of drug therapy	Therapy	Study design	Results
Piracetam	(De Deyn, Reuck, Deberdt, Vlietinck, & Orgogozo, 1997)	Acute stroke	927	12 hours	Stroke	12 g then 4.8 g	Daily	4 weeks then 8 weeks	Routine therapy	P, R, DB, PC	− overall + early subgroup
	(Orgogozo, 1999)	Aphasia									+ aphasia − func − neuro
Priacetam	(Enderby, Broeckx, Hospers, Schildermans, & Deberdt, 1994)	Acute stroke	158	6–9 wks post	Stroke	Unknown	Daily	12 weeks	Routine SLP	P, R, DB, PC	+ 12 wks − 24 wks
Piracetam	(Huber, Willmes, Poeck, Van Vleymen, & Deberdt, 1997)	Aphasia	66	4 weeks to 3 yrs	Stroke	4.8 g	Daily	6 weeks	Intensive controlled SLP	P, DB, PC	± (AAT subtests only)
Piracetam	(Kessler, Thiel, Karbe, & Heiss, 2000)	Aphasia	24	< 14 days	Stroke	4.8 g	BID	6 weeks	Intensive controlled SLP	P, R, DB, PC	± (some subtests

In Study design, P = prospective, DB = double blind, R = randomised; PC = placebo controlled; AB = one agent or placebo A then another B.
In Time of dose, BID = twice daily; TID = three times daily.
In Dose, → indicates escalating dose.
In therapy, PT = physical therapy; SLP = speech therapy; Controlled = "Same" for all subjects.

In pharmacotherapy for post-stroke depression, randomised controlled trials shown positive effects of both nortriptyline (Lipsey, Robinson, Pearlson, Rao, & Price, 1984) and citalopram (Andersen, Vestergaard, & Lauritzen, 1994). In a head-to-head comparison, nortriptyline (62% response) was more effective than fluoxetine (9% response), which did not differ from placebo (24% response) (Robinson et al., 2000). In another study, fluoxetine was no more effective than placebo in the first 3 months post stroke (blinded), but was much better at 18 months (open label) (Fruehwald, Gatterbauer, Rehak, & Baumhackl, 2003).

As noted previously, methylphenidate may effective in as many as 50–80% of stroke patients with depression and may help with functional recovery (Grade et al., 1998). Unfortunately, this finding in a small number of patients has not yet been replicated. Note that the treatment onset of this drug is significantly more rapid than the tricyclics or SSRIs.

The role of anti-depressant drugs in aphasia rehabilitation, apart from their demonstrated role in the treatment of depression *per se*, is not yet clear. Certainly, the data cited above on the effects of depression on recovery, and the role of these drugs in alleviating depression, suggest that they should play a large role in any rehabilitation programme.

DRUGS TO AVOID IN APHASIA RECOVERY

Two basic principles should motivate pharmacological interventions in aphasia: The first and foremost issue is to avoid detrimental agents; only second is the issue of trying to help with beneficial agents. That is, there is pharmacotherapy for aphasia, but also pharmacotherapy *against* aphasia. If some pharmacological manipulation appears to play a role in accelerating or improving recovery, then the opposite manipulation could delay or prevent recovery. Importantly, drugs that can adversely affect aphasia recovery include agents used to treat a number of highly prevalent diseases, particularly in aphasic patients; namely, hypertension, coronary artery disease, seizures, anxiety, psychotic symptoms, and gastrointestinal disturbances.

The first study of the inadvertent pharmacological interference with aphasia recovery was a retrospective review of the medications of 32 patients presenting for language evaluation following stroke (Porch, Wyckes, & Feeney, 1985), which showed that the 19 patients taking medicines performed more poorly on the Porch Index of Communicative Ability (PICA: Porch, 1967) than the 13 who were not taking medicines.

More recently, a single investigator has taken up this important area of research, and has performed a number of studies in both animals and man addressing the effects of common medications taken by people who have strokes (Goldstein, 1993, 1995, 1998a, 2000a, 2000b). His work is generally well controlled and the results are important. This research programme was initiated with the observation that over 80% of all patients were taking some medicine at the time of their stroke, and that 65% were taking multiple medications. Included in this list were such drugs as α adrenergic blockers and benzodiazepines, which are known to impede stroke recovery in animal studies.

This research programme has included both investigations in animal models and clinical studies of patients. An initial report noted that a number of drugs that impair recovery in experimental stroke (e.g., drugs that affect catecholamine or GABA systems) are commonly given to stroke patients for coincident medical problems (Goldstein, 1993). This led to a formal retrospective (chart review) study of patients taking these specific drugs at the time of their strokes (Goldstein, 1995). A total of 96 patient records were reviewed and patients were grouped on whether or not they were taking one or more of the following drugs: clonidine, prazosin, any dopamine receptor antagonist (e.g., neuroleptics), benzodiazepines, phenytoin, or phenobarbital. Statistical analysis revealed that whereas patient demographics and stroke severity were similar between groups, motor recovery time was significantly shorter in the group that was not taking one of these drugs.

Several other drugs have been associated with language difficulties of one type or another and in one context or another. Certainly, the effects of anticholinergic medications on memory function (Koller et al., 2003; Sherman, Atri, Hasselmo, Stern, & Howard, 2003; Taffe, Weed, & Gold, 1999) would suggest avoidance of agents with these effects. Several anticonvulsant medications have potentially serious cognitive effects, including causing or exacerbating aphasia (Wong & Lhatoo, 2000). Two important medications in this respect are vidagibrine, which has both exacerbated existing aphasia (Gil & Neau, 1995) and produced a motor aphasia in a child following seizure control (Jambaque, Chiron, Kaminska, Plouin, & Dulac, 1998). Toparimate has been recently implicated in word-finding problems in a subgroup of epilepsy patients (with left temporal foci) (Mula, Trimble, Thompson, & Sander, 2003).

This work has profound relevance to aphasia rehabilitation as it is currently practised, independent of the explicit biological interventions discussed here. In order to maximise functional recovery, it is important not only to ensure adequate behavioural treatment, but also to ensure the appropriate neurobiological substrate for this treatment (or, more concretely, to ensure that this substrate is not pharmacologically inhibited from responding to the therapy). It is thus advisable for patients in aphasia therapy to avoid drugs that might interfere with catecholaminergic or GABAergic function, or are thought to delay recovery by empirical study. A summary of these potentially deleterious agents is shown in Table 2.

TABLE 2
Drugs with potentially deleterious effects on stroke recovery

Drug (class of agent)	Reason for administration	Neurotransmitter system
Diazepam, Chlordiazepoxide, Lorezepam, etc. (benzodiazepine)	Anxiety	γ aminobutyric acid (GABA) agonist
Clonidine	Hypertension	α_2 adrenergic agonist
Labetalol (predominantly β-blocking but also α_1 antagonist	Hypertension, Coronary artery disease	Partial α_1 adrenergic antagonist
Phenoxybenzamine, prazosin, etc.	Hypertension	α_1 adrenergic antagonist
Haloperidol (butyrophenone), Chlorpromazine (phenothiazine), Quetiapine, etc.	Psychosis	D_2 dopaminergic antagonist
Droperidol (butyrophenone), Metaclopramide (phenothiazine), etc.	Gastrointestinal disturbances	D_2 dopaminergic antagonist
Phenobarbital (barbiturate)	Seizures	γ aminobutyric acid (GABA) agonist
Phenytoin (hydantoin)	Seizures	Not transmitter specific

CONCLUSIONS

Existing studies on biological approaches to the treatment of aphasia do not yet paint an unambiguous picture. Nonetheless, there are increasingly reliable data suggesting a potential beneficial effect of increased central nervous system catecholamines on human motor recovery and aphasia rehabilitation. In the realm of motor system recovery, both human and animal studies suggest that dextro-amphetamine can facilitate recovery when combined with practice. Weaker evidence also suggests that when coupled with practice in oral communication, increasing brain norepinephrine and/or dopamine might facilitate improvement in speech and language impairments after stroke. No data on any agent yet demonstrates effectiveness. Larger multi-centre studies of this question are needed.

Pharmacotherapy should not be used as a replacement for speech therapy, since any biological intervention should be used only in conjunction with individually tailored behavioural therapy, preferably carefully designed adaptive learning approaches. In the published cases where pharmacotherapy improved language functioning in people with aphasia, it was used adjunctively. Importantly, the most valid and useful pharmacological interventions at present are (a) withdrawal of agents than are detrimental to recovery; and (b) institution of agents than can treat major and minor depression. Nevertheless, it is very likely that pharmacotherapy will ultimately play a valuable role as an adjunct to behavioural rehabilitation to speed recovery, improve learning, decrease performance variability, and improve mean performance in patients with mild to moderate language dysfunction from cerebral infarctions.

REFERENCES

Aarsland, D., Larsen, J. P., Reinvang, I., & Aasland, A. M. (1994). Effects of cholinergic blockade on language in healthy young women. Implications for the cholinergic hypothesis in dementia of the Alzheimer type. *Brain, 117*(6), 1377–1384.

Albert, M. L., Bachman, D. L., Morgan, A., & Helm-Estabrooks, N. (1988). Pharmacotherapy for aphasia. *Neurology, 38*(6), 877–879.

Andersen, G., Vestergaard, K., & Lauritzen, L. (1994). Effective treatment of poststroke depression with the selective serotonin reuptake inhibitor citalopram. *Stroke, 25*(6), 1099–1104.

Bakin, J. S., & Weinberger, N. M. (1996). Induction of a physiological memory in the cerebral cortex by stimulation of the nucleus basalis. *Proceedings of the National Academy of Science, USA, 93*(20), 11219–11224.

Baskerville, K. A., Schweitzer, J. B., & Herron, P. (1997). Effects of cholinergic depletion on experience-dependent plasticity in the cortex of the rat. *Neuroscience, 80*(4), 1159–1169.

Bergman, P. S., & Green, M. (1951). Aphasia: Effect of Intravenous Sodium Amytal. *Neurology, 1*, 471–475.

Berthier, M. L., Hinojosa, J., Martin Mdel, C., & Fernandez, I. (2003). Open-label study of donepezil in chronic poststroke aphasia. *Neurology, 60*(7), 1218–1219.

Boyeson, M. G. (1996). Effects of fluoxetine and maprotiline on functional recovery in poststroke hemiplegic patients undergoing rehabilitation therapy [letter; comment]. *Stroke, 27*(11), 2145–2146.

Boyeson, M. G., & Feeney, D. M. (1984). The role of norepinephrine in recovery from brain injury (abstract). *Annual Meeting of the Society for Neuroscience, 10,* 68.

Boyeson, M. G., & Harmon, R. L. (1993). Effects of trazodone and desipramine on motor recovery in brain-injured rats. *American Journal of Physical Medicine and Rehabilitation, 72*(5), 286–293.

Boyeson, M. G., Harmon, R. L., & Jones, J. L. (1994). Comparative effects of fluoxetine, amitriptyline and serotonin on functional motor recovery after sensorimotor cortex injury. *American Journal of Physical Medicine and Rehabilitation, 73*(2), 76–83.

Bracco, L., Tiezzi, A., Ginanneschi, A., Campanella, C., & Amaducci, L. (1984). Lateralization of choline acetyltransferase (ChAT) activity in fetus and adult human brain. *Neuroscience Letters, 50*(1–3), 301–305.

Bragoni, M., Altieri, M., Di Piero, V., Padovani, A., Mostardini, C., & Lenzi, G. L. (2000). Bromocriptine and speech therapy in non-fluent chronic aphasia after stroke. *Neurological Sciences, 21*(1), 19–22.

Brown, R. M., Carlson, A., Ljungren, B. L., Seisjö, B. K., & Snider, S. R. (1974). Effect of ischemia on monoamine metabolism in the brain. *Acta Scandinavica Physiologica, 90,* 789–791.

Castren, E., Zafra, F., Thoenen, H., & Lindholm, D. (1992). Light regulates expression of brain-derived neurotrophic factor mRNA in rat visual cortex. *Proceedings of the National Academy of Science, USA, 89*(20), 9444–9448.

CEBM (Centre for Evidence-Based Medicine). (2003). *Vol. 2003.* University Department of Psychiatry, Warneford Hospital, Headington, Oxford, UK.

Clark, A. N. G., & Mankikar, G. D. (1979). d-Amphetamine in elderly patients refractory to rehabilitation procedures. *Journal of the American Geriatrics Society, 27*(4), 174–177.

Cohen, H. P., Woltz, A. G., & Jacobson, R. L. (1975). Catecholamine content of cerebral tissue after occlusion or manipulation of middle cerebral artery in cats. *Journal of Neurosurgery, 43,* 32–36.

Connors, J. J. III (2002). Interventional stroke therapy: The potential benefit of direct intra-arterial infusion. *Reviews in Cardiovascular Medicine, 3 Suppl 2,* S92–99.

Crisostomo, E. A., Duncan, P. W., Propst, M., Dawson, D. V., & Davis, J. N. (1988). Evidence that amphetamine with physical therapy promotes recovery of motor function in stroke patients. *Annals of Neurology, 23,* 94–97.

Darley, F. L., Keith, R. L., & Sasanuma, S. (1977). The effect of alerting and tranquilizing drugs upon the performance of aphasic patients. *Clinical Aphasiology, 7,* 91–96.

De Deyn, P. P., Reuck, J. D., Deberdt, W., Vlietinck, R., & Orgogozo, J. M. (1997). Treatment of acute ischemic stroke with piracetam. Members of the Piracetam in Acute Stroke Study (PASS) Group. *Stroke, 28*(12), 2347–2352.

De Keyser, J., Sulter, G., & Luiten, P. G. (1999). Clinical trials with neuroprotective drugs in acute ischaemic stroke: Are we doing the right thing? *Trends in Neuroscience, 22*(12), 535–540.

Dixon, C. E., Hamm, R. J., Taft, W. C., & Hayes, R. L. (1994). Increased anticholinergic sensitivity following closed skull impact and controlled cortical impact traumatic brain injury in the rat. *Journal of Neurotrauma, 11*(3), 275–287.

Downhill, J. R. Jr., & Robinson, R. G. (1994). Longitudinal assessment of depression and cognitive impairment following stroke. *Journal of Nervous and Mental Disease, 182*(8), 425–431.

Enderby, P., Broeckx, J., Hospers, W., Schildermans, F., & Deberdt, W. (1994). Effect of piracetam on recovery and rehabilitation after stroke: A double-blind, placebo-controlled study. *Clinical Neuropharmacology, 17*(4), 320–331.

Feeney, D. M., Gonzalez, A., & Law, W. A. (1982). Amphetamine, haloperidol, and experience interact to affect rate of recovery after motor cortex injury. *Science, 217,* 855–857.

Feeney, D. M., & Hovda, D. A. (1983). Amphetamine and apomorphine restore tactile placing after motor cortex injury in the cat. *Psychopharmacology, 79,* 67–71.

Feeney, D. M., & Hovda, D. A. (1985). Reinstatement of binocular depth perception by amphetamine and visual experience after visual cortex ablation. *Brain Research, 342,* 352–356.

Féré, C. (1886). La rééducation des aphasiques. *Revue Générale de Clinique et de Thérapeutique, 785.*

Freund, H. J., Sabel, B. A., & Witte, O. W. (Ed.). (1997). *Brain plasticity.* Philadelphia, PA: Lippencott-Raven Publishers.

Friel, K. M., & Nudo, R. J. (1998). Recovery of motor function after focal cortical injury in primates: Compensatory movement patterns used during rehabilitative training. *Somatosensory and Motor Research, 15*(3), 173–189.

Fruehwald, S., Gatterbauer, E., Rehak, P., & Baumhackl, U. (2003). Early fluoxetine treatment of post-stroke depression—a three-month double-blind placebo-controlled study with an open-label long-term follow up. *Journal of Neurology, 250*(3), 347–351.

Gernsbacher, M. A., & St. John, M. F. (1998). Learning and losing syntax: Practice makes perfect and frequency builds fortitude. In J. L. E. Bourne (Ed.), *Foreign language learning: Psycholinguistic experiments on training and retention* (pp. 231–255). Mawah, NJ: Laurence Erlbaum Associates Inc.

Gil, R., & Neau, J. P. (1995). Rapid aggravation of aphasia by vigabatrin. *Journal of Neurology, 242*(4), 251–252.

Giurgea, C. E., Greindl, M. G., & Preat, S. (1983). Nootropic drugs and aging. *Acta Psychiatrica Belgica, 83*(4), 349–358.

Goldberg, E., Gerstman, L. J., Mattis, S., Hughes, J. E., Sirio, C. A., & Bilder, R. M. Jr. (1982). Selective effects of cholinergic treatment on verbal memory in posttraumatic amnesia. *Journal of Clinical Neuropsychology, 4*(3), 219–234.

Goldstein, L. B. (1993). Basic and clinical studies of pharmacologic effects on recovery from brain injury. *Journal of Neural Transplantation & Plasticity, 4*(3), 175–192.

Goldstein, L. B. (1995). Common drugs may influence motor recovery after stroke: The sygen in acute stroke study investigators [see comments]. *Neurology*, *45*(5), 865–871.

Goldstein, L. B. (1998a). Potential effects of common drugs on stroke recovery. *Archives of Neurology*, *55*(4), 454–467

Goldstein, L. B. (Ed.). (1998b). *Restorative neurology: Advances in pharmacotherapy for recovery after stroke*. Armonk, NY: Futura Publishing Company.

Goldstein, L. B. (1999). Pharmacological approach to functional reorganization: The role of norepinephrine. *Revue Neurologique (Paris)*, *155*(9), 731–736.

Goldstein, L. B. (2000a). Effects of amphetamines and small related molecules on recovery after stroke in animals and man. *Neuropharmacology*, *39*(5), 852–859.

Goldstein, L. B. (2000b). Should antihypertensive therapies be given to patients with acute ischemic stroke? *Drug Safety*, *22*(1), 13–18.

Goldstein, L. B. (2003). Amphetamines and related drugs in motor recovery after stroke. *Physical Medicine and Rehabilitation Clinics of North America*, *14*(1 Suppl), S125–134, x.

Goldstein, L. B., & Bullman, S. (1997). Effects of dorsal noradrenergic bundle lesions on recovery after sensorimotor cortex injury. *Pharmacology, Biochemistry and Behavior*, *58*(4), 1151–1157.

Goldstein, L. B., Miller, G. D., Cress, N. M., Tyson, A. G., & Davis, J. N. (1988). Studies of an animal model for the recovery of function after stroke (abstract). *Annals of Neurology*, *22*, 159–160.

Grade, C., Redford, B., Chrostowski, J., Toussaint, L., & Blackwell, B. (1998). Methylphenidate in early poststroke recovery: A double-blind, placebo-controlled study. *Archives of Physical Medicine and Rehabilitation*, *79*(9), 1047–1050.

Greener, J., Enderby, P., & Whurr, R. (2001). Pharmacological treatment for aphasia following stroke. *Cochrane Database Syst Rev*(4), CD000424.

Grotta, J. C. (1987). Current medical and surgical therapy for cerebrovascular disease. *New England Journal of Medicine*, *317*(24), 1505–1516.

Gupta, S. R., & Mlcoch, A. G. (1992). Bromocriptine treatment of nonfluent aphasia. *Archives of Physical Medicine and Rehabilitation*, *73*, 373–376.

Gupta, S. R., Mlcoch, A. G., Scolaro, C., & Moritz, T. (1995). Bromocriptine treatment of nonfluent aphasia. *Neurology*, *45*(12), 2170–2173.

Gustafson, Y., Nilsson, I., Mattsson, M., Astrom, M., & Bucht, G. (1995). Epidemiology and treatment of post-stroke depression. *Drugs and Aging*, *7*(4), 298–309.

Hacke, W., Kaste, M., Fieschi, C., Toni, D., Lesaffre, E., von Kummer, R. et al. (1995). Intravenous thrombolysis with recombinant tissue plasminogen activator for acute hemispheric stroke. The European Cooperative Acute Stroke Study (ECASS). *Journal of the American Medical Association*, *274*(13), 1017–1025.

Hamm, R. J., O'Dell, D. M., Pike, B. R., & Lyeth, B. G. (1993). Cognitive impairment following traumatic brain injury: The effect of pre- and post-injury administration of scopolamine and MK-801. *Brain Research: Cognitive Brain Research*, *1*(4), 223–226.

Helmuth, L. (2003). Aging. The wisdom of the wizened. *Science*, *299*(5611), 1300–1302.

Hendry, S. H., Schwark, H. D., Jones, E. G., & Yan, J. (1987). Numbers and proportions of GABA-immunoreactive neurons in different areas of monkey cerebral cortex. *Journal of Neuroscience*, *7*(5), 1503–1519.

Hernandez, T. D., & Holling, L. C. (1994). Disruption of behavioral recovery by the anti-convulsant phenobarbital. *Brain Research*, *635*(1–2), 300–306.

Hovda, D. A., & Feeney, D. M. (1984). Amphetamine with experience promotes recovery of locomotor function after unilateral frontal cortex injury in the cat. *Brain Research*, *298*, 358–361.

Huber, W. (1999). The role of piracetam in the treatment of acute and chronic aphasia. *Pharmacopsychiatry*, *32*(Suppl 1), 38–43.

Huber, W., Willmes, K., Poeck, K., Van Vleymen, B., & Deberdt, W. (1997). Piracetam as an adjuvant to language therapy for aphasia: A randomized double-blind placebo-controlled pilot study. *Archives of Physical Medicine and Rehabilitation*, *78*(3), 245–250.

Hughes, J. D., Jacobs, D. H., & Heilman, K. M. (2000). Neuropharmacology and linguistic neuroplasticity. *Brain and Language*, *71*(1), 96–101.

Jacobs, D., Shuren, J., Gold, M., Adair, J., Bowers, D., Williamson, D. et al. (1996). Physostigmine pharmacotherapy for anomia. *Neurocase*, *2*(2), 83–91.

Jacobs, K. M., & Donoghue, J. P. (1991). Reshaping the cortical motor map by unmasking latent intracortical connections. *Science*, *251*(4996), 944–947.

Jambaque, I., Chiron, C., Kaminska, A., Plouin, P., & Dulac, O. (1998). Transient motor aphasia and recurrent partial seizures in a child: Language recovery upon seizure control. *Journal of Child Neurology*, *13*(6), 296–300.

Jenkins, W. M., & Merzenich, M. M. (1987). Reorganization of neocortical representations after brain injury: A neurophysiological model of the bases of recovery from stroke. *Progress in Brain Research, 71,* 241–266.

Johansson, B. B. (2000). Brain plasticity and stroke rehabilitation. The Willis lecture. *Stroke, 31*(1), 223–230.

Kent, T. A., Quast, M., Taglialatela, G., Rea, C., Wei, J., Tao, Z. et al. (1999). Effect of NGF treatment on outcome measures in a rat model of middle cerebral artery occlusion. *Journal of Neuroscience Research, 55*(3), 357–369.

Kessler, J., Thiel, A., Karbe, H., & Heiss, W. D. (2000). Piracetam improves activated blood flow and facilitates rehabilitation of poststroke aphasic patients. *Stroke, 31*(9), 2112–2116.

Kilgard, M. P., & Merzenich, M. M. (1998). Cortical map reorganization enabled by nucleus basalis activity. *Science, 279*(5357), 1714–1718.

Koller, G., Satzger, W., Adam, M., Wagner, M., Kathmann, N., Soyka, M. et al. (2003). Effects of scopolamine on matching to sample paradigm and related tests in human subjects. *Neuropsychobiology, 48*(2), 87–94.

Kondziolka, D., Wechsler, L., & Achim, C. (2002). Neural transplantation for stroke. *Journal of Clinical Neuroscience, 9*(3), 225–230.

Kondziolka, D., Wechsler, L., Gebel, J., DeCesare, S., Elder, E., & Meltzer, C. C. (2003). Neuronal transplantation for motor stroke: from the laboratory to the clinic. *Physical Medicine and Rehabilitation Clinics of North America, 14*(1 Suppl), S153–160, xi.

Kondziolka, D., Wechsler, L., Goldstein, S., Meltzer, C., Thulborn, K. R., Gebel, J. et al. (2000). Transplantation of cultured human neuronal cells for patients with stroke. *Neurology, 55*(4), 565–569.

Lazarus, L. W., Winemiller, D. R., Lingam, V. R., Neyman, I., Hartman, C., Abassian, M. et al. (1992). Efficacy and side effects of methylphenidate for poststroke depression [see comments]. *Journal of Clinical Psychiatry, 53*(12), 447–449.

Lecours, A. R., Lhermitte, F., & Bryans, B. (1983). *Aphasiology.* London: Baillière Tindall.

Linn, L. (1947). Sodium amytal in treatment of aphasia. *Archives of Neurology and Psychiatry, 58,* 357–358.

Lipsey, J. R., Robinson, R. G., Pearlson, G. D., Rao, K., & Price, T. R. (1984). Nortriptyline treatment of post-stroke depression: A double-blind study. *Lancet, 1*(8372), 297–300.

Lutsep, H., & Clark, W. (2001). An update of neuroprotectants in clinical development for acute stroke. *Current Opinion in Investigational Drugs, 2*(12), 1732–1736.

Lyeth, B. G., Ray, M., Hamm, R. J., Schnabel, J., Saady, J. J., Poklis, A. et al. (1992). Postinjury scopolamine administration in experimental traumatic brain injury. *Brain Research, 569*(2), 281–286.

Macklis, J. D. (1993). Transplanted neocortical neurons migrate selectively into regions of neuronal degeneration produced by chromophore-targeted laser photolysis. *Journal of Neuroscience, 13*(9), 3848–3863.

MacLennan, D. L., Nicholas, L. E., Morley, G. K., & Brookshire, R. H. (1991). The effects of bromocriptine on speech and language function in a man with transcortical motor aphasia. *Clinical Aphasiology, 21,* 145–155.

McCloskey, M., & Cohen, N. J. (1989). Catastrophic interference in connectionist networks: The sequential learning problem. In G. Bower (Ed.), *The psychology of learning and motivation* (pp. 109–165). New York: Academic Press.

Merzenich, M. M., Nelson, R. J., Stryker, M. P., Cynader, M. S., Schoppmann, A., & Zook, J. M. (1984). Somatosensory cortical map changes following digit amputation in adult monkeys. *Journal of Comparative Anatomy, 224,* 591–605.

Montanez, S., Kline, A. E., Gasser, T. A., & Hernandez, T. D. (2000). Phenobarbital administration directed against kindled seizures delays functional recovery following brain insult [In Process Citation]. *Brain Research, 860*(1–2), 29–40.

Morris, P. L., Raphael, B., & Robinson, R. G. (1992). Clinical depression is associated with impaired recovery from stroke. *Medical Journal of Australia, 157*(4), 239–242.

Mula, M., Trimble, M. R., Thompson, P., & Sander, J. W. (2003). Topiramate and word-finding difficulties in patients with epilepsy. *Neurology, 60*(7), 1104–1107.

Mulrow, C., & Cook, D. (1998). *Systematic reviews: Synthesis of best evidence for health care decisions.* Philadelphia, PA: American College of Physicians.

Neville, H. J., & Bavelier, D. (1998). Neural organization and plasticity of language. *Current Opinion in Neurobiology, 8*(2), 254–258.

Nudo, R. J., & Friel, K. M. (1999). Cortical plasticity after stroke: Implications for rehabilitation. *Revue Neurologique (Paris), 155*(9), 713–717.

Nudo, R. J., Wise, B. M., SiFuentes, F., & Milliken, G. W. (1996). Neural substrates for the effects of rehabilitative training on motor recovery after ischemic infarct. *Science, 272*(5269), 1791–1794.

Olson, L., Backman, L., Ebendal, T., Eriksdotter-Jonhagen, M., Hoffer, B., Humpel, C. et al. (1994). Role of growth factors in degeneration and regeneration in the central nervous system; clinical experiences with NGF in Parkinson's and Alzheimer's diseases. *Journal of Neurology, 242*(1 Suppl 1), S12–15.

Orgogozo, J. M. (1999). Piracetam in the treatment of acute stroke. *Pharmacopsychiatry, 32* (Suppl 1), 25–32.

Pashek, G. V., & Bachman, D. L. (2003). Cognitive, linguistic and motor speech effects of donepezil hydrochloride in a patient with stroke-related aphasia and apraxia of speech. *Brain and Language, 87*(1), 179–180.

Petersen, R. C. (1977). Scopolamine induced learning failures in man. *Psychopharmacology (Berlin), 52*(3), 283–289.

Porch, B., Wyckes, J., & Feeney, D. M. (1985). Haloperidol, thiazides, and some antihypertensives slow recovery from aphasia (abstract). *Annual Meeting of the Society for Neuroscience, 11*, 52.

Porch, B. E. (1967). *Porch Index of Communicative Ability: Volume 1: Theory and development.* Palo Alto, CA: Consulting Psychologists Press.

Robinson, R. G. (1998). *The clinical neuropsychiatry of stroke: Cognitive, behavioral and emotional disorders following vascular brain injury.* Cambridge: Cambridge University Press.

Robinson, R. G., Kubos, K. L., Starr, L. B., Rao, K., & Price, T. R. (1984). Mood disorders in stroke patients: Importance of location of lesion. *Brain, 107*, 81–93.

Robinson, R. G., Schultz, S. K., Castillo, C., Kopel, T., Kosier, J. T., Newman, R. M. et al. (2000). Nortriptyline versus fluoxetine in the treatment of depression and in short-term recovery after stroke: A placebo-controlled, double-blind study. *American Journal of Psychiatry 157*(3), 351–359.

Robinson, R. G., Shoemaker, W. J., & Schlumpf, M. (1980). Time course of changes in catecholamines following right hemisphere cerebral infarction in the rat. *Brain Research, 181*, 202–208.

Robinson, R. G., Shoemaker, W. J., Schlumpf, M., Valk, T., & Bloom, F. E. (1975). Effect of experimental cerebral infarction in rat brain on catecholamines and behavior. *Nature, 255*, 332–334.

Rocamora, N., Welker, E., Pascual, M., & Soriano, E. (1996). Upregulation of BDNF mRNA expression in the barrel cortex of adult mice after sensory stimulation. *Journal of Neuroscience, 16*(14), 4411–4419.

Sabe, L., Leiguarda, R., & Starkstein, S. E. (1992). An open-label trial of bromocriptine in nonfluent aphasia. *Neurology, 42*, 1637–1638.

Sackett, D., Richardson, W., Rosenberg, W., & Haynes, R. (2000). *Evidence-based medicine: How to practice and teach EBM* (2nd ed.). New York: Churchill Livingstone.

Saija, A., Robinson, S. E., Lyeth, B. G., Dixon, C. E., Yamamoto, T., Clifton, G. L. et al. (1988). The effects of scopolamine and traumatic brain injury on central cholinergic neurons. *Journal of Neurotrauma, 5*(2), 161–170.

Sarno, M. T., Sarno, J. E., & Diller, L. (1972). The effect of hyperbaric oxygen on communication function in adults with aphasia secondary to stroke. *Journal of Speech and Hearing Research, 15*, 42–48.

Schallert, T., Jones, T., Weaver, M., Shapiro, L., Crippens, D., & Fulton, R. (1992). Pharmacologic and anatomic considerations in recovery of function. *Phys Med Rehabil, 6*, 375–393.

Sherman, S. J., Atri, A., Hasselmo, M. E., Stern, C. E., & Howard, M. W. (2003). Scopolamine impairs human recognition memory: Data and modeling. *Behavioural Neuroscience, 117*(3), 526–539.

Singh, A., Herrmann, N., & Black, S. E. (1998). The importance of lesion location in poststroke depression: A critical review. *Canadian Journal of Psychiatry, 43*(9), 921–927.

Small, S. L. (1994). Pharmacotherapy of Aphasia: A Critical Review. *Stroke, 25*(6), 1282-1289.

Small, S. L. (2000). The future of aphasia treatment. *Brain and Language, 71*(1), 227–232.

Small, S. L. (2001). Biological approaches to the treatment of aphasia. In A. Hillis (Ed.), *Handbook on adult language disorders: Integrating cognitive neuropsychology, neurology, and rehabilitation* (pp. 397–411). Philadelphia, PA: Psychology Press.

Small, S. L., & Burton, M. W. (2001). Functional neuroimaging of language. In R. S. Berndt (Ed.), *Handbook of neuropsychology. Vol. 3: Language and aphasia* (2nd ed., pp. 335–351). Amsterdam: Elsevier.

Snyder, E. Y., Yoon, C., Flax, J. D., & Macklis, J. D. (1997). Multipotent neural precursors can differentiate toward replacement of neurons undergoing targeted apoptotic degeneration in adult mouse neocortex. *Proceedings of the National Academy of Science, USA, 94*(21), 11663–11668.

Starkstein, S. E., Bryer, J. B., Berthier, M. L., Cohen, B., Price, T. R., & Robinson, R. G. (1991). Depression after stroke: The importance of cerebral hemisphere asymmetries. *Journal of Neuropsychiatry and Clinical Neuroscience, 3*(3), 276–285.

Starkstein, S. E., & Robinson, R. G. (1989). Affective disorders and cerebral vascular disease. *British Journal of Psychiatry, 154*, 170–182.

Stroemer, R. P., Kent, T. A., & Hulsebosch, C. E. (1995). Neocortical neural sprouting, synaptogenesis, and behavioral recovery after neocortical infarction in rats. *Stroke, 26*(11), 2135–2144.

Stroemer, R. P., Kent, T. A., & Hulsebosch, C. E. (1998). Enhanced neocortical neural sprouting, synaptogenesis, and behavioral recovery with D-amphetamine therapy after neocortical infarction in rats. *Stroke, 29*(11), 2381–2393.

Taffe, M. A., Weed, M. R., & Gold, L. H. (1999). Scopolamine alters rhesus monkey performance on a novel neuropsychological test battery. *Brain Research: Cognitive Brain Research, 8*(3), 203–212.

Tanaka, Y., Miyazaki, M., & Albert, M. L. (1997). Effects of increased cholinergic activity on naming in aphasia. *Lancet, 350*(9071), 116–117.

Task Force on DSM-IV (1994). *Diagnostic and Statistical Manual of Mental Disorders—IV* (Text Revision) (4th ed.). Washington DC: American Psychiatric Association.

The NINDS rt-PA Stroke Study Group (1995). Tissue plasminogen activator for acute ischemic stroke. *New England Journal of Medicine, 333*(24), 1581–1587.

Tsz-Ming, C., & Kaufer, D. (2001). Effects of donepezil on aphasia, agnosia, and apraxia in patients with cerebrovascular lesions [abstract]. *Journal of Neuropsychiatry and Clinical Neurosciences, 13*, 140.

van de Weg, F. B., Kuik, D. J., & Lankhorst, G. J. (1999). Post-stroke depression and functional outcome: A cohort study investigating the influence of depression on functional recovery from stroke. *Clinical Rehabilitation, 13*(3), 268–272.

Vernon, M. W., & Sorkin, E. M. (1991). Piracetam. An overview of its pharmacological properties and a review of its therapeutic use in senile cognitive disorders. *Drugs and Aging, 1*(1), 17–35.

Walker-Batson, D. (2000). Use of pharmacotherapy in the treatment of aphasia. *Brain and Language, 71*(1), 252–254.

Walker-Batson, D., Devous, M. D., Curtis, S., Unwin, D. H., & Greenlee, R. G. (1991). Response to amphetamine to facilitate recovery from aphasia subsequent to stroke. *Clinical Aphasiology, 21*, 137–143.

Walker-Batson, D., Smith, P., Curtis, S., Unwin, H., & Greenlee, R. (1995). Amphetamine paired with physical therapy accelerates motor recovery after stroke. Further evidence. *Stroke, 26*(12), 2254–2259.

West, R., & Stockel, S. (1965). The effect of meprobamate on recovery from aphasia. *Journal of Speech and Hearing Research, 8*, 57–62.

Whitehouse, P. J., Price, D. L., Clark, A. W., Coyle, J. T., & DeLong, M. R. (1981). Alzheimer disease: Evidence for selective loss of cholinergic neurons in the nucleus basalis. *Annals of Neurology, 10*(2), 122–126.

Wong, I. C., & Lhatoo, S. D. (2000). Adverse reactions to new anticonvulsant drugs. *Drug Safety, 23*(1), 35–56.

Xerri, C., Merzenich, M. M., Peterson, B. E., & Jenkins, W. (1998). Plasticity of primary somatosensory cortex paralleling sensorimotor skill recovery from stroke in adult monkeys. *Journal of Neurophysiology, 79*(4), 2119–2148.

Yu, A. J., & Dayan, P. (2002). Acetylcholine in cortical inference. *Neural Networks, 15*(4–6), 719–730.

Zhang, W. R., Kitagawa, H., Hayashi, T., Sasaki, C., Sakai, K., Warita, H. et al. (1999). Topical application of neurotrophin-3 attenuates ischemic brain injury after transient middle cerebral artery occlusion in rats. *Brain Research, 842*(1), 211–214.

Zlokovic, B. V., & Apuzzo, M. L. (1997). Cellular and molecular neurosurgery: Pathways from concept to reality—part II: Vector systems and delivery methodologies for gene therapy of the central nervous system. *Neurosurgery, 40*(4), 805–812; discussion 812–813.

APHASIOLOGY, 2004, *18* (5/6/7), 493–519

Assessing the validity of multiple-choice questions for RAPP story comprehension

Tepanta R. D. Fossett, Malcolm R. McNeil, Patrick J. Doyle, and Hillel Rubinsky

VA Pittsburgh Healthcare System, and University of Pittsburgh, PA, USA

Stephanie Nixon

University of Pittsburgh, PA, USA

William Hula

VA Pittsburgh Healthcare System, and University of Pittsburgh, PA, USA

Jill Brady

University of Pittsburgh, PA, USA

Background: Passage dependency (PD) is a measure of how much information is required to answer test questions based only on information provided in the relevant text (Tuiman, 1974). Prior learning, information included in other test questions or responses, and the ability to eliminate less plausible or irrelevant foils are all factors that may affect PD. The PD of the multiple-choice questions for the auditory story comprehension task in the RAPP software environment has yet to be established.

Aims: The purpose of this experiment was to investigate the validity of newly developed multiple-choice comprehension questions for the story comprehension tasks used in the RAPP software environment.

Methods & Procedures: Participants were 40 young adults without speech or language impairment, 20 of whom heard each of 12 stimulus stories and answered 10 multiple-choice questions with 5 response choices, and 20 who answered the multiple-choice questions but were not exposed to the stimulus stories. Questions concerned information about stated and implied main ideas and details presented in the stories. Based on four pre-determined story forms (three stories each), analyses examined the questions' validity in terms of their PD compared to chance performance and to a pre-established Passage Dependency Index (PDI) criterion (.60). Significant differences in the PDI and in the percentage of correctly answered questions among predetermined forms were also evaluated. Analyses also examined the PD of questions based on the type of information queried both within and among forms.

Outcomes & Results: Results provide support for the validity of the multiple-choice questions without consideration of the nature of the information queried by them. The percentage of correctly answered questions exceeded chance for all story forms, PDIs met or exceeded the pre-established criterion, there were no significant differences in the PDIs among the four forms and there were no significant differences in the percentage of correctly answered questions among the four forms. There were no significant differences in the PDIs among the

Address correspondence to: Tepanta R. D. Fossett, University of Pittsburgh, 4033 Forbes Tower, Pittsburgh, PA 15232, USA. Email: fossett@shrs.pitt.edu

This study was funded by the VA Rehabilitation Research and Development Service, project #B2265R.

http://www.tandf.co.uk/journals/pp/02687038.html   DOI: 10.1080/02687030444000066

four question types by story form or among question types within a form and all PDIs met or exceeded pre-established criteria (except detail implied questions in one form).

Conclusions: These results provide support for the PD of the multiple-choice questions constructed for the four story forms that make up this version of a story-length auditory comprehension task. Results suggest that the questions are not biased relative to the content of the stories and results add to the overall validity of the task.

Auditory comprehension of story length material has been measured in normal language users and persons with aphasia in a variety of ways. Yes/no (true/false) questions (Brookshire & Nicholas, 1997; Goodglass, Kaplan, & Baressi, 2001), story retell procedures (McNeil, Doyle, Fossett, Park, & Goda, 2001; McNeil, Doyle, Park, Fossett, & Brodsky, 2002), and various multiple-choice question tasks (Chapman, Ulatowska, Franklin, Shobe, Thompson, & McIntire, 1997; Ulatowska et al., 2001) have been used to quantify and describe the comprehension process. Doyle, McNeil, Spencer, Goda, Cottrell, and Lustig (1998) developed a software environment Resource Allocation Paradigms of Pittsburgh (RAPP), in which dual-task experiments could be conducted. One such dual task consists of a story comprehension and a visual-motor tracking task. Subsequent to the concurrent tracking and paragraph comprehension tasks participants either retell the auditorily presented story or respond to multiple-choice questions, in order to measure their comprehension of the material. The story comprehension task was developed using stories from the Discourse Comprehension Test (DCT: Brookshire & Nicholas, 1997). However, in order to measure story comprehension with a task more sensitive to a range of comprehension problems than that assessed by the true/false questions of the DCT, a series of multiple-choice questions was developed for each of the 12 stories used in the RAPP paradigm. Although the reliability and validity in the story retell procedure (SRP) has been investigated (McNeil et al., 2001, 2002), the psychometric properties of the multiple-choice question format have not.

The purpose of this experiment was to investigate the validity of newly developed multiple-choice comprehension questions for the story comprehension tasks derived from the DCT (Brookshire & Nicholas, 1997) and used in the RAPP> program. In a previous unpublished investigation in this laboratory, multiple-choice questions for the RAPP stories were developed to increase the sensitivity of the measurement relative to the true/false questions of the original DCT task. An informal assessment of those questions revealed that normal participants were able to answer questions at a substantially greater than chance level even when they had not heard the stories. To ensure that performance on the second version of the multiple-choice questions provides a valid measure of comprehension, we sought to evaluate whether the 10 questions, with five multiple-choice answers each, are based on information presented in the stories or whether unintentional information in the response choices or multiple-choice questions themselves might provide cues to the correct answers. To evaluate this, the passage dependency (Tuiman, 1974), was determined for each of the 12 stories and for each of the four story forms (three stories in each) that compose the comprehension tasks of the RAPP dual-task program. Passage dependency is a measure of how much information in test questions and their alternative answers can be derived only from exposure to the relevant text. Prior learning, information included in other test questions or responses, and the ability to eliminate less plausible or irrelevant foils are all factors that may affect passage dependency. If individuals are able to use information other than that contained in the stimulus to answer test questions without exposure to the stimulus, then those questions are passage-independent and may not be a valid assessment of comprehension for the test material.

The Passage Dependency Index (PDI) is computed by first determining the number of times an item was answered correctly relative to the number of times it was answered. This is calculated for each item for each of the participant groups (those exposed to the stimuli and those not exposed to the stimuli). The result of each of these calculations is a proportion. The proportion obtained on a particular item for the group not exposed to the stimulus is then divided by the proportion obtained for that same item by those exposed to the stimulus. The result is then subtracted from the value of one and the resulting value is the PDI for that question.

A few studies have examined the passage dependency of materials developed for persons with aphasia. Using non-brain damaged participants, Thomas and Jackson (1997) evaluated the passage dependency for multiple-choice questions, for four sets of paragraph-length reading comprehension therapy materials developed for persons with aphasia. Results revealed a relatively large range (.24 to .49) of PDIs for these stimuli. After examination of individual questions, the authors suggested that additional variables such as the relatedness of test questions and plausibility of answer choices may have contributed to low passage dependency. Nicholas, MacLennan, and Brookshire (1986) and Nicholas and Brookshire (1987) evaluated the passage dependency of reading items in various tests of aphasia and in a standardised reading test. Results revealed that most of the items from published tests for aphasia were not passage-dependent. Nicholas and Brookshire (1987) evaluated the passage dependency of questions on the Nelson Reading Test, a test not developed for persons with aphasia, with non-brain-damaged (NBD) adults and persons with aphasia. While the authors acknowledged that they were not aware of any standard acceptable PDI value, they suggested that the obtained value of .44 for persons with aphasia appeared satisfactory, as fewer than half of all the test items could be answered without exposure to the relevant text.

Brookshire and Nicholas (1997) developed a test of paragraph-length comprehension for persons with aphasia, right-hemisphere brain damage, or traumatic brain injury that could be presented with participants either reading or listening to the text and then answering eight yes/no questions. The yes/no questions concerned main ideas stated (M-S), main ideas implied (M-I), details stated (D-S), and details implied (D-I) in the stories. The authors established the PD for each of 10 stories, for 2 combinations of 5 stories and for all 10 stories together. PDI values for individual stories for the auditory version of this test ranged from .35 to .59 and averaged .45 and .47 for the two sets of five stories, with a combined average PDI value of .46 for both sets of stories

The stories in the RAPP dual-task software include the 10 stories used in the DCT (Brookshire & Nicholas, 1997), and the two practice stories. However, the yes/no question format was changed to a 10-question, 5-item multiple-choice format for each of 12 DCT stories, to increase the sensitivity and range of impairment captured by the test. It was reasoned that for participants to answer questions in this format correctly, they would need to have processed information well enough to discriminate among and eliminate plausible but inaccurate response choices. Additionally, in order to increase the test's sensitivity, two questions each were developed to assess stated and implied main ideas, and three questions each were developed to assess stated and implied details. From these stories and questions passage dependency was assessed. This study asked the following experimental questions: (1) Does the percentage of correctly answered questions for each story form differ significantly ($p \leq .05$) from chance (20%) for the Story + Questions and for the Questions Only groups? (2) Does the average PDI equal or exceed .60 for each form? (3) Is there a significant ($p \leq .05$) difference in the PDI among the story forms? (4) Is there a significant ($p \leq .05$) difference in the percentage of correctly answered questions among the four story forms for each group? Secondary experimental questions addressed differences in performance based on the nature of the information queried by the test question—i.e., main idea stated (M-S), main idea implied (M-I), detail stated (D-S), or detail implied (D-I). Definitions for these concepts were those provided by Brookshire and Nicholas (1997). The following secondary experimental questions were asked: (1) Does the percentage of correctly answered questions for each question type, for each story form, differ significantly ($p \le .05$) from chance (20%) for both the Story + Questions and Questions Only groups? (2) Does the average PDI equal or exceed .60 for each question type? (3) Is there a significant ($p \le .05$) difference in the PDIs within each question type among the four forms and among question types within a form? (4) Is there a significant ($p \le .05$) difference in the percentage of correctly answered questions within each question type among the four story forms and among questions types within a story form for the Stories + Questions group?

METHOD

Participants

Participants were 40 normal young adults between the ages of 20 and 40 years ($M = 25.25$, $SD = 6.03$), with 12–23 years of education ($M = 16.02$, $SD = 1.87$) and a negative self-reported history of speech, language, hearing, or neurological impairment. Descriptive participant information is displayed in Table 1. Participants were volunteers from the university community and were pseudo-randomly assigned to one of two groups based on room and scheduling availability. Participants in the Stories + Questions group had a mean age of 27 years ($SD = 7.02$) and a mean education of 16.7 years ($SD = 2.15$).

TABLE 1
Biobraphical and descriptive participant information

	Questions Only group				Stories + Questions group		
Participant	Gender	Age	Education	Participant	Gender	Age	Education
1	F	32	16	1	F	22	16
2	F	21	16	2	M	21	14
3	F	21	14	3	F	21	16
4	F	21	15	4	F	20	14
5	F	22	16	5	F	20	15
6	F	28	17	6	F	28	17
7	F	32	12	7	F	28	18
8	F	22	16	8	F	40	17
9	F	21	15	9	F	25	16
10	F	21	15	10	F	22	16
11	F	22	15	11	F	23	16
12	F	21	15	12	F	23	18
13	F	21	15	13	F	23	16
14	F	20	15	14	F	23	16
15	F	21	15	15	F	23	16
16	F	21	15	16	F	28	15
17	F	21	15	17	F	38	23
18	F	21	15	18	F	38	16
19	F	33	18	19	F	40	18
20	F	28	18	20	M	34	21

Participants in the Questions Only group had a mean age of 23.5 years ($SD = 4.37$) and a mean education of 15.35 years ($SD = 1.27$). Participants were tested in small groups of one to four at times convenient to the participants and examiners.

Stimuli

Details regarding story recordings are reported in McNeil et al. (2001). For this study, stories were presented in sound field at a comfortable loudness level as determined by each participant. Response choices were randomly ordered following development through group consensus of the authors, with attention to response plausibility, homogeneity, length, and grammatical form. Question order for each of the 12 stories was predetermined such that earlier questions did not provide answers or clues to information requested in later questions. Questions and answers are listed in appendix A.

Procedures

For participants in the Story + Questions group, stories were presented auditorily with the pictures that go with each story via the RAPP computer program. Stories were presented in one of six randomised orders. After each story presentation, each of the 10 questions with its five response choices was visually presented on the screen, one at a time, without re-presentation. Participants answered each question by circling their lettered response on answer sheets. Questions and response choices were not printed on the answer sheets.

Participants in the Questions Only group sat at a desktop computer on which were the 120 multiple-choice questions (10 for each of 12 stories). They were presented with the same answer packets as those presented to the Story + Questions group. Participants were instructed to read each question and circle the letter that corresponded with their answer. The participants controlled presentation of subsequent questions, but they were instructed to answer questions in the order in which they appeared and not to go back to a previously answered question.

Analyses

To organise the data for analyses, the percentage of questions answered correctly by each participant, for each story, and then by predetermined story forms (Doyle et al., 2000) was calculated. The percentage of questions answered correctly by each subject for each question type by form was also computed. Because there was an unequal number of questions among question types, the percentage of correctly answered questions for each question type was calculated by dividing the number of correctly answered questions of a particular type by the total possible number of that particular question type in a story form (M-S = 6, M-I = 6, D-S = 9, D-I = 9). After organisation of the data, two passage dependency measures were calculated. First, one sample t-tests were computed to determine if the mean percentage of questions answered correctly for each form and for each of the four question types within and among story forms differed significantly ($p \leq .05$) from the percentage that would be expected by chance (20%), for both experimental conditions. Additionally, the PDI was computed for each question and question type and averaged for each story and story form. After the number and proportion of correct responses for each question was determined for both participant groups, proportions were entered into the PDI equation and a PDI value was obtained for each question. Thus, PDI was calculated as: $1 -$ (proportion correct for the questions only condition, divided by proportion correct for the stories + questions condition). The 10 resulting question PDI values were then averaged to obtain the PDI for a given story, and PDIs for the three stories in a form were averaged to get the PDI value for each of the four forms. PDI values for question types were calculated by averaging the PDI values by form for each question type. PDI was conservatively set at .60 or greater, a value higher than previous referents (Nicholas & Brookshire, 1987; Nicholas et al., 1986). Due to small sample sizes and violation of the normality assumption, the Kruskal-Wallis procedure was used to determine significant PDI differences among forms, among question types within a form, and within question types across forms. Similarly, non-parametric Friedman tests were computed to determine significant differences in the percentage of questions answered correctly among story forms and for each question type among and within forms. Wilcoxon Signed Rank Tests were used to determine significant differences among levels when the Friedman procedure revealed significant results. An alpha level of .05 was used for all statistical tests, except to determine significance for post hoc multiple comparisons. For post hoc multiple comparisons an alpha level of .008 (.05/6) was used to control Type 1 error rate. Observed p-values which have been obtained from tests that use an alpha level of .008 are presented to the third place value.

RESULTS

Results of the Mann-Whitney U tests revealed a significantly ($p \leq .05$) higher age for the Stories + Questions group ($M = 27.0$ years; $SD = 7.01$) compared to the Questions Only group ($M = 23.5$ years; $SD = 4.37$) ($U = 121.00$, $p = .03$). Additionally, the Questions Only group had significantly ($p \leq .05$) fewer years of education ($M = 15.35$; $SD = 1.26$) compared with the Stories + Questions group ($M = 16.7$; $SD = 2.25$) ($U = 109.5$, $p = .01$).

The first experimental question addressed whether the percentage of correctly answered questions for each story form differed significantly ($p \leq .05$) from chance (20%) for the Story + Questions and for the Questions Only groups. A one-sample t-test revealed ($p \leq .05$) differences significant from chance (20%), in the percentage of correctly answered questions for the Stories + Questions group for each of the four story forms (see Table 2 for t- and p-values). Means and standard deviations for the forms were as follows: form A ($M = 88.33$, $SD = 11.07$); form B ($M = 87.45$, $SD = 9.57$); form C ($M = 87.5$, $SD = 10.35$); form D ($M = 86.27$, $SD = 9.80$). The percentage of correctly answered questions for the Questions Only group was not significantly different from chance for forms A ($M = 20.5$, $SD = 13.70$); B ($M = 22.17$, $SD = 16.37$); and D ($M = 23.10$, $SD = 12.31$). However, differences significantly exceeded chance levels for form C ($M = 30.51$, $SD = 14.19$) (See Table 2).

TABLE 2
t test and significance values for differences between percentage correct and chance for Stories + Questions and Questions Only experimental conditions

| Form | Questions Only | | | | Stories + Questions | | | |
	df	t	p	d	df	t	p	d
Form A	59	0.28	.77	0.03	59	47.80	.00*	6.17
Form B	59	1.02	.31	0.13	58	54.10	.00*	7.04
Form C	58	5.68	.00*	0.74	59	50.49	.00*	6.52
Form D	57	1.92	.06	0.25	58	51.89	.00*	6.76

*$p < .05$

The secondary question asked whether the percentage of correctly answered questions for each question type was significantly ($p \leq .05$) different from chance (20%) for the Stories + Questions and Questions Only group (see Table 3 for means and standard deviations for all question types and forms for both groups). Results of t-tests computed for the Stories + Questions group revealed that the percentage of correctly answered questions for each of the four question types was significantly ($p \leq .05$) greater than chance (20%) for all forms (see Table 4). T-test results for the Questions Only group varied among forms for each question type (see Table 4).

The second primary experimental question addressed whether the average PDI equalled or exceeded .60 for each story form. Result revealed average story form PDIs of: .76 (form A); .74 (form B); .61 (form C); and .74 (form D). These values equalled or exceeded the pre-established PDI criteria of .60. Individual story PDIs are reported in Table 5. Only story number two (form C) failed to reach the pre-established PDI criteria. PDIs for all question types for all story forms equalled or exceeded the pre-established PD criteria of .60 with the exception of D-I questions in form C (see Table 6).

The third primary experimental question addressed whether there was a significant difference in the PDI among the story forms. Results of the Kruskal-Wallis procedure revealed no significant ($p \leq .05$) differences in the PDI among the four story forms $H(3, N = 120) = 4.14$, $p = .24$, $\eta^2 = .03$. The following mean ranks were obtained: Form A = 66.73; Form B = 61.65; Form C = 49.77; Form D = 63.85. Results from the secondary analyses regarding significant differences for each question type among the four story forms revealed no statistically significant differences for M-S $H(3, N = 24) = 1.58$, $p = .66$, $\eta^2 = .06$; M-I $H(3, N = 24) = 1.63$, $p = .65$, $\eta^2 = .07$; D-S $H(3, N = 36) = 3.72$, $p = .29$, $\eta^2 = .10$; and D-I $H(3, N = 36) = 2.80$, $p = .42$, $\eta^2 = .08$, questions (see Table 7 for mean ranks for each form within a question type). Additionally, results revealed no significant differences in PDIs among the four question types, within a form: form A $H(3, N = 30) = 4.43$, $p = .21$, $\eta^2 = .15$; form B $H(3, N = 30) = .40$, $p = .93$, $\eta^2 = .01$; form C $H(3, N = 30) = 2.04$, $p = .56$, $\eta^2 = .07$; and form D $H(3, N = 30) = 2.59$, $p = .45$, $\eta^2 = .08$ (see Table 8 for mean ranks within a form for each question type).

TABLE 3
Means and standard deviations for each question type for each form for both participant groups

Form	MI-S		MI-I		DT-S		DT-I	
	Mean	SD	Mean	SD	Mean	SD	Mean	SD
Questions Only								
A	17.5	14.78	29.16	11.93	12.77	11.55	27.77	17.47
B	15.83	14.78	23.33	13.67	23.33	13.44	19.44	12.93
C	25.83	15.74	37.5	16.99	22.22	15.71	34.99	14.98
D	30.83	21.13	29.16	16.99	16.66	13.24	19.44	14.36
Mean percent total	**22.50**	16.61	**29.79**	14.90	**18.75**	13.49	**25.41**	14.94
Story + Question								
A	97.49	6.10	93.33	12.56	83.88	16.7	78.89	13.44
B	98.33	5.13	93.33	9.97	92.22	8.9	71.66	16.70
C	97.49	6.10	85.83	9.78	89.44	11.66	80.55	12.93
D	97.5	8.15	89.16	16.46	80.55	13.42	77.78	14.41
Mean percent total	**97.70**	6.37	**90.41**	12.19	**86.52**	12.67	**77.22**	14.37

TABLE 4
t test and significance values for differences between percentage correct and chance for question types for Stories + Questions and Question Only experimental conditions

Question type	FORM	Question Only				Stories + Questions			
		df	t	d	p	df	t	d	p
MI-S	A	19	−0.75	−0.16	.45	19	56.75	12.70	.00*
	B	19	−1.26	−0.28	.22	19	68.27	15.26	.00*
	C	19	1.65	0.37	.11	19	56.75	12.70	.00*
	D	19	2.29	0.51	.03*	19	42.49	9.50	.00*
MI-I	A	19	3.43	0.76	.00*	19	26.09	5.83	.00*
	B	19	1.09	0.24	.28	19	32.89	7.35	.00*
	C	19	4.60	1.03	.00*	19	30.08	6.73	.00*
	D	19	2.41	0.53	.02*	19	18.78	4.20	.00*
DT-S	A	19	−2.79	−0.62	.01*	19	17.10	3.82	.00*
	B	19	1.10	0.24	.28	19	36.28	8.11	.00*
	C	19	0.63	0.14	.53	19	26.62	5.95	.00*
	D	19	−1.12	−0.25	.27	19	20.17	4.51	.00*
DT-I	A	19	1.99	0.44	.06	19	19.59	4.38	.00*
	B	19	−0.19	−0.04	.84	19	13.83	3.05	.00*
	C	19	4.47	1.00	.00*	19	20.93	4.68	.00*
	D	19	−0.17	−0.03	.86	19	17.92	4.00	.00*

*$p \leq .05$

TABLE 5
PDI values for each form and each of the 12 stories

Story form	Story												Form PDI
	3	8	10	5	6	12	2	7	11	1	4	9	
A	0.78	0.80	0.70										0.76
B				0.70	0.69	0.84							0.74
C							0.48	0.71	0.65				0.61
D										0.71	0.73	0.79	0.74

TABLE 6
PDI values for all question types for each form

	Main idea stated	Main idea implied	Detail stated	Detail implied
Form A	0.84	0.71	0.85	0.66
Form B	0.77	0.76	0.75	0.67
Form C	0.72	0.61	0.75	0.39
Form D	0.70	0.67	0.85	0.71

TABLE 7

Mean PDI rank for each question type among
the four story forms

	Question type			
Form	MI-S	MI-I	DT-S	DT-I
A	15.50	13.83	21.89	17.67
B	12.33	14.75	14.11	20.44
C	11.00	16.33	10.33	14.11
D	11.17	11.08	21.67	21.78

TABLE 8

Mean PDI rank for question types within each
story form

	Form			
Question type	A	B	C	D
MI-S	18.08	16.58	16.42	13.83
MI-I	13.83	16.58	14.17	11.58
DT-S	19.17	14.11	18.44	18.61
DT-I	11.22	15.44	12.83	16.11

The fourth experimental question addressed differences in the percentage of correctly answered questions among the four story forms for each of the participant groups. Results of the Friedman procedure revealed no significant ($p \leq .05$) differences in the percentage of correctly answered questions among the forms (form A: $M = 88.33$, $SD = 11.07$; form B: $M = 87.45$, $SD = 9.57$; form C: $M = 87.50$, $SD = 10.35$; and form D: $M = 86.27$, $SD = 9.80$), for the Stories + Question group $\chi^2(3, N = 58) = 1.90$, $p = .59$, $W = .01$ (see Figure 1). There were, however, significant differences in the percentage of correctly answered questions among story forms (form A: $M = 21.05$, $SD = 13.71$; form B: $M = 22.28$, $SD = 16.69$; form C: $M = 31.22$, $SD = 13.76$; form D: $M = 22.45$, $SD = 12.71$) for the Questions Only group $\chi^2(3, N = 57) = 16.51$, $p = .00$, $W = .09$. Results of the Wilcoxon Signed Ranks test revealed significantly fewer correctly answered questions for form A than for form C ($T = -4.25$, $p = .000$), for form B than for form C ($T = -3.12$, $p = .002$), and for form D than for form C ($T = -3.34$, $p = .001$). No significant differences were obtained between forms A and B ($T = -0.45$, $p = .651$), forms A and D ($T = -0.46$, $p = .644$), and forms B and D ($T = -0.10$, $p = .919$). As form C was significantly different from all other forms in the Questions Only group, an independent samples t-test was computed to determine whether there were significant differences for form C between the Stories + Questions and Questions Only groups. Results revealed that the Questions Only group produced significantly fewer correct answers, $t(38) = 24.69$, $p = .00$, $d = 1.91$ ($M = 30.25$, $SD = 8.65$), than the Stories + Questions group ($M = 87.50$, $SD = 5.71$) on form C. The secondary question asked whether there were significant differences in the percentage of correctly answered questions for each question type for the Stories + Questions group. Results for question type data *within* each form for the Stories + Questions group are presented first, followed by question type data analysed for each question type *among*

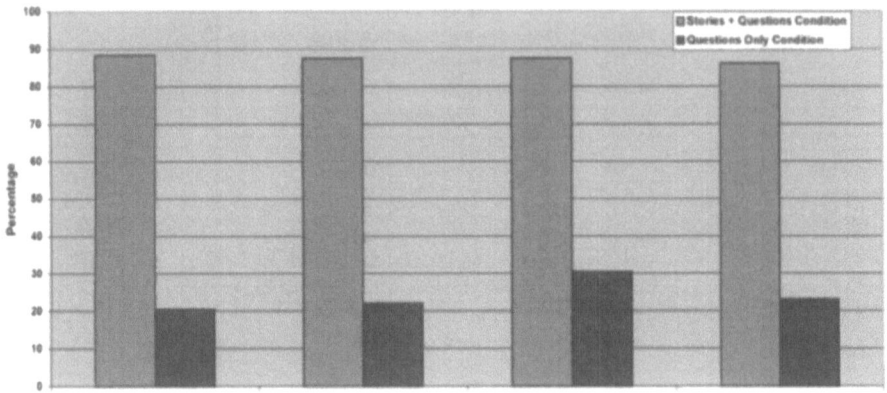

RAPP Story Forms

Figure 1. Percentage of correctly answered multiple choice questions for each RAPP story form.

forms. Average percent and standard deviations for all question types for all forms are summarised in Table 3.

Stories + Questions group for question types within form

Results of the Friedman test computed to examine differences in the percentage of correctly answered questions within each story form among question types for the Stories + Questions group revealed significant differences among question types within forms A $\chi^2(3, N = 20) = 28.13$, $p = .00$, $W = .46$; B $\chi^2(3, N = 20) = 29.64$, $p = .00$, $W = .49$; C $\chi^2(3, N = 20) = 19.08$, $p = .00$, $W = .31$; and D $\chi^2(3, N = 20) = 28.35$, $p = .00$, $W = .47$ (see Table 9 for question type mean ranks for each of the forms). Results of the Wilcoxon Signed Ranks Test varied for question types within forms and are presented in Table 10. In general, several question types were significantly different from one another for each story form, with the direction of differences generally in the expected directions with M-S > M-I, D-S and D-I; M-I > D-S and D-I, and D-S > D-I (see Table 3 and Figure 2).

Stories + Questions group for question types among forms

Results of the Friedman analysis revealed no significant differences in the percentage of correctly answered questions among forms for M-S questions $\chi^2(3, N = 20) = .42$, $p = .93$, $W = .00$ (see Table 3 for question type means among the forms and Table 9 for question type mean ranks). The percentage of correctly answered M-I questions was significantly different among forms $\chi^2(3, N = 20) = 8.40$, $p = .03$, $W = .14$. There was a significant difference among forms for the D-S question type, $\chi^2(3, N = 20) = 8.93$, $p = .03$, $W = .14$, but results were not significantly different among forms for D-I questions, $\chi^2(3, N = 20) = 4.51$, $p = .21$, $W = .07$ (see Table 11 for results of the Wilcoxon Signed Ranks Test). Although there were significant differences among forms for the M-I and D-S question types, results of the Wilcoxon Signed Ranks test revealed no significant differences for any simple contrasts between forms for either question type (see Table 11).

TABLE 9

(a) Mean rank for percentage of questions answered
correctly by question type *within* each form

	Story + Questions			
	Form			
Question type	A	B	C	D
MI-S	3.28	3.28	3.40	3.50
MI-I	3.00	2.75	2.17	2.83
DT-S	2.15	2.63	2.58	1.95
DT-I	1.58	1.35	1.85	1.73

(b) Mean rank for each question type for percentage of
questions answered correctly *among* forms

	Story + Questions			
	Question type			
Form	MI-S	MI-I	DT-S	DT-I
A	2.45	2.85	2.40	2.65
B	2.55	2.72	2.92	2.10
C	2.45	1.95	2.72	2.83
D	2.55	2.47	1.95	2.42

TABLE 10

Wilcoxon test and significance values for differences between percentage correct for question
types within a form for the Stories + Questions condition

	Forms							
	A		B		C		D	
Question type	T	p	T	p	T	p	T	p
MI-S–MI-I	−1.41	.157	−1.73	.083	−3.27	.001*	−2.12	.033
MI-S–DT-S	−3.13	.002*	−2.27	.023	−2.36	.018	−3.66	.000*
MI-S–DT-I	−3.75	.000*	−3.76	.000*	−3.66	.000*	−3.65	.000*
MI-I–DT-S	−2.71	.007*	−0.37	.710	−1.33	.182	−1.73	.082
MI-I–DT-I	−2.75	.006*	−3.43	.001*	−1.19	.234	−2.16	.031
DT-S–DT-I	−1.39	.162	−3.41	.001*	−2.12	.033	−0.7	.481

*$p < .008$

Questions Only group

Results of the Friedman analysis revealed significant differences among story forms for
the percentage of correctly answered questions $\chi^2(3, N = 57) = 16.51, p = .00, W = .09$ for
the Questions Only group. Mean ranks for forms were as follows: Form A = 2.28, form B
= 2.32, form C = 3.06, form D = 2.33. There was a significant difference among form C
and all other forms: A and C ($T = -4.25, p = .000$); B and C ($T = -3.12, p = .002$); and

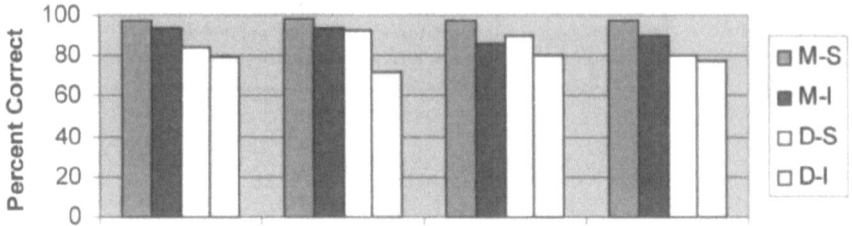

Story Form

Figure 2. Stories + Questions group: Mean percent for question types for each story form.

TABLE 11
Wilcoxon test and significance values for differences between percentage correct for
question types among forms for the Stories + Questions condition

	Question type							
	M-S		M-I		D-S		D-I	
Forms	T	p	T	p	T	p	T	p
A–B	—	—	−0.18	0.850	−2.38	0.017	—	—
A–C	—	—	−1.95	0.051	−1.92	0.055	—	—
A–D	—	—	−1.09	0.272	−0.98	0.327	—	—
B–C	—	—	−2.51	0.012	−0.96	0.334	—	—
B–D	—	—	−0.56	0.570	−2.4	0.016	—	—
C–D	—	—	−0.57	0.563	−1.93	0.053	—	—

C and D ($T = -3.34$, $p = .001$). No other significant differences were revealed among the other forms: A and B ($T = -0.45$, $p = .651$), A and D ($T = -0.46$, $p = .644$), B and D ($T = -0.10$, $p = .919$).

A post-hoc analysis designed to examine question difficulty was completed by determining if there were significant differences in the proportions of respondents answering questions correctly for each question type for the Stories + Question group. Data were analysed using the Kruskal-Wallis procedure and the Mann-Whitney U test was used to test for significant differences between question types. Results revealed significant differences among the question types $H(3, N = 30) = 9.54$, $p = .02$, $\eta^2 = .32$ for form A, with mean ranks of M-S = 23.75, M-I = 18.25, D-S = 12.28, D-I = 11.39, and for form B $H(3, N = 30) = 9.07$, $p = .02$, $\eta^2 = .31$, with mean ranks of M-S = 22.08, M-I = 18.83, D-S = 14.89, D-I = 9.50. There were no significant differences among question types for form C $H(3, N = 30) = 4.62$, $p = .201$, $\eta^2 = .15$; (M-S = 20.83, M-I = 18.08, D-S = 12.89, and D-I = 12.83); or form D $H(3, N = 30) = 6.55$, $p = .088$, $\eta^2 = .22$, (M-S = 23.00, M-I = 14.17, D-S = 15.06, D-I = 11.83). Although the Kruskal-Wallis procedure revealed significant differences among the question types for form A, no significant differences were revealed with the post-hoc Mann-Whitney test; M-S − M-I ($U = 8.0$, $p = .132$), M-S − D-S ($U = 7.0$, $p = .018$), M-S − D-I ($U = 7.5$, $p = .018$), M-I − D-S ($U = 12.5$, $p = .088$), M-I − D-I ($U = 15.0$, $p = .181$), and D-S − D-I ($U = 35.0$, $p = .666$). Similar results were obtained for form B, again with no significant differences between simple contrasts; M-S $-$ M-I ($U = 14.5$, $p = .589$), M-S $-$ D-S ($U = 11.5$, $p = .066$), M-S $-$ D-I ($U = 6.5$, $p = .012$), M-I $-$ D-S ($U = 19.5$, $p = .388$), M-I $-$ D-I ($U = 11.0$, $p = .066$), and D-S $-$ D-I ($U = 23.0$, $p = .136$).

DISCUSSION

This study examined the passage dependency of newly developed multiple-choice questions that were designed to assess auditory comprehension of paragraph-length passages. Analyses examined the questions' validity in terms of their passage dependency compared to chance performance and to a pre-established PDI criterion. Differences in the PDI and in the percentage of correctly answered questions among predetermined forms were also evaluated. These same analyses were also used to examine the passage dependency of the questions based on the type of information queried by a question both within and among forms. Additionally, a measure of question type difficulty was computed to provide further insight into the validity of the multiple-choice questions.

The results of the primary analyses that examined the multiple-choice questions without consideration of the nature of the information queried by them support the passage dependency of the questions that make up the four story forms for the RAPP version of the DCT. The percentage of correctly answered questions exceeded chance for all four story forms, PDIs met or exceeded the pre-established criterion, there were no significant differences in the PDIs among the four forms, and there were no significant differences in the percentage of correctly answered questions among the four story forms. While calculation of the PDI measure necessarily includes performance results from participants who heard the stories preceding the questions and participants who only received the questions, it was determined that the percentage of correctly answered questions should be compared with chance across forms for the Questions Only group. The results revealed that participants in the Questions Only group were able to answer the questions on form C at significantly greater than chance level, and that the percentage of correctly answered questions on all other forms for the Questions Only group was significantly different from that of form C. To determine if there were significant differences in the performance of both groups on form C, a post-hoc analysis was completed. The results revealed that although participants in the Questions Only group were able to answer the questions at greater than chance level, their percentage of correctly answered questions on form C was significantly worse than the performance of participants who had heard the stories. These findings might be interpreted to suggest that the multiple-choice questions on form C may be less passage-dependent or less well-constructed than the multiple-choice questions on the other forms. Because significant differences remained between the two groups in the percentage of correctly answered questions, and because the PDI criterion was met or exceeded, it is concluded that these newly developed multiple-choice questions are sufficiently passage-dependent when question type is not considered.

According to Brookshire and Nicholas (1997), explicitness and saliency are two factors that may affect discourse comprehension. Saliency is described as whether information is considered to be a main idea or a detail, while explicitness relates to whether information has been stated or only implied in the presented information. Brookshire and Nicholas (1984; 1997) reported that both non-brain-damaged (NBD) persons and persons with aphasia comprehended and retained main idea information better than details. Similar findings were reported by Welland, Lubinski, and Higgenbotham (2002) in a study examining discourse comprehension in persons with dementia of the Alzheimer Type. However, findings regarding the effect of explicitness on comprehension are less consistent. Results have at times demonstrated a significant effect on performance (Welland et al., 2002) and have not at other times (Brookshire & Nicholas, 1984). Questions in the DCT were developed with saliency and explicitness incorporated into their structure. In the present study these factors were also incorporated during the development of the multiple-choice questions, and question type categorisation was determined by group discussion and consensus of the investigators. Thus, in addition to analyses of the multiple-choice questions in general, secondary analyses were performed to evaluate the validity and passage dependency of the multiple-choice questions relative to question type for the Stories + Questions group. It was reasoned that these analyses would provide further information regarding the passage dependency and validity of these specific question types. For the Stories + Questions group, question type analyses revealed that all question types were answered significantly better than chance for all forms. All PDIs met or exceeded pre-established criteria (except D-I questions in form C) and there were no significant differences in the PDIs among the four question types by story form or among question types within a form. There were significant differences in the percentage of correctly answered questions for question types among forms for M-I and D-S question types. While post hoc tests of simple contrasts failed to locate these differences, omnibus tests revealed differences between specific form combinations for each of these question types. Additional studies, with larger samples sizes, will assess the reliability of this finding. There were no significant differences among forms for M-S or for D-I questions. There were significant differences in the percentage of correctly answered questions among question types *within* a form for each of the four forms. These results were mixed for the forms, with only form A demonstrating results that showed significant differences between both stated and implied main ideas and stated and implied details. Some expected significant differences in saliency (main idea vs detail) were not obtained for form B and form C. There were, however, some differences in explicitness within each level of saliency. Form D revealed significant differences between M-S questions and both levels of explicitness for detail questions, but not for M-I questions for either level of explicitness. The within-form findings for the Story + Questions group suggests that following replication on larger numbers and assessment with relevant pathological groups, these multiple-choice questions may need to be re-evaluated relative to their sensitivity for detecting these expected category differences. Alternatively, these results might be interpreted as reflecting age/education-related processing differences. The majority of the participants in this study were young undergraduate or graduate students enrolled in communication disorders courses at a major university. The other studies reviewed examining explicitness and saliency used older normal participants. It is possible that because our participants were young and highly educated, the lack of observed differences in saliency and explicitness resulted from a diminished challenge in linguistic complexity or structure in the discourse stimuli for these particular participants.

Conclusions

These results provide support for the passage dependency of the multiple-choice questions constructed for the four story forms that make up the RAPP version of the DCT. These results provide potential users with confidence that the questions are not biased relative to the content of the story and add to the overall establishment of the validity of this version of the DCT. Despite the significant difference from chance for the Questions Only group for form C and the lower than criterion PDI for the D-I questions in form C, we do not suggest that the multiple-choice questions for that form need further modification, as performance on that form for the Questions Only group remained significantly different from the Stories + Questions group. Further investigations should address the validity of these questions with older non-brain-damaged persons and a variety of pathological populations (left- and right-brain-damaged persons, patients with traumatic brain injury, dementia, etc.). Additionally, the validity of this task may be enhanced by correlations with other methods of examining comprehension such as the SRP (McNeil et al., 2001). Although this study examined a variable that addresses the validity of the multiple-choice questions task, it should be noted for future investigations that the reliability of these questions remains to be demonstrated. In summary, the results of this study support the validity of the multiple-choice question task as a way to measure auditory comprehension for the RAPP version of the DCT.

REFERENCES

Brookshire, R. H., & Nicholas, L. E. (1984). Comprehension of directly and indirectly stated main ideas and details in discourse by brain-damaged and non-brain-damaged listeners. *Brain and Language, 21*, 21–36.

Brookshire, R. H., & Nicholas, L. E. (1997). *Discourse Comprehension Test*. Minneapolis, Minnesota: BRK Publishers.

Chapman, S. B., Ulatowska, H. K., Franklin, L. R., Shobe, A. E., Thompson, J. L., & McIntire, D. D. (1997). Proverb interpretation in fluent aphasia and Alzheimer's disease: Implications beyond abstract thinking. *Aphasiology, 11*, 337–350.

Doyle, P. J., McNeil, M. R., Park, G. H., Goda, A. J., Rubenstein, E., Spencer, K. et al. (2000). Linguistic validation of four parallel forms of a story retelling procedure. *Aphasiology, 14*, 537–549.

Doyle, P. J., McNeil, M. R., Spencer, K. A., Goda, A. J., Cottrell, K., & Lustig, A. P. (1998). The effects of concurrent picture presentations on retelling of orally presented stories by adults with aphasia. *Aphasiology, 12*, 561–574.

Goodglass, H., Kaplan, E., & Baressi, B. (2001). *Boston Diagnostic Aphasia Examination*. (3rd ed.). Philadelphia: Lippincott Williams & Wilkins.

McNeil, M. R., Doyle, P. J., Fossett, T. R. D., Park, G. H., & Goda, A. J. (2001). Reliability and concurrent validity of the information unit scoring metric for the story retelling procedure. *Aphasiology, 15*, 991–1006.

McNeil, M. R., Doyle, P. J., Park, G. H., Fossett, T. R. D., & Brodsky, M. B. (2002). Increasing the sensitivity of the Story Retell Procedure for the discrimination of normal elderly subjects from persons with aphasia. *Aphasiology, 16*, 815–822.

Nicholas, L. E., & Brookshire, R. H. (1987). Error analysis and passage dependency of test items from a standardized test of multiple-sentence reading comprehension for aphasic and non-brain-damaged adults. *Journal of Speech and Hearing Disorders, 52*, 358–366.

Nicholas, L. E., MacLennan, D. L., & Brookshire, R. H. (1986). Validity of multiple-sentence reading comprehension tests for aphasic adults. *Journal of Speech and Hearing Disorders, 51*, 82–87.

Thomas, C. A. & Jackson, S. T. (1997). The validity of reading comprehension therapy materials. *Journal of Communication Disorders, 30*, 231–243.

Tuiman, J. J. (1974). Determining the passage dependency of comprehension questions in 5 major tests. *Reading Research Quarterly, 2*, 206–223.

Ulatowska, H. K., Wertz, R. T., Chapman, S. B., Hill, C. L., Thompson, J. L., Keebler, M. W. et al. (2001). Interpretation of fables and proverbs by African Americans with and without aphasia. *American Journal of Speech-Language Pathology, 10*, 40–50.

Welland, R. J., Lubinski, R., & Higginbotham, D. J. (2002). Discourse Comprehension Test performance of elders with dementia of the Alzheimer Type. *Journal of Speech, Language, and Hearing Research, 45*, 1175–1187.

APPENDIX A

Story 1: Baseball

1. The game was played about:
D-I   a. 2:00
      b. 12:00
      c. 7:00
      d. 4:00
      e. 9:00

2. When George got to his seat, he:
D-S   a. Bought a hot dog
      b. Pretended to play baseball
      c. Put on a baseball cap
      d. Wanted a better seat
      e. Put film in his camera

3. George told everyone around him that:
M-S   a. He planned to catch a home run ball
      b. He was a sports announcer
      c. His son was a famous baseball star
      d. He deserved a better seat
      e. He had played baseball in high school

4. The batter:
D-S   a. Struck out
      b. Hit a ground ball
      c. Hit a foul ball
      d. Hit a home run
      e. Walked

5. During the game, George:
M-I   **a. Missed the ball**
      b. Caught the ball
      c. Pretended to catch the ball
      d. Got hit by the ball
      e. Threw the ball back

6. George tried to catch the baseball:
D-I   a. At the beginning of the game
      b. In the middle of the game
      c. Before the game
      d. At the end of the game
      e. After the game

7. The ball was found by:
D-I   a. Hotdog vender
      b. George
      c. A security guard
      d. A bat boy
      e. A recruiter

8. George was approached by a:
M-S   a. Baseball scout
      b. Doctor
      c. Baseball player
      d. Man with the circus
      e. Hotdog vendor

9. The man gave George
D-S   **a. A business card**
      b. An autographed baseball
      c. A ride to the hospital
      d. Help getting up
      e. A hotdog

10. George wanted the man to:
M-I   a. Bring him a hotdog
      b. Sign his baseball
      c. Help him back to his seat
      d. Recruit him for a team
      e. Take him to the hospital

Story 2: Fire

1. Mrs. Wilson lived:
M-S   **a. Alone**
      b. In her daughter's house
      c. With her son
      d. With her sister
      e. In a nursing home

2. Mrs. Wilson lived in:
D-S   a. Alabama
      b. Kansas
      c. Kentucky
      d. Arkansas
      e. Iowa

3. Mrs. Wilson's son wanted her to:
D-S   a. Buy a smaller house
      b. Move in with him
      c. Hold onto the family farm
      d. Move into a nursing home
      e. Rent an apartment

4. Lightening struck the:
M-I   a. Garage
      b. Neighbor's house
      c. Barn
      d. House
      e. Neighbor's tree

5. Mrs. Wilson realized there was a fire when she:
D-I   a. Saw the lightening strike
      b. Smelled smoke
      c. Heard the fire alarm
      d. Looked out her window
      e. Got a phone call

6. The telephone was:
D-I   a. By the back door
      b. In the bedroom
      c. In the living room
      d. By the window
      e. In the kitchen

7. The fire was put out by:
M-I   a. The fire sprinklers
      b. The neighbors
      c. Mrs. Wilson
      d. The firemen
      e. The rain

8. The firemen arrived:
D-S   a. After the fire was out
      b. As Mrs. Wilson left for her neighbors
      c. While Mrs. Wilson was on the phone
      d. After Mrs. Wilson called the fire department
      e. Too late to save the barn

9. The fire department was notified by:
M-S   a. Mrs. Wilson's son
      b. The telephone operator
      c. The fire alarm
      d. Mrs. Wilson's neighbors
      e. Mrs. Wilson

10. In the barn there were:
D-I   **a. Cows**
      b. Chickens
      c. Horses
      d. Pigs
      e. Sheep

Story 3: Loan

1. Neil asked his parents to:
D-S   **a. Lend him their car**
      b. Give him some money
      c. Sign some forms
      d. Take him out to eat
      e. Give him some advice

2. Neil wanted to:
M-I   a. Pay off his loan
      b. Join the army
      c. Get married
      d. Stay in school
      e. Start a business

3. Neil needed money:
M-S   a. To repay student loans
      b. For tuition
      c. For rent
      d. To buy a ring
      e. For a computer

4. In an attempt to get money, Neil:
M-S   a. Sold his car
      b. Got a job
      c. Went to the bank
      d. Asked his parents
      e. Applied for a scholarship

5. Neil went to the bank:
D-I   a. With his fiancé
      b. In the morning
      c. In the afternoon
      d. At lunchtime
      e. With his parents

6. The woman asked Neil:
D-S   a. About his monthly expenses
      b. About his marital status
      c. For his parents' signatures
      d. To fill out a form
      e. About his grades

7. Neil was:
D-I   a. Determined
      b. Optimistic
      c. Impatient
      d. Lazy
      e. Nervous

8. Neil said he ate a:
D-S   a. Pickle sandwich
      b. Macaroni sandwich
      c. Mayonnaise sandwich
      d. Lettuce sandwich
      e. Cheese sandwich

9. The woman thought Neil's lunch was:
D-I   a. Tasty
      b. Expensive
      c. Healthy
      d. Not enough
      e. Strange

10. The woman:
M-I   a. Offered to cook for Neil
      b. Asked Neil to leave
      c. Turned Neil down
      d. Changed her mind
      e. Called Neil's parents

Story 4: Painting

1. Fred and Ben had a business in:
M-S   a. Gardening
      b. Siding
      c. Carpentry
      d. Painting
      e. Roofing

2. Fred and Ben were:
D-S   a. Neighbors
      b. Brothers
      c. Friends
      d. Cousins
      e. Father and son

3. Mrs. Foster called the men on:
D-I   a. Saturday
      b. Sunday
      c. Wednesday
      d. Thursday
      e. Monday

4. Mrs. Foster found out about the painters from:
D-I   a. The local hardware store
      b. The newspaper
      c. Signs
      d. Friends
      e. Yellow pages

5. Mrs. Foster was their:
M-S   a. 100th customer
      b. Best customer
      c. 1st customer
      d. 500th customer
      e. Least favorite customer

6. Fred and Ben were painting a:
D-I   **a. Two-story house**
      b. Garage
      c. Fence
      d. One-story house
      e. Barn

7. Mrs. Foster asked Fred and Ben to:
M-I   a. Paint her house on Saturday
      b. Help choose a paint color
      c. Give her a discount
      d. Meet with her by Tuesday
      e. Paint her house quickly

8. Mrs. Foster needed the house painted for:
D-S   **a. Her daughter's wedding**
      b. Her 50th anniversary party
      c. An open house
      d. Her husband's birthday
      e. Her 25th anniversary party

9. The man came around the house at about:
D-S   a. 5 p.m.
      b. 3 p.m.
      c. 1 p.m.
      d. 2 p.m.
      e. 4 p.m.

10. Fred and Ben:
M-I   a. Ran out of paint
      b. Used the wrong color of paint
      c. Painted the house too late
      d. Painted the wrong house
      e. Painted the windows shut

Story 5: Water

1. The story took place:
D-I a. In the fall
     b. In the summer
     c. In the morning
     d. At lunchtime
     e. In the winter

2. Joe had just finished:
D-S **a. Shoveling the walk**
     b. Mowing the grass
     c. Fixing a sandwich
     d. Watching TV
     e. Raking the leaves

3. Betty was:
M-S a. Taking a nap
     b. Reading a book
     c. Cooking dinner
     d. Knitting a sweater
     e. Sewing a dress

4. Joe was:
D-S a. Fixing the sink
     b. Watching TV
     c. Listening to the radio
     d. Reading the newspaper
     e. Taking a nap

5. Joe and Betty:
D-I **a. Had children**
     b. Were sitting in different rooms
     c. Had pets
     d. Wre arguing
     e. Were just married

6. Joe was:
D-I a. Angry
     b. Impatient
     c. Hungry
     d. Sick
     e. Depressed

7. Joe asked his wife to bring him:
M-S a. The newspaper
     b. The remote control
     c. Some food
     d. A cup of coffee
     e. An aspirin

8. Betty made a:
D-S a. Cup of hot chocolate
     b. Tuna sandwich
     c. Pot of coffee
     d. Cheese sandwich
     e. Ham sandwich

9. Joe finished:
M-I a. Making a sandwich
     b. Reading the newspaper
     c. Drinking a cup of coffee
     d. Drinking a cup of water
     e. Eating the sandwich

10. Betty wanted:
M-I a. To get things for Joe
     b. To finish knitting the sweater
     c. Joe to get things for her
     d. To finish baking her cookies
     e. Joe to make her a sandwich

Story 6: Snow

1. Don was waiting at the:
M-S   a. Restaurant
       b. Doctor\s office
       c. Airport
       d. Hotel
       e. Train station

2. Don was traveling in:
D-I   a. July
       b. November
       c. January
       d. March
       e. December

3. Don was going to see his:
D-S   **a. Brother**
       b. Son
       c. Friend
       d. Grandparents
       e. Sister

4. They were supposed to leave:
D-I   a. At night
       b. In the evening
       c. In the morning
       d. At noon
       e. In the afternoon

5. People were told:
M-S   **a. To wait for the next plane**
       b. The flight was cancelled
       c. There were extra seats available
       d. To return to the ticket counter
       e. To get a refund

6. Don was:
M-I   a. Relieved not to get on the plane
       b. Looking forward to seeing his brother
       c. Eager to hear his name called
       d. Anxious to perform surgery
       d. Late getting to the airport

7. The number of people who had to wait was:
D-S   a. Five
       b. Seven
       c. Two
       d. Twelve
       e. Ten

8. Don was flying to:
D-S   a. Baltimore
       b. Denver
       c. Orlando
       d. Detroit
       e. Seattle

9. The woman:
M-I   a. Asked if Don was a surgeon
       b. Wanted Don's ticket
       c. Lied to Don
       d. Gave Don a ticket
       e. Did not believe Don's story

10. Don had been waiting for about:
D-I   a. Two hours
       b. Thirty minutes
       c. Three hours
       d. One hour
       e. Forty-five minutes

Story 7: Garage Sale

1. Several women had:
M-S a. A baby shower
     b. A tea party
     c. A garage sale
     d. A fundraiser
     e. An auction

2. The women had:
M-I **a. Collected many items**
     b. Given away many prizes
     c. Brought many gifts
     d. Bought a few items
     e. Nothing left for sale

3. The women put a sign up at:
D-S a. A high school
     b. A community center
     c. A church
     d. An antique store
     e. A shopping center

4. The weather that day was:
D-I a. Windy
     b. Hot
     c. Rainy
     d. Cloudy
     e. Cold

5. The women were drinking:
D-S a. Water
     b. Lemonade
     c. Iced tea
     d. Coffee
     e. Fruit punch

6. The man was driving a:
D-S **a. Truck**
     b. Van
     c. Station wagon
     d. Jeep
     e. Car

7. The man was:
D-I a. Widowed
     b. Engaged
     c. Single
     d. Married
     e. Divorced

8. The mattress was:
M-S a. Too expensive
     b. In bad condition
     c. Too small
     d. In good condition
     e. Too big

9. The man:
D-I a. Could not afford the mattress
     b. Decided he did not want the mattress
     c. Forgot to take the mattress
     d. Got the mattress for free
     e. Paid too much for the mattress

10. The man did not want his father-in-law to:
M-I **a. Stay for a long time**
     b. Tell him what to do
     c. Ask for money
     d. Complain about the bed
     e. Pay for the mattress

Story 8: Gas

1. Jim was:
D-S   a. A mailman
      b. An insurance salesman
      c. A paint salesman
      d. A repairman
      e. A real estate agent

2. Jim was driving:
M-S   a. On an interstate
      b. Through the city
      c. Near his home
      d. Through the suburbs
      e. Through the country

3. It was a:
D-I   a. Cold, cloudy day
      b. Hot, sunny day
      c. Cold, rainy night
      d. Warm, rainy night
      e. Cool, sunny evening

4. While waiting, Jim:
D-S   a. Listened to the radio
      b. Took a nap
      c. Ate a snack
      d. Sat down under a tree
      e. Checked the oil

5. Jim's car stopped running:
D-I   a. On his way home at night
      b. After he had made many stops
      c. Early in the day
      d. On his way to lunch
      e. During a bad rainstorm

6. Jim decided to:
M-S   a. Cancel an appointment
      b. Walk to get help
      c. Call a tow truck
      d. Get a ride to town
      e. Call his boss

7. The car Jim was driving was:
D-I   **a. Fairly new**
      b. Rented
      c. Rarely driven
      d. Just repaired
      e. Very old

8. Jim's car:
M-I   a. Had a dead battery
      b. Was leaking oil
      c. Had a bad transmission
      d. Was out of gas
      e. Was overheated

9. While walking, Jim stopped to:
D-S   a. Use a pay phone
      b. Fill the gas can
      c. Flag down a passing car
      d. Ask a young lady for help
      e. Talk to an old man

10. The gas station was:
M-I   **a. Over two miles**
      b. About a mile
      c. Just around the bend
      d. Closed that day
      e. Out of gas

Story 9: Tickets

1. Harry was pulled over in:
D-I   a. July
    b. April
    c. September
    d. January
    e. December

2. Harry was driving a:
D-S   **a. Van**
    b. Station wagon
    c. Sports car
    d. Truck
    e. Motorcycle

3. Harry was going to the:
M-S   a. Mall
    b. Cleaners
    c. Hospital
    d. Post office
    e. Bank

4. The policeman asked Harry:
M-S   a. Where he was going
    b. For his registration
    c. To get out of his car
    d. For his driver's license
    e. If he needed help

5. Harry had:
D-I   a. No proof of insurance
    b. Lost his wallet
    c. Left his license at home
    d. Lost his registration
    e. Many cards in his wallet

6. Harry's license was:
D-S   **a. Expired for a month**
    b. From another state
    c. Suspended
    d. Stolen
    e. Not in his wallet

7. The policeman said that Harry had:
M-I   a. Been tailgating
    b. Made an illegal turn
    c. Been speeding
    d. Run a stop sign
    e. Run a red light

8. Harry had been driving:
D-S   a. 55 miles per hour
    b. 35 miles per hour
    c. 60 miles per hour
    d. 25 miles per hour
    e. 40 miles per hour

9. Harry did not see the:
D-I   a. Red light
    b. No parking sign
    c. Stop sign
    d. Speed limit
    e. Other car

10. Harry was not able to:
M-I   a. Get a parking space
    b. Find his license
    c. Make it on time
    d. Find the cleaners
    e. Drive anymore

Story 10: Library

1. Henry went to the:
M-S a. Bank
     b. Hospital
     c. Bookstore
     d. Library
     e. Airport

2. On that day, it was:
D-I   **a. Raining**
     b. Hot
     c. Snowing
     d. Windy
     e. Pleasant

3. The woman Henry spoke to:
D-S a. Had long hair
     b. Wore glasses
     c. Had gray hair
     d. Wore a skirt
     e. Wore a sweater

4. When Henry approached the woman, she was:
D-S a. Talking on the phone
     b. Helping a customer
     c. Reading a book
     d. Shelving books
     e. Sorting papers

5. Henry had trouble:
M-I   **a. Remembering**
     b. Talking
     c. Concentrating
     d. Seeing
     e. Learning

6. The woman was:
M-I   a. Pleased
     b. Disappointed
     c. Irritated
     d. Furious
     e. Relieved

7. The woman:
D-I   a. Asked Henry to leave
     b. Filled out a report
     c. Took back the book
     d. Called the supervisor
     e. Took away Henry's privileges

8. The book was:
M-S a. Replaced
     b. Returned
     c. Damaged
     d. Lost
     e. Found

9. Henry had been:
D-I   a. Away at school
     b. On a business trip
     c. On a cruise
     d. At home
     e. On vacation

10. Henry left the book in:
D-S a. Florida
     b. Mexico
     c. California
     d. Bermuda
     e. Puerto Rico

Story 11: Tightrope

1. George was a:
D-S a. Television reporter
    b. Circus performer
    c. Bookkeeper
    d. Stuntman
    e. Bachelor

2. George was planning to cross Niagara Falls:
M-S a. In an airplane
    b. In a hot air balloon
    c. In a canoe
    d. With a hang glider
    e. On a tightrope

3. George had:
M-I a. Seen this stunt on TV
    b. Tried this stunt once before
    c. Done this stunt many times before
    d. Seen this stunt at the circus
    e. Never done this stunt before

4. George was:
D-I a. Single
    b. Divorced
    c. Married
    d. Widowed
    e. Engaged

5. George's wife tried to convince him:
M-S a. Wear a life vest
    b. Not to walk over the falls on a tightrope
    c. Practice more for the stunt
    d. Wear a helmet
    e. Not to row across the falls

6. The crowd consisted of almost:
D-S **a. 1,000 people**
    b. 2,000 people
    c. 5,000 people
    d. 500 people
    e. 5,000 people

7. Going across the falls took George:
D-I **a. Twenty minutes**
    b. Thirty minutes
    c. Ten minutes
    d. Five minutes
    e. Forty-five minutes

8. After going across the falls, George was:
D-S a. Greeted by the crowd
    b. Interviewed by a television reporter
    c. Arrested by the police
    d. Yelled at by his wife
    e. Interviewed by a newspaper reporter

9. George forgot to make arrangements for:
D-I a. His family
    b. The celebration
    c. The media interview
    d. Medical support
    e. His car

10. By walking across the falls, George wanted to:
M-I a. Win a bet
    b. Earn money
    c. Gain fame
    d. Feel good about himself
    e. Prove his courage

Story 12: Sandwich

1. Sam traveled by:
D-S   a. Bicycle
       b. Subway
       c. Bus
       d. Car
       e. Motorcycle

2. The story took place:
D-S   a. In a mall
       b. Downtown
       c. At a high school
       d. In the summer
       e. In the fall

3. After running his errands, Sam went to:
M-S   **a. Eat lunch**
       b. Meet with students
       c. A bus stop
       d. His office
       e. Meet his wife

4. Sam was:
D-I   a. Recently married
       b. Young
       c. Divorced
       d. Middle-aged
       e. Old

5. Sam wanted to eat at a restaurant that was:
D-I   **a. Quiet**
       b. Cheap
       c. Quick
       d. Nearby
       e. Familiar

6. Sam went into a restaurant that:
M-I   a. Was crowded with teenagers
       b. Had a sign in the window
       c. Was close to his office
       d. He ate at regularly
       e. Had a senior discount

7. Sam ordered a:
M-S   a. Grilled cheese sandwich
       b. Goat sandwich
       c. Rabbit sandwich
       d. Buffalo sandwich
       e. Turkey sandwich

8. When Sam placed his order, the waitress:
D-I   a. Suggested something else
       b. Was shocked by it
       c. Put it in right away
       d. Wrote it down wrong
       e. Asked the cook about it

9. Sam tried to order a sandwich that would:
M-I   a. Taste good
       b. Arrive very quickly
       c. Prove the sign wrong
       d. Be healthy
       e. Be inexpensive

10. The price of the sandwich was:
D-S   a. $1.49
       b. $.99
       c. $2.99
       d. $1.99
       e. $2.09

APHASIOLOGY, 2004, *18* (5/6/7), 521–542

Using resource allocation theory and dual-task methods to increase the sensitivity of assessment in aphasia

Malcolm R. McNeil, Patrick J. Doyle, William D. Hula, and Hillel J. Rubinsky

VA Pittsburgh Healthcare System Geriatric Research Education & Clinical Center and University of Pittsburgh, PA, USA

Tepanta R. D. Fossett

University of Pittsburgh, PA, USA

Christine T. Matthews

VA Pittsburgh Healthcare System Geriatric Research Education & Clinical Center and University of Pittsburgh, PA, USA

Background: Quantifying the severity of language impairment and measuring change in language performance over time are two important objectives in the assessment of aphasia. The notion of cognitive effort as understood from a resource allocation perspective provides a potentially useful complement to traditional constructs employed in aphasia assessment.
Aims: The series of experiments described in this paper used resource allocation theory and dual-task methodology (1) to assess whether a language comprehension task (Story Retell Procedure) and a visual-manual tracking task trade performance under dual-task conditions, and (2) to investigate the potential utility of these methods in clinical assessment of aphasia. In Experiment 1, the validity of a difficulty manipulation of the SRP was investigated. In Experiments 2 and 3, the reliability and validity of the visual-manual tracking task were evaluated. Experiment 4 investigated whether the two tasks trade performance under dual-task conditions.
Methods & Procedures: In Experiment 1, 20 normal participants listened to and retold stories presented by a normal speaker and speakers with mild, moderate, and severe aphasia. Participants' comprehension performance was measured by calculating the amount of information retold per unit time. In Experiment 2, root mean square (RMS) tracking error data were collected under fixed joystick displacement conditions. In Experiment 3, 20 normal participants performed single-task tracking across 12 trials at each of three difficulty levels, and performance was evaluated in terms of RMS error. In Experiment 4, three groups of 20 normal individuals performed the tracking task while listening to stories told by the normal speaker and speakers with aphasia. Story retell performance was evaluated between subjects across three tracking difficulty levels and tracking performance was evaluated within subjects across story difficulty (normal, mild, moderate, and severe aphasia).
Outcomes & Results: The results of Experiments 1–3 supported the reliability and validity of the difficulty manipulations for the story retell and tracking tasks. In Experiment 4, tracking performance was found to vary significantly across story difficulty, with subjects demonstrating better tracking performance while listening to stories told by a mildly aphasic

---

Address correspondence to: Malcolm R. McNeil, Professor and Chair, Department of Communication Science & Disorders, University of Pittsburgh, 4033 Forbes Tower, Pittsburgh, PA 15260, USA. Email: mcneil@csd.pitt.edu

---

© 2004 by Taylor & Francis.
http://www.tandf.co.uk/journals/pp/02687038.html
DOI: 10.1080/02687030444000138

speaker than during stories told by a speaker with moderate aphasia. There was no effect of tracking difficulty on story comprehension as measured by subsequent story retell performance.

Conclusions: The results provide qualified support for both a resource allocation view of language performance in normal individuals and the potential utility of these methods in the assessment of aphasia. These conclusions, however, are mitigated by the finding of only a unidirectional (as opposed to bidirectional) performance trade, and by the fact that the effect of story difficulty on tracking performance was observed across only two levels of aphasia severity.

One of the significant challenges of clinical aphasiology is the task of measuring severity of deficits and change in the language performance of persons with aphasia in terms that are meaningful to them and to their communication partners. Measures that do this typically include the assessment of spoken language as one component. Language samples are typically obtained through such procedures as stimulus repetition (Porch, 1981), picture description tasks (Kertesz, 1982), personal and procedural narratives (Nicholas & Brookshire, 1993), structured interviews (Goodglass, Kaplan, & Barresi, 2001), retelling of fables (Rochon, Saffran, Berndt, & Schwartz, 2003; Saffran, Berndt, & Schwartz, 2003), video narration (Dollaghan, Campbell, & Tomlin, 1990), and discourse simulations (Doyle, Thompson, Oleyar, Wambaugh, & Jackson, 1994). Performance is quantified in a variety of ways; including behaviour counts (Nicholas & Brookshire, 1993, 1995), rating scales (Goodglass et al., 2001), questionnaires (Sarno, 1969), and multidimensional scoring systems (Holland, 1980; Porch, 1981). The nature and severity of the spoken language deficit is judged based on these pre-determined behaviours. As part of these judgements each of the pre-selected behaviours is either assumed to be of equal importance and summed to form a frequency of error type, or is assigned a weight or value as in multidimensional rating scales. The untested assumptions about the individual contributions of error types threaten the interpretation of test results, because of their unknown impact on such constructs as information transfer, overall communication handicap, and the burden placed on communication partners of individuals with aphasia.

Some assessment instruments seek to measure communication handicap by having clinicians or communication partners rate the burden placed on communication partners (Goodglass et al., 2001), compare the pre- and post-morbid ability of the person with aphasia to perform in certain communication situations (Lomas, Pickard, Bester, Elbard, Finlayson, & Zoghaib, 1989), or rate the amount of assistance required by the person with aphasia to accomplish certain tasks (Frattali, Thompson, Holland, Wohl, & Ferketic, 1995).

An alternative way of approaching this measurement problem is to attempt to quantify more directly the effort expended by interlocutors when they communicate with persons with aphasia. Such a procedure would be particularly useful for demonstrating and quantifying change in the level of communication handicap experienced by speakers with aphasia in instances where traditional measures of such constructs as auditory comprehension or information transfer are insensitive. These traditional measures may be insensitive for a variety of reasons. All people, including partners of individuals with aphasia, bring to the task of communication a variety of strengths, weaknesses, and strategies. Such factors as hearing loss, familiarity with a given person's speech, and motivation conspire to affect information transfer in multifarious ways, make tenuous the assumption that treatment of aphasic language impairment will benefit all of the patient's interlocutors to the same extent. A procedure that would allow reliable measurement of the effort expended by communication partners, in addition to information transfer, would have the added benefit of taking into consideration the strengths, weaknesses, and strategies emerging from the communication dyad tested. It might also prove more sensitive to severity differences among patients and more responsive to change in either member of the dyad.

The resource allocation view of attention (Hirst & Kalmar, 1987; Kahneman, 1973; McNeil, Odell, & Tseng, 1991; Navon & Gopher, 1979) provides one of the more enduring and useful frameworks for approaching effort as a psychological construct. Within resource allocation models, the terms attention, processing resources, capacity, and cognitive effort are used interchangeably to refer to a source of fuel or activation for cognitive operations that can be flexibly allocated within and among processing domains. Kahneman (1973), in his early, influential formulation of the theory, proposed that attention (or effort) is limited in capacity and that its availability and allocation are influenced by a variety of factors including arousal, momentary and enduring disposi-tions, goals, priorities, and evaluation of task demands. The various resource allocation models differ in many respects, most notably on the issue of whether there is a single, undifferentiated reservoir of attentional resources (Kahneman, 1973) or whether there are multiple pools that are more or less dedicated to specific processes or domains (Gopher, Brickner, & Navon, 1982; Navon & Gopher, 1979, 1980; Wickens, 1984). The feature that they all share, however, is the notion of attention as a capacity that can be distributed among cognitive processes in a graded fashion.

Most studies supporting or employing resource allocation models have been dual-task experiments in which decrements in the performance of one task have been taken as an indicator of processing load incurred by a second, concurrently performed task (Arvedson & McNeil, 1987; Brown, 1978; Campbell & McNeil, 1985; Erickson, Goldinger, & LaPointe, 1996; Gopher et al., 1982; Granier, Robin, Shapiro, Peach, & Zimba, 2000; Hirst & Kalmar, 1987; McLeod, 1977; Murray, 2000; Murray, Holland, & Beeson, 1997a, 1997b, 1998; Navon, 1990; Payne, Peters, Birkmire, Bonto, Anastasi, & Wenger, 1994; Slansky & McNeil, 1997; Tseng, McNeil, & Milenkovic, 1993; Wickens, 1976, 1986). Dual-task experiments can be grouped into three broad categories, depending on the specific methods involved. The simplest method, single-to-dual task comparison, requires that the task(s) of interest be performed in isolation and concurrently with a secondary task. Performance decrements should be observed in the dual-task condition and when they are, sharing of a limited-capacity resource is typically inferred. This subtraction method has been productively employed in investigations of language pro-cessing in aphasia (Erickson et al., 1996; Murray, 2000; Murray et al., 1997a, 1997b, 1998), as well as of attention in general (Wickens, 1976), but it has substantial short-comings when used in isolation to provide evidence for resource sharing. Among these are the assumptions that concurrent task demands are linear and additive combinations of the separate single-task demands and that equal attentional capacity is available in both single and dual-task conditions (Navon & Gopher, 1979). According to Kahneman (1973), the quantity of resources a person has available may fluctuate from moment to moment according to factors that include task demands. If one proposes that a person might recruit additional resources in a more demanding dual-task condition than in a less demanding single-task condition, then inferring secondary task resource demands from primary task performance decrements is problematic at best. At the very least, a failure to observe decrements in the dual-task condition should not necessarily lead to the con-clusion that the two tasks do not share processing resources.

A second and even more problematic assumption of the single-to-dual-task com-parison method holds that the structures and processes recruited for single-task performance are the same as those recruited during dual-task conditions (Navon & Gopher, 1979). This assumption, which is similar to the one that underlies the subtraction method in functional imaging studies, holds that the set of structures and processes utilised in dual-task performance is equivalent to the combination of the sets used in the performance of each task in isolation. It implicitly denies consideration of any qualitative changes in how the cognitive architecture is mobilised to complete the tasks concurrently versus in isolation. Primarily because of these two suspect assumptions, attempts to quantify effort or gather data supporting resource models of attention using only the single-to-dual-task subtraction method are problematic and unlikely to be successful.

A second dual-task procedure, the voluntary effort allocation method, avoids making the problematic assumptions discussed above by having subjects perform both tasks in all experimental conditions. In this method, subjects perform two concurrent tasks with explicit instructions to vary their allocation of effort between them according to the experimental condition (Arvedson & McNeil, 1987; Gopher et al., 1982; Matthews & Margetts, 1991; Navon, 1990; Slansky & McNeil, 1997; Wickens & Gopher, 1977). These instructions may take the form of allocation ratios stated as percentages of total effort, qualitative instructions to vary emphasis, or relative performance targets. For example, in one condition a subject may be instructed to give 75% effort to Task A and 25% to Task B, and then to give 50% effort to both tasks in another condition, and finally to give 25% effort to Task A and 75% to Task B. Changing allocation ratios in this way is intended to induce a trade-off between the two tasks, and performance on one may be plotted on coordinate axes against performance on the other, resulting in a performance operating characteristic or curve (POC). In theory, the POC describes the limits of joint performance on the two tasks, given the assumption that all available resources are allocated between the two tasks (Navon & Gopher, 1979).

While the voluntary effort allocation method represents an improvement over the single-to-dual-task subtraction method, it has been criticised by Navon (1984) on the grounds that observed performance trading between the two tasks may be the result of subject biases and attempts to please the experimenter by meeting performance expectations.

Given the limitations of the single-to-dual-task subtraction and voluntary effort allocation methods reviewed above, a third dual-task procedure has been described in the literature and used to investigate resource models of attention. This method is referred to here as the concurrent task difficulty manipulation method. In this procedure, subjects perform two concurrent tasks and the difficulty (or some other parameter) of each task is systematically and independently manipulated (Campbell & McNeil, 1985; Hirst & Kalmar, 1987; McLeod, 1977; Payne et al., 1994; Wickens, 1986; Wickens, Kramer, Vanasse, & Donchin, 1983). This method may be used in concert with the voluntary effort allocation method, in which case it assumes the same limitations, or it may be used exclusively with equal priority instructions. Assuming that the combined demand of the two tasks challenges the available supply of resources, and that these resources are shared, increasing the difficulty of one task should cause a performance decrement in both tasks. Of course the most interesting and useful effect is the effect of a Task A difficulty manipulation on the performance of Task B. Within a single resource model, this performance trade should be bidirectional, i.e., Task A manipulation should affect performance on Task B and vice versa (Kahneman, 1973). Within a multiple-resource model, a bidirectional effect will be observed only if the difficulty manipulations employed for both tasks affect resource pools utilised by both tasks (Navon & Gopher, 1979, 1980).

Within this theoretical framework, Doyle and McNeil (1998) developed the Resource Allocation Paradigms of Pittsburgh (RAPP). RAPP is a dual-task software environment designed to assess the relative processing resources (cognitive effort) utilized by individuals in processing and comprehending the spoken language of persons with varying competencies and performance levels, such as those with and without aphasia.

The current study had two primary goals, one theoretical and the other applied. First, it sought to investigate whether a resource view of attention could be productively used to describe the performance of non-brain-injured subjects in the domains of language and visual-manual tracking. Second, a method for quantifying the effort expended by normal listeners in comprehending stories told by speakers with varying degrees of aphasia was assessed. To this end, a story comprehension task and a visual-manual tracking task were employed in a dual-task procedure in which the difficulty of each task was independently manipulated. The investigation involved four experiments, each of which is described below. Experiments 1, 2, and 3 describe the rationale for the task choices, as well as experiments designed to validate their respective difficulty manipulations, and Experiment 4 details the methods and findings of the dual-task investigation, which used the two previously validated single tasks.

EXPERIMENT 1
VALIDATING DIFFERENT SEVERITY LEVELS IN APHASIC STORY RETELLS

The rationale for selecting auditory discourse comprehension as the language task of interest in this investigation was based on several factors. First, when people communicate in everyday life, they do so most often in multiple-sentence messages that occur within some context. Listening to and comprehending connected speech is a relatively continuous task that is a closer approximation to naturally occurring discourse than comprehending isolated sentences or words, and the latter may not be predictive of the former in some circumstances (Brookshire & Nicholas, 1997).

Second, overt motor responses are not required for auditory comprehension to proceed normally, as they are for performing language production tasks. This ability for task processing to occur without the need for overt on-line responses is desirable in designing a dual-task experiment because it minimises the opportunity for structural and computational, as opposed to capacity, interference (Kahneman, 1973; McNeil et al., 1991). This distinction, which is discussed in more detail below in Experiment 2, refers to dual-task performance decrements that occur when two tasks compete for physical structures or specific and dedicated mental computations, as opposed to those resulting from competition for shareable attention capacity. The choice of the auditory language comprehension and visual-manual tracking tasks was based on the assumption that they would eliminate structural and computational interference while allowing the opportunity to observe capacity interference.

The connected language comprehension stimuli selected for this study were the stories from the Discourse Comprehension Test (DCT: Brookshire & Nicholas, 1997). These stories are controlled for a number of important variables, including number of words, number of sentences, mean sentence length, number of subordinate clauses, number of T-units ("one main clause with all the subordinate clauses and nonclausal phrases attached to or embedded in it"; Paul, 2001, p. 514), ratio of clauses to T-units, listening difficulty, and number of unfamiliar words. Originally, an attempt was made to develop multiple-choice questions for each story as an off-line measure of information transfer that would be more sensitive than the yes-no questions published with the DCT, but preliminary findings indicated that they were psychometrically inadequate (McNeil & Doyle, unpublished data). An alternative procedure that requires subjects to provide verbal reproductions of the stories was then developed. In this Story Retell Procedure (SRP) (McNeil, Doyle, Fossett, Park, & Goda, 2001), the verbal reproductions are scored for information content and efficiency using the *percent information unit per minute* (%IU/Min) (McNeil, Doyle, Park, Fossett, & Brodsky, 2002) a metric derived from Nicholas and Brookshire's *correct information unit* (CIU) (Brookshire & Nicholas, 1997) for use specifically with these stimulus stories. It should be noted that the SRP uses not only the 10 stories comprising the DCT as originally published, but also the 2 practice stories, for a total of 12 stimulus stories.

The conceptual and psychometric development of the resulting instrument, the Story Retell Procedure (SRP) and its associated metric, the %IU/Min, has been described in a series of recent publications. Evidence has been presented to support the SRP's validity as a language sampling procedure and the linguistic equivalence of four alternate forms, comprising three stories each (Doyle et al., 2000). Further, the %IU/Min has been demonstrated to have acceptable alternate forms and inter-rater reliability (Hula, McNeil, Doyle, Rubinsky, & Fossett, 2003; McNeil et al., 2001), concurrent validity with traditional measures of both verbal production and auditory comprehension (McNeil et al., 2001), and the ability to discriminate between normal speakers and persons with aphasia with reasonable sensitivity (McNeil et al., 2002).

Experiment 1 was designed to establish the SRP as a language task whose difficulty could be manipulated by having the stimulus stories presented by speakers with a range of language impairment from none to severe aphasia. This modification of the SRP was accomplished by selecting three speakers with aphasia from the subject sample of a prior validation study (McNeil et al., 2001) to represent mild, moderate, and severe degrees of aphasia. The aphasia severity categorisations were based on their overall scores on the Porch Index of Communicative Ability (PICA: Porch, 1981) and Revised Token Test (RTT: McNeil & Prescott, 1978) and further validated perceptually by 20 normal listeners' direct magnitude estimation judgements (McNeil et al., 1999). The story retells produced by these speakers with aphasia, as well as readings of the original DCT stories by a normal speaker, were grouped into the four three-story forms that had previously shown psychometric equivalence (Doyle et al., 2000; McNeil et al., 2001). These story forms from these four speakers constituted the stimuli for the present experiment.

The specific objective of this experiment was to further validate the different difficulty levels of the stories that would serve as stimuli in the subsequent dual-task experiment. In other words, it was asked whether or not normal listeners demonstrate reduced story comprehension, as indexed by %IU/Min produced in retells of stories told by a normal speaker and speakers with aphasic language impairments of different severities.

Method

Participants. A total of 20 temporarily able-bodied subjects ranging in age from 42 to 74 years (mean = 55, SD = 10) participated in the study. All participants met the following selection criteria: Negative self-reported history of neurological, communication, or psychiatric disorders; age between 40 and 75 years, passing a pure tone hearing screening at 35 dB HL in one ear at .5, 1, 2, and 4 KHz; 20/80 vision or better measured with the reduced Snellen chart; performance above the 5th percentile for normal individuals on the Short Porch Index of Communicative Ability (SPICA: DiSimoni, Keith, & Darley, 1980) and the Revised Token Test (RTT) (McNeil & Prescott, 1978); performance at or above the 5th grade level on the reading subtest of the Wide Range Achievement Test-3 (Wilkinson, 1993); no greater than two points decline from the Immediate to the Delayed Story Recall Task from the Arizona Battery of Communication Disorders of Dementia) (ABCD: Bayles & Tomoeda, 1993); a minimum of 12 years of education. Subjects were recruited from the local community by means of fliers posted in public places, presentations to senior citizens' organisations, and by word of mouth. Subjects were paid $15 for their participation.

Procedure. The stimuli consisted of four different story forms, consisting of three stories each, which were produced by each of four different speakers: one normal speaker and three with varying degrees of aphasia. As described above, the speakers with aphasia were categorised as having mild, moderate, and severe aphasia according to standardised test scores and these rankings were validated by direct magnitude estimation (McNeil et al., 1999). Table 1 presents the clinical characteristics of the speakers with aphasia and Table 2 presents the average %IUs and %IU/Min present in the stories at each difficulty level. Each story form was quasi-randomly assigned such that no subject heard a given form more than once, and each subject heard one form produced by each of the four speakers. Following presentation of each story, subjects were instructed to immediately retell the story in their own words, following the standardised procedures of the SRP (McNeil et al., 2001). The resulting language samples were digitally recorded and later scored for %IU/Min, also using standardised procedures. An IU was defined as "... an identified word, phrase, or acceptable alter-

TABLE 1
Clinical characteristics of the speakers with aphasia who provided story retell stimuli for Experiments 1 and 4

Subject	Age	MPO	RTT %ile	RCPM	PICA OA %ile	PICA Verbal %ile
Mild	52	17	92	36	87	91
Moderate	55	30	63	32	75	71
Severe	71	94	5	22	43	37

TABLE 2
Information content and efficiency of stimulus stories in percent information units (%IU) and percent information units per minute (%IU/Min)

	%IU	%IU/Min
Normal	100	64
Mild aphasia	48	40
Moderate aphasia	23	11
Severe aphasia	13	8

native from the story stimulus that is intelligible and informative and that conveys accurate and relevant information about the story'' (McNeil et al., 2001, p. 994). To derive the %IU/Min score for each retell, the number of IUs was first tallied, and then divided by the number of IUs available in the original story (as published in the *DCT*), giving %IU.[1] This measure of information transfer was then divided by the number of minutes taken to produce the retell, giving %IU/Min, a metric of the efficiency of information transfer.

Results

A significant main effect [$F(3, 57) = 162.27$; $p < .01$] of story form was obtained using a single-factor repeated measures ANOVA. Post-hoc pair-wise comparisons using the Bonferroni adjustment showed significant differences between the mild, moderate, and severe story forms generated by the persons with aphasia, as well as between the normal, moderate, and severe story forms. No significant difference was found between the normal and mild aphasic story forms. The %IU/Min produced by each subject after listening to each of the story levels are presented in Table 3.

Discussion

Three levels of story difficulty were validated by this experiment. There was a significant difference between the mild, moderate, and severe story forms, as well as the normal, moderate, and severe story forms, according to the %IU/Min measure of information transfer efficiency. As such, this experiment demonstrated that the difficulty of the SRP may be varied across three levels by presenting stimulus stories produced by speakers with differing severity of aphasic language impairment.

The lack of a significant difference between the normal and mild story forms may be attributable to the fact that the mildly aphasic story productions were not very impaired in terms of grammar and organisation. Consider data taken from an earlier study on the SRP (Doyle et al., 2000) in which these speakers with aphasia served as subjects: 96% of the clauses in the mild stories were produced correctly, compared to 100%, 77%, and 75% for the normal, moderate, and severe stories, respectively. Also, the mild stories contained only 3.6 mazes per minute—words or partial words that are unintelligible in a known context (e.g., He went to the "frangus"), nonword fillers (e.g., um, er, uh), repetitions, revisions, and word fragments—compared to 0, 6.8, and 10.7 mazes per minute for the normal, moderate, and severe stories.

---

[1] The story retell data were also analysed by calculating %IU/Min relative to the number of information units available in the different stimulus stories produced by the speakers with different severity levels of aphasia (and the normal speaker). These analyses resulted in a different rank ordering of performance across conditions with subjects scoring more relative %IU/Min in the Moderate and Severe conditions. This occurred because, when subjects were presented with less information, they were able to recall a greater proportion of it. In some cases subjects' retells even contained more information than was in the aphasic-produced stimulus story because of their ability to fill in omitted information from context. We elected not to pursue these analyses because they produced unpredictable patterns of results that were unlikely to assist in the interpretation of data from the subsequent dual-task experiment (Experiment 4). This speculation was subsequently borne out, as the re-ordering of the story difficulty conditions along the lines of this relative %IU/Min analysis would not have helped to clarify the effects of story difficulty on tracking performance, and would not have changed the nonsignificant effect of tracking difficulty on story retell performance.

TABLE 3
%IU/Min produced by individual subjects at each
story difficulty level in Experiment 1

Subject	Normal	Mild aphasia	Moderate aphasia	Severe aphasia
1	51.7	47.6	35.1	15.5
2	50.3	44.2	25.5	16.7
3	42.1	50.9	25.0	11.3
4	57.8	50.1	36.7	12.2
5	66.4	53.4	40.8	27.6
6	52.1	59.9	32.6	18.2
7	43.0	55.7	38.0	18.6
8	61.0	65.8	41.3	11.9
9	46.1	39.8	27.4	14.3
10	50.6	50.5	39.4	14.7
11	44.9	54.4	36.7	17.8
12	32.2	49.7	36.5	9.9
13	51.5	50.5	39.8	13.4
14	41.9	38.9	26.3	19.0
15	49.2	48.8	36.5	24.1
16	42.0	40.0	22.7	17.6
17	63.2	43.7	43.1	19.8
18	53.2	54.3	33.0	19.9
19	52.2	45.5	23.8	15.3
20	51.4	41.9	33.7	20.7
Mean	50.14	49.28	33.70	16.93
SD	8.12	6.94	6.40	4.38

EXPERIMENTS 2 AND 3:
RELIABILITY OF A VISUAL-MANUAL TRACKING TASK

The literature on attention and motor control contains many dual-task studies in which visual-manual tracking has been used to induce or measure processing load in a variety of concurrent tasks, including non-verbal auditory discrimination (Backs, 1997; McLeod, 1977; Wickens, 1976), auditory verbal memory search, (Payne et al., 1994), typing (Gopher et al., 1982), mathematical reasoning (McLeod, 1977; Payne et al., 1994), speech production (Lively, Pisoni, Van Summers, & Bernacki, 1993), and auditory sentence processing (Granier et al., 2000). Visual-manual tracking was chosen as a concurrent task in the present dual-task investigation for multiple reasons. First, the continuous nature of the task makes it suitable for inducing and measuring processing load in a task requiring auditory comprehension of connected speech such as the SRP. More discrete concurrent tasks, such as visual lexical decision or form discrimination, could potentially invite subjects to allocate resources exclusively to the auditory comprehension task during inter-stimulus intervals, and to only periodically share capacity between the tasks (McLeod, 1977).

Second, visual-manual tracking has previously been shown to trade performance, and thus presumably share resources with auditory language tasks. Granier and colleagues (2000) found differences in tracking performance associated with the time course of sentence processing, with subjects demonstrating poorer tracking performance during the beginning and the end of subject-verb-object sentences than during the middle, and performance that was poorer still during post-sentence processing and answering yes-no comprehension questions. They concluded that visual-manual tracking was sensitive to the cognitive load imposed not only by off-line sentence comprehension processes, but also to demands incurred by (presumably) less automatic and more integrative on-line processes. Payne and colleagues (1994) demonstrated a performance trade between an unstable manual tracking task and an auditory Sternberg task, which required subjects to recognise spoken words from target lists of varying sizes. Subjects demonstrated less accurate and slower responses to the verbal memory search task as tracking difficulty was increased. The same study also showed an effect of Sternberg task difficulty on tracking performance, but, interestingly, the effect was in an unexpected direction, with tracking error decreasing as memory set size increased from 2 to 4.

Third, visual-manual tracking was selected as a concurrent task because it avoids structural interference when the distinction is drawn between structural and capacity interference in explaining dual-task performance decrements. According to Kahneman (1973), structural interference is a more peripheral phenomenon that results when two tasks compete for the same perceptual or effector organs. McNeil et al. (1991) further suggested that computational interference, as distinct from both structural and capacity interference, may result from competition between two tasks for the same mental representations, processing stages, or other cognitive machinery. Capacity interference, on the other hand, involves competition for resources that can be allocated flexibly between two tasks that employ independent structures and computations. When capacity interference occurs, performance changes are related to task difficulty and the intensive aspect of attention demand, rather the structural requirements. Navon and Gopher (1979) have discussed similar distinctions as *concurrence cost* versus *resource cost*. In their formulation, concurrence cost encompasses not only Kahneman's (1973) notion of structural interference, but also the state of affairs in which concurrent tasks create conditions detrimental for one another, such as increased demand on mechanisms that organise, schedule, and coordinate dual-task performance. They also pointed out that, in practice, many concurrent task pairs will present some combination of central capacity interference and non-central structural or computational interference when the terms are defined as above.

The goal of Experiments 2 and 3 was to demonstrate the reliability and validity of the motor tracking task in the RAPP software for the purposes of demonstrating performance trading in subsequent dual-task investigations. The objective of Experiment 2 was to demonstrate that the software produces target waveforms of equivalent difficulty across tracking trials. The objectives of Experiment 3 were (1) to demonstrate that three a priori chosen levels of difficulty produce reliable differences in tracking performance; (2) to describe performance changes across repeated trials for the purpose of determining how much single-task practice to give subjects in a subsequent dual-task study in order to minimise performance changes in that study due to practice and learning; and (3) to determine the reliability of tracking performance measures across repeated trials.

EXPERIMENT 2
TARGET WAVEFORM RELIABILITY UNDER FIXED DISPLACEMENT CONDITIONS

Method

Procedure. The RAPP software displays an uneven line that scrolls across the computer screen from left to right, with a circle and crosshairs whose position is controlled manually by a joystick. For the current set of experiments, the software was installed on a Dell Latitude computer with a 366 MHz processor and 128K RAM. The joystick was a Saitek Cyborg.

The target waveform is composed of a sequence of waveform segments, or wavelets, chosen from a pre-generated set of 1000 segments. Each wavelet is defined by five points or vertices, which describe the amplitude of the waveform. The points have been calculated so that each of the 1000 wavelets has the same mean and standard deviation amplitude. The starting set of vertices for each run was randomly chosen from the set of predefined wavelets. The amplitude of the displayed waveform can be adjusted from 100% to 10% in 10% steps. Two factors control the rate at which the waveform moves horizontally across the screen, the speed at which the waveform scrolls across the screen and the horizontal distance between the vertices. For the current experiments, a constant scroll speed of 15 twips[2] per ms was utilised, the waveform amplitude was set to 100%, and the distance between points was adjusted to give 10, 20, or 50 vertices per minute in the Easy, Moderate, and Hard tracking conditions. Figure 1 provides a visual example of the target waveforms produced at each of the three difficulty levels.

In order to confirm that the software produces target waveforms of consistent difficulty at each of three pre-selected difficulty levels, tracking error data were collected by generating a series of waveforms and fixing the value of the crosshair position at

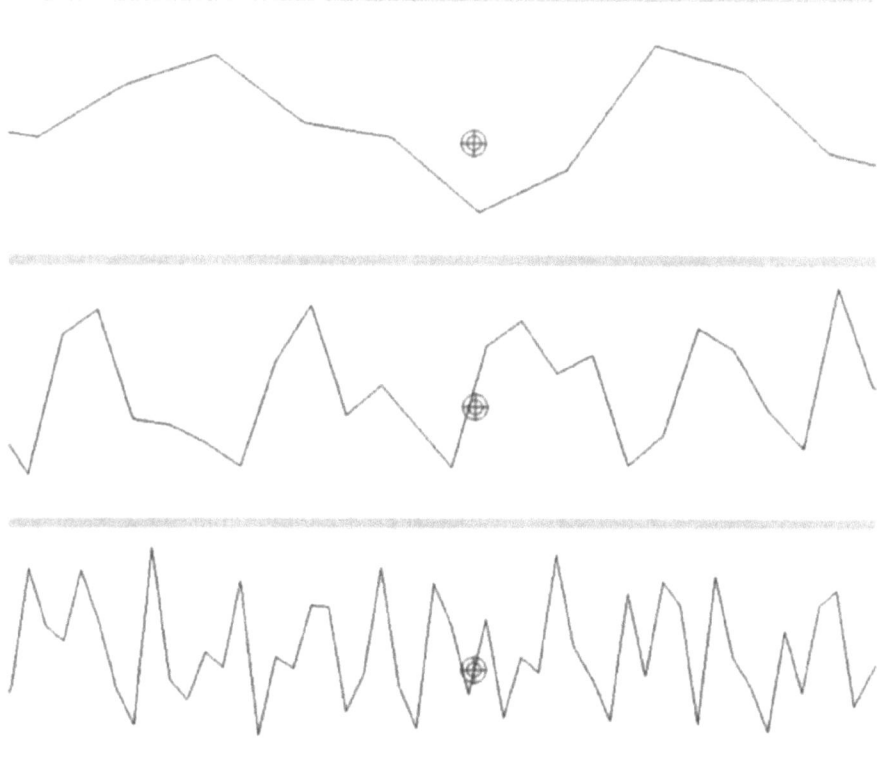

Figure 1. Examples of the target waveform for the RAPP visual-manual tracking task at the Easy, Moderate, and Hard difficulty levels.

---

[2] A twip is a standardised pixel, defined as 1/1140th of a logical inch.

maximum forward displacement. The waveform trials were equal in length and number to the trials that were administered to subjects in a subsequent dual-task experiment in which the manual tracking task was paired with a story listening and retelling task. Four groups of three trials were collected for each of 20 hypothetical subjects at each of the three difficulty levels. Individual trials were approximately 90 seconds in length.

Analysis.   RMS tracking error was calculated for each tracking trial using the following formula, where T_i is the position of the target waveform for a given sample i, and x_i is crosshair position for the same sample, and n is the number of samples in a given trial:

$$RMS\ error = \sqrt{\left(\sum_i (T_i - x_i)^2\right) \div n}$$

Conceptually, RMS tracking error is roughly equivalent to the total area between the curves described by the target waveform and the subject's tracking response (Schmidt & Lee, 1999). It is a measure of total error that includes both bias (in terms of the current task, a tendency to respond consistently above or below the target) and variability in responding. The RMS tracking error values calculated for each tracking trial were averaged across three-trial sequences to yield four values for 20 subjects at each of the tracking difficulty levels. The means for three-trial blocks were examined because this was to be the unit of analysis of interest in the subsequent dual-task investigation.

Results and discussion

To address the question of waveform reliability independent of subject response, the tracking error values obtained from trials where the crosshair position was fixed at maximum displacement were entered into a 2-way ANOVA with a design analogous to the one to be used in the subsequent dual-task experiment: one four-level repeated factor of trial block and one between-subjects factor of tracking difficulty level. Neither main effect [$F(3, 171) = 1.107$ for trial block; $F(2, 57) = .611$ for difficulty level, $p > .3$ for both] nor their interaction [$F(6, 171) = .432$, $p > .8$] was significant, supporting the assumptions that (1) the target waveform stimulus used in subsequent visual-manual tracking experiments is of consistent difficulty across trials, and (2) differences across tracking conditions can confidently be attributed to differences in subject performance, and not to stimulus variability. The overall mean tracking error with fixed maximum joystick displacement was 1892 twips and mean differences in tracking error across trial blocks and difficulty levels ranged from 0 to 4 twips.

The objective of this experiment was to investigate whether the target waveform produced by the RAPP software produces a visual-manual tracking task of equivalent difficulty across trials, independent of human response. This was done by examining the differences in tracking error across repeated trials with the crosshair position fixed at its maximum displacement. This particular analysis revealed no differences across repeated trials in terms of RMS or variable tracking error, supporting the contention that target waveforms are of equivalent difficulty across trials of lengths equivalent to those used in the subsequent dual-task experiment.

EXPERIMENT 3
TRACKING PERFORMANCE ACROSS DIFFICULTY LEVELS AND TRIALS

Method

Subjects.   A total of 20 participants (13 women, 7 men) between the ages of 40 and 74 (mean = 51, SD = 15) who met the same selection criteria as used in Experiment 1 took part in this experiment. Subjects were recruited by the same methods and were reimbursed $15 for their participation.

Procedure.   Informed consent and screening measures were administered in a 60-minute session. In a second 120-minute session, conducted within a week of the first, 36 two-minute single-task tracking trials (12 each at the easy, moderate, hard tracking difficulty levels) were presented. The order of the 36 tracking trials was determined such that each sequence of three tracking trials contained one trial at each difficulty level in pseudorandom order. This was accomplished by randomly selecting without replacement from the six possible orderings of the three difficulty levels in six cycles. The time between tracking trials was approximately 30 seconds, and subjects were given a 5-minute rest after trial 12 and again after trial 24; or, stated differently, after the 4th and 8th trials had been completed for each of the three difficulty levels. Subjects were instructed to use the joystick with their dominant hand to keep the crosshairs as close to the line as possible at all times, and they were discouraged from resting their wrist on the table as they tracked.

Analysis.   RMS tracking error was calculated for each 2-minute tracking trial.

Results

To address the questions of the validity of the difficulty levels and performance across repeated trials by human subjects, the RMS error values for each 2-minute tracking trial were entered into an ANOVA with two repeated factors: Difficulty (3 levels) and trial (12 levels). Because the data violated the sphericity assumption, the Huynh-Feldt correction for degrees of freedom was used. The analysis revealed a significant main effect of difficulty [$F(1.15, 21.87) = 602.19, p < .001$] and trial [$F(7.41, 140.82) = 42.53, p < .001$], as well as a significant interaction [$F(12.66, 240.45) = 5.052, p < .001$]. Given the presence of the interaction, post hoc analysis was carried out using the Bonferroni correction for multiple comparisons ($\alpha = .05$) to test for simple main effects of difficulty at each trial and of trial at each difficulty level. Inspection of Figure 2 reveals large differences in tracking error across difficulty levels, with all three pairwise comparisons demonstrating statistical significance at all levels of the trial factor. Analysis of the effect of trial at the hard tracking level revealed that trial 6 was the earliest trial that did not differ reliably from any of the subsequent six trials at that level, with performance at trials 1–5 all being significantly worse than at trial 9. For the moderate and easy tracking levels, trial 5 was the earliest trial that did not differ significantly from any of the seven subsequent trials at each of those levels, again demonstrating more error on trials 1–4 than on trial 9.

The standard error of measurement was also calculated for three-trial blocks within each difficulty level, using trials 7–12 at each level. Three-trial block means were used in this calculation because this was to be the unit of analysis in a subsequent dual-task experiment. The results of this analysis are presented in Table 4.

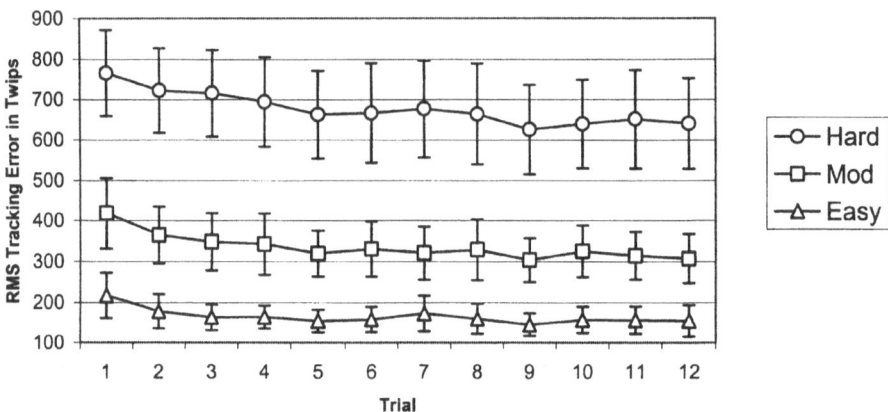

Figure 2. RMS tracking error across the 12 trials at each of the three difficulty levels in Experiment 2. Error bars indicate +/− 1 SD.

TABLE 4
Standard error of measurement for RMS tracking
error in twips in single-task three-trial blocks

	Hard	Moderate	Easy
SEM	22.6	16.3	11.5

Discussion

The first objective of this experiment was to confirm that three levels of difficulty chosen for the tracking task do indeed result in differences in tracking performance. Analysis of tracking error data provided by human trackers showed large and reliable differences across the three difficulty levels chosen for this investigation. This suggests that these levels of the tracking task represent a potentially appropriate difficulty manipulation for induction of performance trade-offs in a concurrently performed task.

The second objective was to determine the amount of practice with this particular task that should be given to subjects preceding a subsequent dual-task experiment in order to minimise performance changes across dual-task conditions due to practice and learning. To accomplish this, mean performance for each trial at each difficulty level, beginning with trial 1, was compared to subsequent trials at that difficulty level until the first trial that did not differ significantly from any subsequent trials was found. This criterion was chosen because it was hypothesised that performance improvements that might not be detectable by comparing adjacent trials might, however, become apparent across a number of trials. For the hard tracking level, the first trial that met this condition was trial 6. For both the moderate and easy levels, trial 5 was the first that did not differ from subsequent trials. Thus, it was concluded that four or five single-task practice trials should be sufficient to minimise learning effects in subsequent dual-task studies with these specific tracking difficulty levels.

It is worth noting that at each difficulty level, the best average performance was obtained on trial 9 (equivalent to trials 25–27 of 36 across all conditions), and indeed in the comparisons described above, trial 9 was the only subsequent trial found to be significantly different from trial 6 for the hard condition and trial 5 for the easy and moderate conditions. A similar trend was noted for subjects to perform better on trial 5 at each level (trials 13–15 overall) than on the trials immediately preceding or following them.

We attribute these performance patterns to the fact that subjects were given a full 5-minute rest immediately prior to trials 13 and 25 of the total 36 trials. In the motor learning literature this recovery of performance following a rest period is known as the reminiscence effect. This effect has been attributed to the distinction between massed practice, where the rest time between trials is less than the time spent practising on each trial, and distributed practice, in which the rest between trials is longer than the practice trials themselves (Schmidt & Lee, 1999). In their review, Schmidt and Lee suggest that subjects receiving massed practice on pursuit rotor tasks perform worse during practice than subjects receiving distributed practice, and demonstrate less learning on retention tests.

The final objective of this study was to describe the reliability of the RMS tracking error dependent variable in terms of its standard error of measurement. It is notable that the between-subjects variability on this motor tracking task, as displayed by the standard deviation error bars in Figure 2, is large relative to the SEM values and also relative to the mean trial-to-trial differences in performance. This suggests that performance differences between individuals may be large relative to performance differences attributable to experimental conditions, such as different amounts of practice or dual-task manipulations. For this reason, examination of within-subjects effects is likely to be the most appropriate when investigating hypotheses regarding the effects of dual-task processing load on performance of this task.

To summarise, Experiments 2 and 3 provided support for the following conclusions: the RAPP tracking software produces a target waveform of consistent difficulty across repeated trials at a given difficulty level; the three a priori chosen levels of task difficulty studied here result in reliable differences in performance; and performance improvement due to practice in a single session will be negligible after four to five trials at each of the three difficulty levels.

EXPERIMENT 4
DUAL-TASK COST SHARING

Experiment 1 provided support for the validity of the difficulty manipulation of the SRP, and Experiments 2 and 3 demonstrated the reliability of the target waveform in the visual-manual tracking task and its differential difficulty manipulations. Experiment 3 investigated whether these two tasks demonstrate cost sharing under dual-task conditions. It was hypothesised that by independently manipulating the difficulty of these two concurrent tasks, a performance trade could be demonstrated, such that increasing the difficulty of one task would result in a performance decrement in the other. Such a finding would be consistent with the view that these computations share limited attentional resources and would also suggest that this dual-task procedure could be used to index the spoken language handicap in aphasia by quantifying, not only information transfer, but also the amount of effort expended by communication partners of aphasic persons in comprehending their connected spoken language.

Method

Participants.   A total of 60 healthy individuals (44 females, 16 males) aged between 40 and 75 years (mean = 58, SD = 10) who were recruited by the same methods and met the same selection criteria as those used in Experiment 1, served as participants. None of the individuals participating in Experiment 4 had taken part in any prior studies of the SRP. Each participant was paid $50 for completing the study.

Procedure.   The dual-task procedure involved simultaneous presentation of the SRP and visual-motor tracking tasks described above using the RAPP software program.

To minimise practice effects on tracking performance, immediately preceding the dual-task procedure, subjects performed 12 two-minute single-task tracking trials, four at each of the three tracking difficulty levels used in Experiment 2. The order of presentation of tracking difficulty levels during the 12 single-task trials was determined such that each sequence of three trials contained one trial from each difficulty level in pseudorandom order, as was done in Experiment 3.

For the dual-task conditions, the 60 subjects were randomly assigned to the three tracking difficulty levels, producing three groups of 20 subjects each. Each group performed the tracking task at one of the three difficulty levels while listening to one story form (three stories) from each of the four story difficulty levels (normal speaker and speakers with mild, moderate, and severe aphasia). At the end of each story, the subjects stopped tracking and immediately retold the story in their own words. Subjects were instructed to do their best and to devote equal effort to both tasks. Their retellings were digitally recorded by the RAPP software and later scored off-line for %IUs/Min, using the methods described in Experiment 1.

Results

In order to evaluate concurrent performance costs, two two-way ANOVAs were computed, one each with RMS tracking error and %IUs/Min as the dependent variable. For both analyses, story severity was a within-groups factor and tracking difficulty was a between-groups factor.

For the analysis of tracking performance, the results showed a significant ($p < .05$) main effect for both tracking level [$F(2, 57) = 57.62$] and story level [$F(3, 171) = 3.52$] with no significant interaction [$F(6, 171) = 1.44$]. Post-hoc analyses for both main effects were carried out at $p < .05$ using the Bonferroni adjustment for multiple comparisons. As expected, tracking performance decreased significantly as tracking difficulty increased. The analysis of the effect of story difficulty level revealed significantly better tracking performance during the "Mild" compared to the "Moderate" stories across all three tracking levels. No other comparisons reached statistical significance. The dual-task tracking data are presented numerically by tracking and story level in Table 5, and they are presented graphically, averaged across tracking levels in Figure 3.

The effects of tracking and story difficulty on story retell performance are shown in Figure 4. The main effect for story level was significant [$F(3, 171) = 319.85$]. As in Experiment 1, story retell performance was significantly different ($p < .05$; using the Bonferroni adjustment for multiple comparisons) among the three aphasic story levels (i.e., performance decreased as story difficulty increased) but not between the "Normal" and "Mild" story forms. Neither tracking difficulty level [$F(2, 57) = 1.631$], nor the interaction between story and tracking difficulty levels [$F(6, 171) = 1.226$] resulted in statistically significant changes in %IUs/Min story retell performance.

TABLE 5
Means, standard deviations, and standard errors of the mean for dual-task RMS
tracking error in twips*

Story level	Easy			Moderate			Hard		
	Mean	SD	SE	Mean	SD	SE	Mean	SD	SE
Normal	158	43	10	333	165	37	547	128	29
Mild aphasia	153	48	11	313	152	34	540	130	29
Moderate aphasia	156	43	10	333	132	30	566	137	31
Severe aphasia	149	40	9	336	174	39	556	121	27

*A twip is a standardised pixel, defined as 1/1140th of a logical inch.

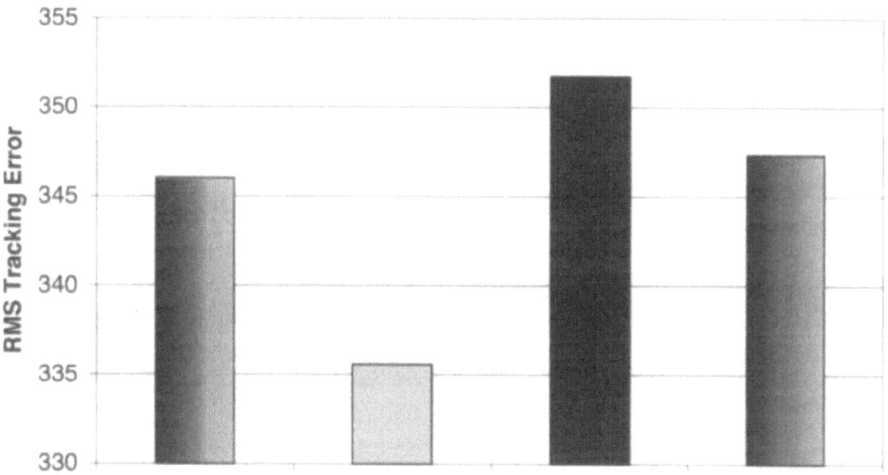

Story Level

Figure 3. Dual-task tracking performance by story difficulty level, averaged across tracking difficulty levels. As indicated by the shading in the bars, RMS tracking error was significantly greater in the Moderate Aphasia than the Mild Aphasia condition ($p < .05$), and no other comparisons were significant.

Discussion

In this study, participants were required to simultaneously perform two tasks that were proposed to be computationally independent but which shared limited attentional resources under demanding conditions. It was hypothesised that a trade-off of these resources between the two tasks would affect performance on both tasks. As predicted, tracking performance was found to be significantly better under the "Mild" compared to the "Moderate" aphasic story retell condition. This finding provides qualified support for the validity of these dual tasks for augmenting the measurement of normal persons' comprehension of connected language in persons with aphasia, in addition to those captured by traditional measures of aphasic language performance. The performance

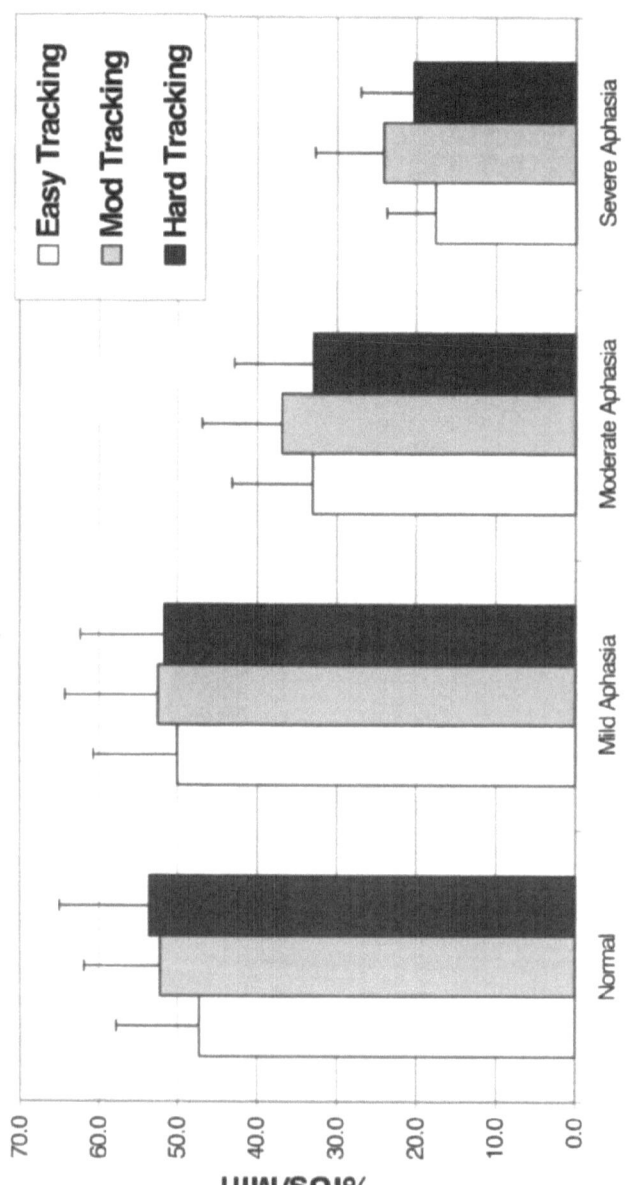

Figure 4. Dual-task story retell performance by story and tracking difficulty level.

interaction between these language comprehension and visual-manual tracking tasks also provides qualified support for resource allocation theory. Each of these qualified conclusions will be examined in turn.

The finding of a tracking performance decrement during stories told by a moderately aphasic speaker compared to stories told by a mildly aphasic speaker suggests that dual-task procedures may be used to index effort experienced by communication partners of individuals with aphasia. However, the tasks used in the present study appear to be inadequate for that purpose. First, an effect of story difficulty on tracking performance was demonstrated only across a limited severity range, from Mild aphasia to Moderate aphasia. The Normal and Severe aphasia story conditions did not show a differential effect on tracking, in spite of having resulted in significantly different %IUs/Min on retell compared to the Mild and Moderate stories. The reasons for this are not entirely clear. Perhaps, because of uncontrolled stimulus variables such as rate of presentation of new information and overall amount of information content, the attention demands of these particular story difficulty levels were not as disparate as originally presumed, based on the single-task %IUs/Min measure and normal listeners' DME judgements. For example, the Severe stimulus stories contained an average of 13% of the information units present in the Normal stories, and were delivered with an efficiency of 8%IU/Min. The overall reduced information content and the slow rate of delivery of information may have counteracted the effects of the aphasic errors and diminished content in the stories, resulting in no net change in attention demand compared to the other stories. Given the fact that participants in Experiment 1 produced fewer %IU/Min in response to the Severe stories than in response to any of the other story levels, the above speculation suggests that, in the case of the SRP, single-task performance may not be a useful measure of resource demand as indexed by dual-task performance.

Second, and more importantly, it is apparent that the dual-task procedures employed in this study will not be clinically useful because of the small effect size of aphasia severity on tracking performance. While the effect was statistically reliable, with 44 of 60 subjects demonstrating performance differences in the predicted direction, the average differences in RMS tracking error were only 26, 20, and 2 twips, respectively at the Hard, Moderate, and Easy tracking levels. These differences amount to slightly more than one standard error of measurement, as determined in Experiment 2, at the Hard and Moderate tracking levels, and considerably less than one SEM at the Easy level. A much larger effect size would be necessary in order for these methods to be clinically useful, especially on an individual basis.

The conclusions that can be drawn from the present investigation regarding resource allocation theory and the role of attention and effort in language processing, while somewhat more positive than the clinical implications of our methods, are still mitigated by the finding of a unidirectional performance trade. Although an effect of story difficulty (aphasia severity) on tracking performance was found, there was no effect of tracking difficulty on story retell performance, as most versions of resource allocation theory might predict (McNeil et al., 1991; Murray, 1999). Both methodological and theoretical factors may have contributed to this negative finding. One relevant feature of the method was the fact that SRP performance was measured off-line and, as such, may have been subject to a variety of strategies not related to on-line story comprehension during concurrent performance of the tracking task. It is also possible that the tracking task provided a more fine-grained index of the resource demand than the SRP task (D. Swinney, personal communication, 2003). The redundancy of connected language might have made it possible for subjects to divert attention away from the SRP task for brief periods while maintaining performance, while the tracking task may have required a more constant investment of resources in order to minimise error.

From a theoretical perspective, the finding of a unidirectional performance trade could result from concurrent performance of two tasks that share partially overlapping sets of resource pools (Navon & Gopher, 1980). The tracking difficulty manipulation may not have challenged the shared pools, while the story difficulty manipulation did. For example, the two tasks might share a resource pool subserving perceptual computations and it might be that it was this particular pool from which the story manipulation recruited additional resources. On the other hand, the tracking difficulty manipulation may have affected a motor-specific pool not utilised by the story comprehension task. Indeed, prior dual-task studies using event-related potential methods have shown that manipulating the frequency of the target waveform in a visual-manual tracking task degrades performance without placing additional load on perceptual and central processing, as measured by P300 amplitude elicited by an oddball secondary task (Backs, 1997; Isreal, Chesney, Wickens, & Donchin, 1980). This speculation could be investigated by introducing new difficulty manipulations into the tracking task, such as order of control, that place greater load on perceptual or central processes (Backs, 1997; Sirevaag, Kramer, Coles, & Donchin, 1989; Wickens et al., 1983).

Another potential theoretical explanation for this finding may be that the tracking levels selected for this study were not "attention-demanding" enough to interfere with story listening and retell. Subjects may have benefited from spatial and/or temporal prediction (Rosenbaum, 1980; Schmidt & Gordan, 1977) created by being able to view the upcoming wave. It is also possible that providing subjects with 12 single-task practice trials prior to the dual-task condition may have led to some automaticity (Brown, 1998; Brown & Carr, 1989) and too few resource demands in the subsequent tracking task. To test the first two alternative explanations, new studies are planned which will increase tracking task difficulty and use a smaller viewing window to reduce tracking-wave predictability (and presumably increase attentional demands).

REFERENCES

Arvedson, J. C., & McNeil, M. R. (1987). Accuracy and response times for semantic judgments and lexical decisions with left and right hemisphere lesions. *Clinical Aphasiology*, *17*, 188–200.

Backs, R. W. (1997). Psychophysiological aspects of selective and divided attention during continuous manual tracking. *Acta Psychologica*, *96*, 167–191.

Bayles, K. A., & Tomoeda, C. K. (1993). *Arizona Battery for Communication Disorders of Dementia*. Tucson, AZ: Canyonlands Publishing, Inc.

Brookshire, R. H., & Nicholas, L. E. (1997). *Discourse comprehension test* (2nd ed.). Minneapolis, MN: BRK Publishers.

Brown, I. D. (1978). Dual task methods of assessing workload. *Ergonomics*, *21*, 221–224.

Brown, S. W. (1998). Automaticity versus timesharing in timing and dual-task performance. *Psychological Research*, *61*, 71–81.

Brown, T. L., & Carr, T. H. (1989). Automaticity in skill acquisition: Mechanisms for reducing interference in concurrent performance. *Journal of Experimental Psychology: Human Perception and Performance*, *15*, 686–700.

Campbell, T. F., & McNeil, M. R. (1985). Effects of presentation rate and divided attention on auditory comprehension in children with acquired language disorder. *Journal of Speech and Hearing Research*, *28*, 513–520.

DiSimoni, F. G., Keith, R. L., & Darley, F. L. (1980). Prediction of PICA overall score by short versions of the test. *Journal of Speech and Hearing Research*, *23*, 511–516.

Dollaghan, C., Campbell, T. F., & Tomlin, R. (1990). Video narration as a language sampling context. *Journal of Speech and Hearing Disorders*, *55*, 582–590.

Doyle, P. J., & McNeil, M. R. (1998). *Quantifying spoken language handicap in aphasia.* Demonstration exhibit, First National Meeting of the VA Rehabilitation Research & Development Service, Washington, DC.

Doyle, P. J., McNeil, M. R., Spencer, K. A., Goda, A. J., Park, G., Lustig, A. et al. (2000). Linguistic validation of four parallel forms of a story retelling procedure. *Aphasiology, 14,* 537–549.

Doyle, P. J., Thompson, C. K., Oleyar, K. S., Wambaugh, J. L., & Jackson, A. V. (1994). The effects of setting variables on conversational discourse in normal and aphasic adults. *Clinical Aphasiology, 22,* 135–144.

Erickson, R. J., Goldinger, S. D., & LaPointe, L. L. (1996). Auditory vigilance in aphasic individuals: Detecting nonlinguistic stimuli with full or divided attention. *Brain and Cognition, 30,* 244–253.

Frattali, C. M., Thompson, C. K., Holland, A. L., Wohl, C. B., & Ferketic, M. M. (1995). *The American Speech-Language-Hearing Association functional assessment of communication skills for adults (ASHA FACS).* Rockville, MD: American Speech-Language Hearing Association.

Goodglass, H., Kaplan, E., & Barresi, B. (2001). *The assessment of aphasia and related disorders* (3rd ed.). Baltimore, MD: Lippincott, Williams, & Wilkins.

Gopher, D., Brickner, M., & Navon, D. (1982). Different difficulty manipulations interact differently with task emphasis: Evidence for multiple resources. *Journal of Experimental Psychology: Human Perception and Performance, 8,* 146–157.

Granier, J. P., Robin, D. A., Shapiro, L. P., Peach, R. K., & Zimba, L. D. (2000). Measuring processing load during sentence comprehension: Visuomotor tracking. *Aphasiology, 14,* 501–513.

Hirst, W., & Kalmar, D. (1987). Characterizing attentional resources. *Journal of Experimental Psychology: General, 116,* 63–81.

Holland, A. L. (1980). *Communicative abilities in daily living.* Baltimore: University Park Press.

Hula, W. D., McNeil, M. R., Doyle, P. J., Rubinsky, H. J., & Fossett, T. R. D. (2003). The inter-rater reliability of the Story Retell Procedure. *Aphasiology, 17,* 523–528.

Isreal, J. B., Chesney, G. L., Wickens, C. D., & Donchin, E. (1980). P300 and tracking difficulty: Evidence for multiple resources in dual-task performance. *Psychophysiology, 17,* 259–273.

Kahneman, D. (1973). *Attention and effort.* Englewood Cliffs, NJ: Prentice-Hall.

Kertesz, A. (1982). *Western Aphasia Battery.* New York: Grune & Stratton.

Lively, S. E., Pisoni, D. B., Van Summers, W., & Bernacki, R. H. (1993). Effects of cognitive workload on speech production: Acoustic analyses and perceptual consequences. *Journal of the Acoustical Society of America, 93,* 2962–2973.

Lomas, J., Pickard, L., Bester, S., Elbard, H., Finlayson, A., & Zoghaib, C. (1989). The communicative effectiveness index: Development and psychometric evaluation of a functional communication measure for adult aphasia. *Journal of Speech and Hearing Disorders, 54,* 113–124.

Matthews, G., & Margetts, I. (1991). Self-report arousal and divided attention: A study of performance operating characteristics. *Human Performance, 4,* 107–125.

McLeod, P. (1977). A dual task response modality effect: Support for multiprocessor models of attention. *Quarterly Journal of Experimental Psychology, 29,* 651–667.

McNeil, M. R., Doyle, P. J., Fossett, T. R. D., Park, G. H., & Goda, A. J. (2001). Reliability and concurrent validity of the information unit scoring metric for the story retelling procedure. *Aphasiology, 15,* 991–1006.

McNeil, M. R., Doyle, P. J., Goda, A. J., Park, G. H., Szwarc, L., Spencer, K. et al. (1999). *Normal listeners' severity judgments and comprehension of aphasic discourse: Validating a dual-task instrument for the assessment of spoken language handicap.* Poster presentation to the VA Rehabilitation Research and Development Conference, Washington, DC.

McNeil, M. R., Doyle, P. J., Park, G. H., Fossett, T. R. D., & Brodsky, M. B. (2002). Increasing the sensitivity of the Story Retell Procedure for the discrimination of normal elderly subjects from persons with aphasia. *Aphasiology, 16,* 815–822.

McNeil, M. R., Odell, K., & Tseng, C. H. (1991). Toward the integration of resource allocation into a general theory of aphasia. *Clinical Aphasiology, 21,* 21–39.

McNeil, M. R., & Prescott, T. E. (1978). *Revised Token Test.* Austin, TX: Pro-Ed.

Murray, L. L. (1999). Attention and aphasia: Theory, research, and clinical implications. *Aphasiology, 13,* 91–111.

Murray, L. L. (2000). The effects of varying attentional demands on the word retrieval skills of adults with aphasia, right hemisphere brain damage, or no brain damage. *Brain and Language, 72,* 40–72.

Murray, L. L., Holland, A. L., & Beeson, P. M. (1997a). Accuracy monitoring and task demand evaluation in aphasia. *Aphasiology, 11,* 401–414.

Murray, L. L., Holland, A. L., & Beeson, P. M. (1997b). Auditory processing in individuals with mild aphasia: A study of resource allocation. *Journal of Speech, Language, and Hearing Research, 40,* 792–808.

Murray, L. L., Holland, A. L., & Beeson, P. M. (1998). Spoken language of individuals with mild fluent aphasia under focused and divided-attention conditions. *Journal of Speech, Language, and Hearing Research, 41,* 213–227.

Navon, D. (1984). Resources: A theoretical soup stone? *Psychological Review, 91,* 216–234.

Navon, D. (1990). Exploring two methods for estimating performance tradeoff. *Bulletin of the Psychonomic Society, 28,* 155–157.

Navon, D., & Gopher, D. (1979). On the economy of the human processing system. *Psychological Review, 86,* 214–255.

Navon, D., & Gopher, D. (1980). Task difficulty, resources, and dual-task performance. In R. S. Nickerson (Ed.), *Attention and performance* (pp. 297–315). Hillsdale, NJ: Lawrence Erlbaum Associates Inc.

Nicholas, L. E., & Brookshire, R. H. (1993). A system for quantifying the informativeness and efficiency of the connected speech of adults with aphasia. *Journal of Speech and Hearing Research, 36,* 338–350.

Nicholas, L. E., & Brookshire, R. H. (1995). Presence, completeness, and accuracy of main concepts in the connected speech of non-brain-damaged adults and adults with aphasia. *Journal of Speech and Hearing Research, 38,* 145–156.

Paul, R. (2001). *Language disorders from infancy through adolescence.* St. Louis, MO: Mosby.

Payne, D. G., Peters, L. J., Birkmire, D. P., Bonto, M. A., Anastasi, J. S., & Wenger, M. J. (1994). Effects of speech intelligibility level on concurrent visual task performance. *Human Factors, 36,* 441–475.

Porch, B. (1981). *Porch index of communicative ability.* Palo Alto, CA: Consulting Psychologists Press.

Rochon, E., Saffran, E. M., Berndt, R. S., & Schwartz, M. F. (2003). Qualitative analysis of aphasic sentence production: Further development and new data. *Brain and Language, 72,* 193–218.

Rosenbaum, D. A. (1980). Human movement initiation: Specification of arm, direction, and extent. *Journal of Experimental Psychology: General, 109,* 444–474.

Saffran, E. M., Berndt, R. S., & Schwartz, M. F. (2003). The quantitative analysis of agrammatic production: Procedure and data. *Brain and Language, 37,* 440–479.

Sarno, M. T. (1969). *The functional communication profile.* New York: Howard A. Rusk Institute of Rehabilitation Medicine, New York University Medical Center.

Schmidt, R. A., & Gordan, G. B. (1977). Errors in motor responding, "rapid" corrections, and false anticipations. *Journal of Motor Behavior, 9,* 101–111.

Schmidt, R. A. & Lee, T. D. (1999). *Motor control and learning: A behavioral emphasis* (3rd ed.). Champaign, IL: Human Kinetics.

Sirevaag, E. J., Kramer, A. F., Coles, M. G., & Donchin, E. (1989). Resource reciprocity: An event-related brain potentials analysis. *Acta Psychologica, 70,* 77–97.

Slansky, B. L., & McNeil, M. R. (1997). Resource allocation in auditory processing of emphatically stressed stimuli in aphasia. *Aphasiology, 11,* 461–472.

Tseng, C. H., McNeil, M. R., & Milenkovic, P. (1993). An investigation of attention allocation deficits in aphasia. *Brain and Language, 45,* 276–296.

Wickens, C. D. (1976). The effects of divided attention on information processing in manual tracking. *Journal of Experimental Psychology: Human Perception and Performance, 2,* 1–13.

Wickens, C. D. (1984). Processing resources in attention. In R. Parasuraman & D. R. Davies (Eds.), *Varieties of attention* (pp. 63–102). New York: Academic Press.

Wickens, C. D. (1986). The effects of control dynamics on performance. In K. R. Boff, L. Kaufman, & J. P. Thomas (Eds.), *Handbook of perception and human performance* (pp. 1–60). New York: Wiley & Sons.

Wickens, C. D., & Gopher, D. (1977). Control theory measures of tracking as indices of attention allocation strategies. *Human Factors, 9,* 365.

Wickens, C. D., Kramer, A., Vanasse, L., & Donchin, E. (1983). Performance of concurrent tasks: A psychological analysis of the reciprocity of information-processing resources. *Science, 221,* 1080–1082.

Wilkinson, G. S. (1993). *Wide Range Achievement Test-3.* Wilmington, DE: Wide Range, Inc.

APHASIOLOGY, 2004, 18 (5/6/7), 543–554

Anomia in patients with left inferior temporal lobe lesions

Sharon M. Antonucci and Pélagie M. Beeson

University of Arizona, USA

Steven Z. Rapcsak

University of Arizona, and Southern Arizona VA Health Care System, USA

Background: Damage to left inferior temporal cortex has been associated with naming deficits resulting either from impaired access to phonological word forms (pure anomia) or from degraded semantic knowledge (semantic anomia). Neuropsychological evidence indicates that pure anomia may follow damage to posterior inferior temporal cortex (BA 37), whereas semantic anomia is associated with damage to more anterior temporal lobe regions (BA 20, 21, 38). By contrast, some investigators have suggested that it is the overall severity of anomia, rather than the nature of the underlying cognitive impairment, that is affected by the anterior extent of the lesion.
Aims: To examine the naming performance of patients with left inferior temporal lobe damage and determine whether anterior extension of the lesion influences the nature and/or the severity of the naming impairment.
Methods & Procedures: Eight participants with focal damage to left inferior temporal cortex completed a battery of language measures that included confrontation naming, semantic processing, and single-word reading and spelling. Degree and type of anomia was examined relative to anterior lesion extension using both visual inspection and statistical analyses.
Outcomes & Results: Naming performance ranged from unimpaired to severely defective, with only two participants demonstrating an additional mild impairment of semantic knowledge. The underlying mechanism of anomia seemed to be degraded access to phonological word forms in all participants, regardless of lesion configuration. The severity of the naming impairment was positively correlated with anterior extension of the lesion towards the temporal pole, although additional analyses suggested that these findings were significantly influenced by participant age. Naming was not correlated with performance on the nonverbal semantic task or any other demographic variable.
Conclusions: The behavioural and neuroanatomical findings provide modest support for the hypothesis that a relationship exists between anterior lesion extension and the severity of concomitant anomia in patients with left inferior temporal lobe damage. The data suggest that such lesions may disconnect relatively preserved semantic knowledge from regions critical for access to phonological word forms. However, additional research is needed to discern to what extent age and individual variability temper these effects.

Address correspondence to: Sharon M. Antonucci, Department of Speech & Hearing Sciences, University of Arizona, P.O. Box 210071, Tucson, AZ 85721-0071, USA. Email: sharonnj@u.arizona.edu

The authors wish to thank Maya Henry and Ranjini Rajeevan for their assistance with data collection and analysis and Argye Hillis MD for her helpful comments. This work was supported in part by the Small Grants Program in Imaging and Imaging Science from the State of Arizona.

http://www.tandf.co.uk/journals/pp/02687038.html   DOI: 10.1080/02687030444000219

It is well established that the left perisylvian language areas play a critical role in spoken naming of objects and pictures (Benson, 1979; Benson & Geschwind, 1985; Goodglass, 1993). Language contributions made by extrasylvian regions of the left hemisphere are less well understood; however, impaired lexical retrieval (i.e., anomia) is frequently reported following damage to left inferior temporal cortex (middle and inferior temporal gyri and ventrally adjacent fusiform gyrus) (Benson, 1979; Damasio, Grabowski, Tranel, Hichwa, & Damasio 1996; De Renzi, Zambolin, & Crisi, 1987). Focal damage to the left inferior temporal lobe most commonly results from vascular events in the distribution of the posterior cerebral artery (PCA). When De Renzi and colleagues (1987) examined a consecutive series of patients with left PCA infarcts, 10 of 16 exhibited anomia accompanied by alexia and, in some cases, agraphia. Damasio and colleagues (1996) also identified a subset of anomic patients with lesions in inferior temporal regions. Other evidence suggesting involvement of this area in naming comes from pre-surgical studies of epileptic patients, wherein transient anomia was induced by electrical stimulation to the left inferior temporal cortex and the fusiform gyrus (Burnstine et al., 1990; Luders et al., 1991).

Neuropsychological case reports suggest some variability regarding the nature and severity of anomia associated with damage to the left inferior temporal lobe. Several detailed case studies have documented lesions to left posterior inferior temporal cortex involving Brodmann area (BA) 37 that resulted in anomia with preserved semantic knowledge (Foundas, Daniels, & Vasterling, 1998; Raymer et al., 1997). Similar to those reported by Damasio et al. (1996), these patients typically made errors in the form of semantically appropriate circumlocutions, suggesting relatively intact conceptual representations and preserved phonological abilities. Such lexical retrieval deficits have been characterised as representing a disconnection between semantic knowledge and phonological word forms (Damasio et al., 1996; Foundas et al., 1998; Raymer et al., 1997; Whatmough & Chertkow, 2002). Word retrieval difficulties also have been documented following damage to more anterior temporal regions (BA 20, 21, 38) from a variety of lesion aetiologies including temporal lobectomy (Bell, Davies, Hermann, & Walters, 2000; Biederman, Gerhardstein, Cooper, & Nelson, 1997; Glosser & Donofrio, 2001; Hermann et al., 1999), herpes encephalitis (Pietrini, Nertempi, Vaglia, Revello, & Pinna, 1988; Schmolck, Kensinger, Corkin & Squire, 2002; Warrington & Shallice, 1984) and semantic dementia (Hodges, Patterson, Oxbury & Funnell, 1992; Lambdon Ralph, McClelland, Patterson, Galton & Hodges, 2001; Mummery, Patterson, Price, Ashburner, Frackowiak, & Hodges, 2000) The naming difficulties in many of these cases occurred in the context of general semantic impairment, suggesting that anomia following anterior temporal lobe damage may reflect a different underlying mechanism from the lexical retrieval deficits documented in patients with more posterior lesions. Consistent with this hypothesis, patients with semantic anomia following anterior temporal lobe damage typically demonstrate concomitant deficits of single word comprehension and they tend to produce semantic naming errors (bench–chair).

These neuropsychological findings are complemented by functional neuroimaging studies in normal individuals demonstrating the participation of left inferior temporal lobe regions in naming (for review, see Binder & Price, 2001). In particular, left posterior inferior temporal cortex (BA 37) has been shown to be active during lexical retrieval tasks including verbal fluency and picture naming (Freidman et al., 1998; Moore & Price, 1999; Mummery, Patterson, Hodges & Wise, 1996; Murtha, Chertkow, Beauregard & Evans, 1999; Price, Moore, Humphreys, Frackowiak & Friston, 1996). Although it is difficult to isolate semantic processing from lexical retrieval, there is evidence to suggest that a region medial and anterior to left BA 37, located primarily within BA 20, is specifically involved in conceptual processing (Binder & Price, 2001; D'Esposito et al., 1997; Martin, Haxby, Lalonde, Wiggs, & Ungerleider, 1995; Vandenberghe, Price, Wise, Josephs, & Frackowiak, 1996;). Thus, there is some convergence between neuropsychological and functional imaging studies to suggest that within the left inferior temporal lobe, semantic and lexical retrieval operations are subserved by distinct cortical regions distributed along the anterior-posterior axis.

It has also been proposed that the anterior extent of left inferior temporal lesions influences the overall severity of anomia, without necessarily altering the nature of the underlying functional deficit. Sakurai and colleagues (Sakurai, Sakai, Sakuta, & Iwata, 1994) made note of the variability in the anterior extension of left inferior temporal lesions in a series of Japanese individuals who showed a common impairment for writing kanji symbols. They found that patients with damage restricted to BA 37 evidenced little or no impairment of spoken naming, whereas patients with damage extending into the anterior part of the middle/inferior temporal gyri (BA 20,21) and the parahippocampal gyrus demonstrated severe anomia. Although not examined in detail, the word retrieval deficit of these patients was characterised as a pure anomia, presumably reflecting a disruption in the flow of information between semantic representations and phonological word forms. To our knowledge, similar investigations have not been carried out in English-speaking individuals.

The purpose of this study was to examine whether the anterior extent of left inferior temporal lobe lesions plays a critical role in determining the nature and/or severity of anomia. Specifically, we wanted to learn whether patients with more anterior temporal lobe lesions demonstrate a qualitatively different type of naming impairment (i.e., semantic anomia) or whether they simply exhibit a more severe form of pure anomia.

METHOD

Eight right-handed men with lesions restricted to left inferior temporo-occipital cortex participated in this study. Seven of the participants had experienced strokes in the left posterior cerebral artery (PCA) territory, and one participant (TF) had a temporal lobe haematoma associated with anticoagulation treatment. As shown in Table 1, participants ranged in age from 49 to 86 years and were at least 2 months post onset (range = 2 months to 3 years, 4 months). All participants spoke English as their primary language, and at the time of testing they were classified as either "anomic" or "non-aphasic" based on their performance on the Western Aphasia Battery (WAB: Kertesz, 1982) (see Table 1).

Visual confrontation naming was assessed with the Boston Naming Test (BNT: Kaplan, Goodglass, & Weintraub, 1983). Naming errors were recorded so that they could be characterised as semantically appropriate description (i.e., meaningful circumlocution), no response, empty circumlocution, semantic error, visually and semantically related error, or phonemic paraphasia (see Table 2). Differentiation between empty circumlocutions and semantically meaningful circumlocutions was based on a judgement of the communicative effectiveness of responses; specifically, whether an uninformed listener could derive the name of the item from the participant's description. As such, self-referential responses (e.g., pretzels: "I love 'em"; wreath: "I used to make them and sell them") that did not convey any descriptive information were coded as empty circumlocutions. In addition to examining performance on the BNT, information regarding lexical retrieval was available from the WAB subtest for object naming. Semantic

TABLE 1
Participant demographic information and performance on assessment measures

	TF	EM	FS	MS	CC	RB	RN	MH
Gender	male	male	male	male	male	male	male	male
Handedness	R	R	R	R	R	R	R	R
Age (years)	74	74	80	86	68	61	60	49
Education (years)	16	12	16	16	10	12	12	16
Time post onset (months)	8	3	8	13	26	40	2	4
WAB Aphasia Quotient	89*	91.6*	84.8*	95	92.4*	95.8	98.4	100
– auditory word recognition	60/60	60/60	58/60	60/60	56/60	60/60	60/60	60/60
– object naming	46/60	42/60	48/60	53/60	54/60	60/60	60/60	60/60
WAB Aphasia Type†	Anomic	Anomic	Anomic	N-A	Anomic	N-A	N-A	N-A
Boston Naming Test (BNT)	16/60*	16/60*	25/60*	36/60*	37/60*	41/60*	45/60*	60/60
Pyramids & Palm Trees (P&PT)	47/52	45/52*	47/52	51/52	42/52*	48/52	52/52	49/52

† "N-A" indicates a score equated with non-asphasic on the WAB.
* Indicates impaired performance.

TABLE 2
Example errors on the *BNT*

Error type	Example of participant response	Target
Semantically appropriate description	"find them in the desert ... ancient Egypt had them"	pyramid
	"to sleep on or lay down on"	hammock
No response/empty circumlocution	'it's ... it's"	seahorse
	"I know what it is ... sure"	globe
Semantic error	"seagull"	pelican
Visual/semantic error	"flower"	mushroom
	"ledger"	scroll

knowledge was probed with the picture version of the Pyramids and Palm Trees Test (P&PT: Howard & Patterson, 1992), which required participants to recognise the semantic association between two pictures in the presence of a distractor item. The picture version of this test was used to avoid potential difficulties due to reading impairment. As a further measure of semantic processing, single word comprehension scores were available from the auditory word recognition subtest of the WAB.

Although not the focus of this report, acquired impairments of single-word reading and spelling were documented for all participants (see Rapcsak & Beeson, in press, for details). Reading was slow and prone to visual errors, with some participants exhibiting letter-by-letter reading. With regard to spelling, all participants demonstrated a profile consistent with lexical agraphia in that regular word spelling was more accurate than irregular word spelling, and errors were typically phonologically plausible (e.g., "cough"–coff).

Lesion localisation was performed using clinical, structural MRI head scans available for each participant. Lesion maps were generated using the region of interest tool in MRIcro software (Rorden & Brett, 2000). To better match the horizontal orientation of the clinical scans, which were typically parallel to the orbitomeatal line, the MRIcro template was reoriented −15 degrees in pitch from the standard AC–PC (anterior commissure–posterior commissure) plane. The change in pitch shifts the axial plane so that the z values were measured where x and y = 0. The lesions for each participant were manually drawn onto the MRIcro slices by one investigator and then examined and revised by the two other investigators until consensus was reached. Lesions were mapped onto common axial slices at 5–6 mm intervals, with three slices reflecting the regions of greatest overlap in the ventral temporal and occipital lobes at z = −17, −22, and −27 (see Figures 1 and 2). The sagittal view in Figure 2 provides an indication of the anterior-posterior and superior-inferior extent of these three regions. As shown in Figure 2, regions of lesion overlap for all eight participants are designated with an X. Using the MRIcro software, lesion extent was measured using Talairach coordinates along the y

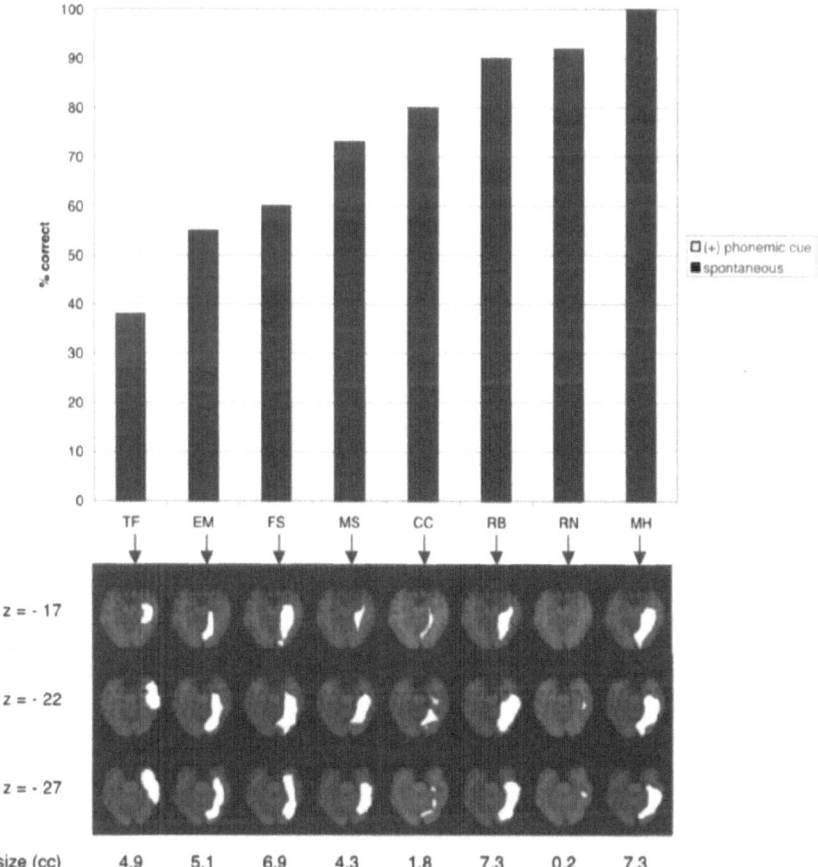

Figure 1. Performance on the Boston Naming Test and schematic representation of respective participant brain lesions (top row of axial slices is superior to bottom row).

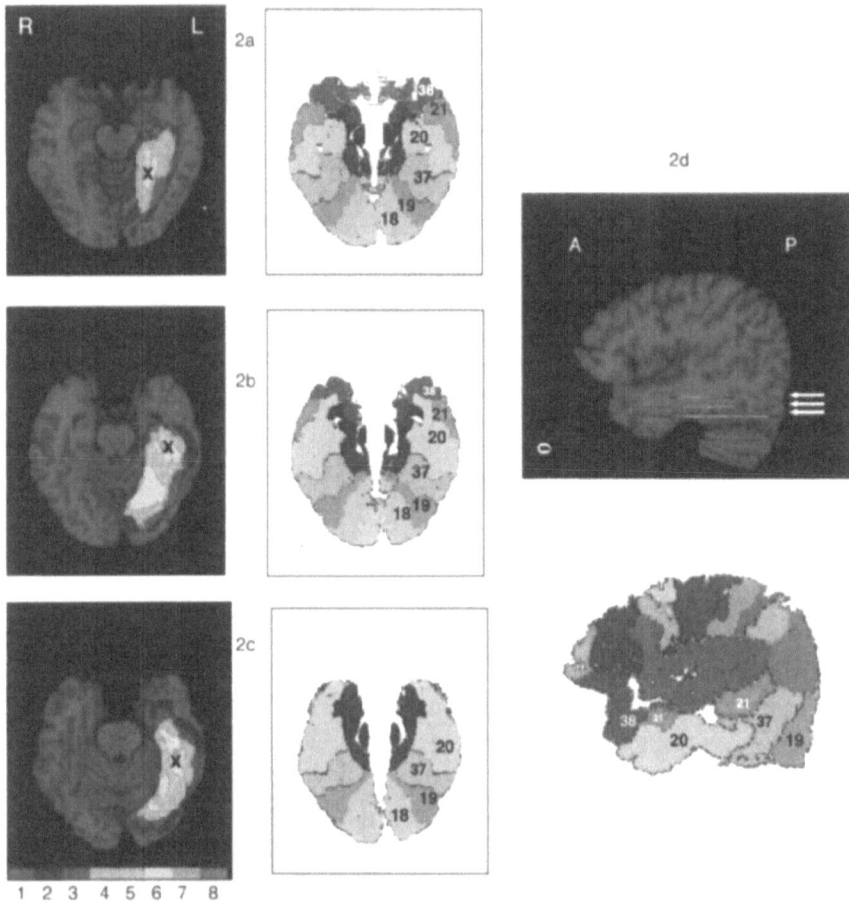

Figure 2. Regions of lesion overlap and associated Brodmann areas. The axial plane was shifted −15 degrees pitch from AC-PC orientation to better match the plane of the clinical scans. With Talairach x and y coordinates set at 0, z = −17 (Figure 2a), z = −22 (Figure 2b) and z = −27 (Figure 2c). Colourbar indicates number of participants' lesion overlap, with regions of greatest overlap marked with an X. Horizontal striations delineated by white arrows in Figure 2d (x = 46, y and z = 0) reflect inferior-superior lesion extent. A colour version of this figure is available online at: http://www.tandf.co.uk/journals/online/0268-7038.asp

(anterior-posterior) plane. An estimate of lesion volume in the ventral temporo-occipital region was calculated by summing the lesion volumes for each slice.

RESULTS

Scores on the BNT ranged from 16 to 60 (out of 60), with seven of the eight participants demonstrating impaired naming. As show in Figure 1, those seven individuals were responsive to phonemic cueing on roughly 18% of the items. During word retrieval failures, all participants frequently indicated that they recognised the pictured item by providing relevant semantic information (e.g., pyramid: ''it's in Egypt''; abacus: ''they used to use it to count''). These semantically appropriate circumlocutions made up the largest proportion of errors for five participants, with ''no response/empty circumlocution'' being the most frequent error type for EM, while RB responded with a roughly equal number of semantically appropriate and empty circumlocutions (see Figure 3). Phonological errors or paraphasias were not produced by any of the participants. Visual misidentification of target items was rare, as demonstrated by the small number of errors that were coded as visual/semantic (see Figure 3). Furthermore, there was no evidence of impaired object recognition on the auditory word recognition subtest of the WAB, nor was there evidence of visual misperception on the object naming subtest of the WAB in that none of the individuals benefited from the provision of tactile cues when they were unable to retrieve item names based on visual presentation alone. There were relatively few semantic errors made on the BNT and, as shown in Table 1, all participants demonstrated preserved or mildly impaired semantic knowledge on the P&PT. Furthermore, on the few occasions that a semantic error was made, participants frequently demonstrated awareness that their responses were incorrect (e.g., MS beaver: "skunk, that's good enough"; RN yoke: "bridle, no, that's not it . . . neck brace?"). Finally, the majority of patients achieved perfect scores on the auditory word recognition subtest of the *WAB*, indicating the absence of significant word comprehension impairment.

The mapping of individual lesions confirmed that brain damage was concentrated in the ventral temporal and occipital lobes encompassing BAs 21, 20, 37, 19, 18, and 17. Individual lesions are shown on the three axial cuts with the greatest lesion overlap (z = -17, z = -22 and z = -27) in Figure 1. Seven of eight participants had damage to BA 37 (all but RN), and all eight had damage to BA 20. Extension into medial temporal lobe regions (BA 36, 28) was also observed in the majority of participants. The most anterior lesion extension was noted in TF, who sustained damage from a haematoma that extended towards the left temporal pole affecting BA 21 and 38. Lesion volumes ranged from 0.2 cc for RN to 7.3 cc for RB and MH (see Figure 1). As shown in Figure 2, the area of greatest lesion overlap for all 8 participants was in the left fusiform gyrus at the border between BA 37 and 20.

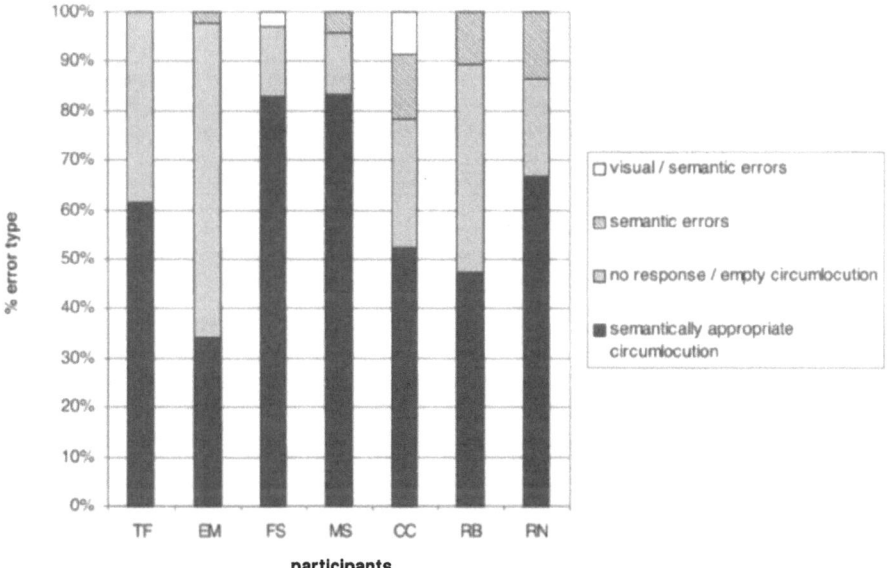

Figure 3. Percentage of error types made by each participant on the Boston Naming Test.

Performance on the BNT is presented along with lesion maps for each of the participants in Figure 1. Results were ordered from most impaired to least impaired naming performance. Visual inspection comparing site of lesion with degree of anomia suggests a progression in naming impairment with increasingly anterior lesion extension, with the exception of MH, who demonstrated unimpaired naming ability despite a sizeable lesion in BA 37 and BA 20 (see Figure 1). To address the fundamental question regarding the relationship between anterior lesion extension and degree of anomia, the y-coordinates reflecting the anterior extent of the lesion for each participant for the three axial slices of interest were correlated with participants' BNT scores. As shown in Table 3, a significant correlation was observed for the most inferior slice (z = −27) and was close to reaching significance for the middle slice (z = −22), with no significant correlation observed for the most superior slice (z = −17). Performance on the BNT was not correlated with the estimate of total lesion volume in the inferior temporal area (see Table 3).

To determine the potential influence of other variables, BNT scores and anterior lesion extension were also correlated with demographic variables and with performance on the semantic test (P&PT). Neither time post onset, education, nor semantic knowledge was significantly correlated with BNT performance (see Table 3) or anterior lesion extension (all p-values > .075). There was also no significant correlation between performance on the P&PT semantic test and anterior lesion extent, r = .289, p = .244. As Table 3 shows, the only significant correlation observed was between age and BNT scores, in the direction of younger participants performing better than older participants. The observed age effect was apparently influenced by the performance of MH who, at age 49, was our youngest participant by more than a decade. MH sustained a large left inferior temporal lobe lesion (encompassing both BAs 20 and 37), yet he demonstrated unimpaired naming on the BNT. Age-span studies of performance

TABLE 3
BNT correlations with lesion information, demographic variables and semantic test

Variable	Analysis with all participants (n = 8)		Analysis with age-education corrected scores for all participants (n = 8)[1]		Analysis with age-education corrected scores excluding MH (n = 7)[1]	
	r-value	p-value	r-value	p-value	r-value	p-value
Demographic variables						
Age	−.73	.019*	—	—	—	—
TPO (months)	+.13	.376	−.25	.274	+.17	.355
Education (years)	−.03	.468	—	—	—	—
P&PT	+.42	.153	+.38	.179	−.15	.378
Lesion information						
Anterior extent z = −27	−.75	.016*	−.46	.127	−.85	.007*
Anterior extent z = −22	−.61	.054†	−.31	.227	−.78	.018*
Anterior extent z = −17	+.17	.346	+.02	.481	−.02	.481
Lesion volume (cc)	−.01	.491	+.22	.299	−.52	.113

[1] Age and education-corrected BNT scores: $A\&E\text{-}MSS_{BNT} = K + (W_1 * \text{Age-corrected } MSS_{BNT}) - (W_2 * \text{Education})$ (From Ivnik et al., 1996, cited in Mitrushina et al., 1999, p. 126); where $K = 3.32$; $W_1 = 1.07$; $W_2 = 0.34$; Education in years.
* significant correlation.
† marginally significant correlation.

on the BNT suggest that a slight age effect may be present even within the normal population, particularly after the age of 70 years (Albert, Heller, & Milberg, 1988; Tombaugh & Humbley, 1997), with level of education appearing to be a mitigating factor that may have even more influence both across and within age groups. To address this issue, all correlations were also performed using BNT standard scores that were corrected for both age and education. These scores were calculated using the formula reported by Ivnik and colleagues (Ivnik, Malec, Smith, Tangalos, & Peterson, 1996, reported in Mitrushina, Boone, & D'Elia, 1999, p. 126). As shown in Table 3, when age- and education-corrected BNT scores were used, the significant correlation between naming performance and anterior lesion extension was not sustained. However, when the youngest participant, MH, was excluded, significant correlations were observed between naming performance and anterior lesion extension in both the inferior slice, $r = -.85$, $p = .007$, and the middle slice $r = -.78$, $p = .018$. We also examined lesion extent specifically within anterior (BA 20/21) and posterior inferior temporal cortex (BA 37) in relation to age- and education-corrected scores on the BNT. For the seven participants (without MH), there was a stronger correlation with the extent of damage to BA 20/21, $r = -.569$, $p = .091$, than to BA 37, $r = -.135$, $p = .386$. Although not statistically significant, these findings are consistent with the proposed relationship between anterior lesion extent and severity of anomia.

DISCUSSION

In this study, we examined the naming performance of individuals with left inferior temporal lobe damage. Seven out of eight participants demonstrated anomia of varying degrees of severity. Analysis of performance on assessment tasks suggests that the cognitive mechanism of anomia in all participants was disrupted access to the phonological lexicon rather than loss of semantic knowledge. Only two of the eight participants demonstrated mild semantic impairment on a test of nonverbal semantic knowledge (P&PT), and none of the participants demonstrated impairment of auditory word comprehension on the WAB. Furthermore, performance on the semantic knowledge measure was not correlated with performance on the BNT. All participants were able to provide semantic information in an attempt to self-cue word retrieval during confrontation naming tasks and during conversation. Analysis of naming errors on the BNT provides additional evidence of well preserved semantic knowledge, as participants were consistently able to provide appropriate semantic information for items they could not name and, in the few instances when semantic errors were produced, participants often indicated awareness that their responses were inaccurate. Finally, it should be noted that patient TF who had the most severe anomia and whose lesion extended all the way to the temporal pole did not produce any semantic naming errors.

These behavioural observations are of particular interest with respect to the lesion sites in our patients. While seven of the eight participants sustained damage to posterior inferior temporal cortex (BA 37), all eight evidenced anterior lesion extension into BA 20/21. These more anterior cortical sites have been previously associated with semantic knowledge in functional neuroimaging studies (D'Esposito et al., 1997; Martin et al., 1995; Moore & Price, 1999), and damage to these brain regions gives rise to semantic anomia (Graham, Patterson, & Hodges, 1995; Hodges et al., 1992; Mummery, Patterson, Wise, Vandenberghe, Price, & Hodges, 1999; Pietrini et al., 1988; Schmolck et al., 2002; Warrington & Shallice, 1984). As such, it may appear contradictory that the naming deficit of our patients with anterior temporal lobe involvement did not appear to be semantic in nature. However, our patients had only partial damage to anterior temporal lobe structures and it is possible that more substantial compromise of semantic networks is required for semantic anomia to occur. Consistent with this hypothesis, some patients with semantic dementia initially show anomia without significant semantic impairment, with single-word comprehension deficits and semantic naming errors appearing later in the course of the illness concomitant with the relentless progression (and bilateral spread) of the cortical degenerative process (Graham et al., 1995; Lambdon Ralph et al., 2001; Mummery et al., 1999). It should also be noted that some of the temporal lobe regions that are frequently involved in semantic dementia (i.e., temporal pole, anterolateral temporal cortex) (Mummery et al., 2000) were largely spared in our patients, whose lesions primarily involved ventromedial temporal cortex. Finally, although anterior lesion extension did not seem to be associated with significant semantic deficit in our patients, it needs to be acknowledged that our assessment battery did not include rigorous tests of semantic knowledge, and it is possible that more subtle semantic impairments remained undetected.

As it appears from our data that the naming impairment in our patients was not related to a loss of semantic knowledge, we next examine whether anterior lesion extension was associated with increasingly severe anomia indicating progressively greater disruption of functional connections between semantic and phonological representations. While anterior lesion extension was significantly correlated with our participants' raw scores on the measure of naming performance, this correlation was not sustained when age- and education-corrected BNT scores were used. The age effect in our results seems to be largely mediated by the influence of our youngest participant by more than a decade, MH, who performed perfectly on the BNT despite having sustained a sizeable lesion encompassing portions of both left BA 37 and 20. When MH was excluded from the analyses, the relationship between degree of naming impairment and anterior lesion extension became significant for both the inferior and middle slices. It is not clear whether MH's intact naming performance reflects age-related differences in neural plasticity or whether it is attributable to individual variability in cortical language organisation. However, a review of the left PCA cases presented by De Renzi et al. (1987) similarly showed preserved performance for object and picture naming in the individual who was substantially younger than all other participants. These findings, in conjunction with studies of naming performance in the normal ageing population (Albert et al., 1988; Tombaugh & Humbley, 1997), indicate that participant age is likely a mitigating factor that should be taken into consideration when examining the effect of lesion variables on naming performance.

Our findings contribute to the growing literature that attempts to distinguish the roles of distinct left inferior temporal lobe regions in various lexical-semantic language tasks. We found that damage localised to left inferior temporal cortex (including BAs 37 and 20) resulted in anomia, which appeared to be caused by a disconnection between semantic knowledge and phonological word forms. While regions within anterior temporal cortex may function to support conceptual representations within a larger semantic network, our data suggest that limited unilateral damage to these cortical areas does not significantly degrade semantic knowledge. Furthermore, our data provide preliminary indication that the anterior extension of inferior temporal lobe lesions may influence the severity of anomia in these patients. Investigations with larger groups of participants, including age-specific patient cohorts, are required to elucidate further the specific functional role of different left temporal lobe regions in name retrieval.

REFERENCES

Albert, M. S., Heller, H. S., & Milberg, W. (1988). Changes in naming ability with age. *Psychology and Aging*, *3*(2), 173–178.

Bell, B. D., Davies, K. G., Hermann, B. P., & Walters, G. (2000). Confrontation naming after anterior temporal lobectomy is related to age of acquisition of object names. *Neuropsychologia*, *38*(1), 83–92.

Benson, D. F. (1979). Neurologic correlates of anomia. In H. Whitaker (Ed.), *Studies in neurolinguistics* (Vol. 4). New York: Academic Press.

Benson, D. F., & Geschwind, N. (1985). The aphasia and related disturbances. In A. B. Baker & R. J. Joynt (Eds.), *Clinical neurology (Vol. 1)*. Philadelphia: Harper & Row.

Biederman, I., Gerhardstein, P. C., Cooper, E. C., & Nelson, C. A. (1997). High level object recognition without an anterior inferior temporal lobe. *Neuropsychologia*, *35*(3), 271–287.

Binder, J., & Price, C. J. (2001). Functional neuroimaging of langauge. In R. Cabeza & A. Kingstone (Eds.), *Handbook of functional neuroimaging of cognition* (Ch. 7). Cambridge, MA: MIT Press.

Burnstine, T. H., Lesser, R. P., Hart, J. Jr., Uematsu, S., Zinreich, S., Drauss, G. L. et al. (1990). Characterization of the basal temporal language area in patients with left temporal lobe epilepsy. *Neurology*, *40*, 966–970.

Damasio, H., Grabowski, T. J., Tranel, D., Hichwa, R. D., & Damasio, A. R. (1996). A neural basis for lexical retrieval [published erratum appears in *Nature*, Jun 27 1996; *381*(6595): 810]. *Nature*, *380*(6574), 499–505.

De Renzi, E., Zambolin, A., & Crisi, G. (1987). The pattern of neuropsychological impairment associated with left posterior cerebral artery infarcts. *Brain*, *110*, 1099–1116.

D'Esposito, M., Detre, J. A., Auguirre, G. K., Stallcup, M., Alsop, D. C., Tippet, L. J. et al. (1997). A functional MRI study of mental image generation. *Neuropsychologia*, *35*(5), 725–730.

Foundas, A. L., Daniels, S. K., & Vasterling, J. J. (1998). Anomia: Case studies with lesion localization. *Neurocase*, *4*, 35–43.

Freidman, L., Kenny, J. T., Wise, A. L., Wu, D., Stuve, T. A., Miller, D. A. et al. (1998). Brain activation during silent word generation evaluated by functional MRI. *Brain and Language*, *64*, 231–256.

Glosser, G., & Donofrio, N. (2001) Differences between nouns and verbs after anterior temporal lobectomy. *Neuropsychology*, *15*(1), 39–47.

Goodglass, H. (1993). *Understanding aphasia*. San Diego, CA: Academic Press, Inc.

Graham, K., Patterson, K., & Hodges, J. R. (1995). Progressive pure anomia: Insufficient activation of phonology by meaning. *Neurocase*, *1*, 25–38.

Hermann, B. P., Perrine, K., Chelune, G. J., Barr, W., Loring, D. W., Strauss, E. et al. (1999). Visual confrontation naming following left anterior temporal lobectomy: A comparison of surgical procedures. *Neuropsychology*, *13*(1), 3–9.

Hodges, J. R., Patterson, K. E., Oxbury, S., & Funnell, E. (1992). Semantic dementia. *Brain*, *115*, 1783–1806.

Howard, D., & Patterson, K. (1992). *The Pyramids and Palm Trees Test*. Windsor, UK: Thames Valley Test Company.

Ivnik, R. J., Malec, J. F., Smith, G. E., Tangalos, E., & Peterson, R. C. (1996). Neuropsychological tests' norms above age 55: COWAT, BNT, MAE, Token, WRAT-R reading, AMNART, STROOP, TMT, & JLO. *The Clinical Neuropsychologist*, *10*(3), 262–278.

Kaplan, E., Goodglass, H., & Weintraub, S. (1983). *The Boston Naming Test*. Philadelphia: Lea & Febiger.

Kertesz, A. (1982). *The Western Aphasia Battery*. New York: Grune & Stratton.

Lambdon Ralph, M. A., McClelland, J. L., Patterson, K., Galton, C. J., & Hodges, J. R. (2001). *Journal of Cognitive Neuroscience*, *13*(3), 341–356.

Luders, H., Lesser, R. P., Hahn, J., Dinner, D. S., Morris, H. H., Wyllie, E. et al. (1991). Basal temporal language area. *Brain*, *114*, 743–754.

Martin, A., Haxby, J. V., Lalonde, F. M., Wiggs, C. L., & Ungerleider, L. G. (1995). Discrete cortical regions associated with knowledge of color and knowledge of action. *Science*, *270*, 102–105.

Mitrushina, M. N., Boone, K. B., & D'Elia, L. F. (1999). Handbook of normative data for neuropsychological assessment. New York: Oxford University Press.

Moore, C. J., & Price, C. J. (1999). Three distinct ventral occipitotemporal regions for reading and object naming. *NeuroImage*, *10*, 181–192.

Mummery, C. J., Patterson, K., Hodges, J. R., & Wise, R. J. S. (1996). Generating "tiger" as an animal name or a word beginning with T: Differences in brain activation. *Proceedings of the Royal Society of London*, *263*, 989–995.

Mummery, C. J., Patterson, K., Price, C. J., Ashburner, J., Frackowiak, R. S. J., & Hodges, J. R. (2000). A voxel-based morphometry study of semantic dementia: Relationship between temporal lobe atrophy and semantic memory. *Annals of Neurology*, *47*, 36–45.

Mummery, C. J., Patterson, K., Wise, R. J. S., Vandenberghe, R., Price, C. J., & Hodges, J. R. (1999). Disrupted temporal lobe connections in semantic dementia. *Brain, 122*, 61–73.

Murtha, S., Chertkow, H., Beauregard, M., & Evans, A. (1999). The neural substrate of picture naming. *Journal of Cognitive Neuroscience, 11*, 399–423.

Pietrini, V., Nertempi, P., Vaglia, A., Revello, M. G., & Pinna, V. (1988). Recovery from herpes simplex encephalitis: Selective impairment of specific semantic categories with neuroradiological correlation. *Journal of Neurology, Neurosurgery and Psychiatry, 51*, 1284–1293.

Price, C. J., Moore, C. J, Humphreys, G. W., Frackowiak, R. S. J., & Friston, K. J. (1996). The neural regions sustaining object recognition and naming. *Proceedings of the Royal Society of London, 263*, 1501–1507.

Rapcsak, S. Z., & Beeson, P. M. (in press). The role of the left posterior inferior temporal cortex in spelling. *Neurology*.

Raymer, A. M., Foundas, A. L., Maher, L. M., Greenwald, M. L., Morris, M., Rothi, L. J. G., & Heilman, K. M. (1997). Cognitive neuropsychological analysis and neuroanatomic correlates in a case of acute anomia. *Brain and Language, 58*, 137–156.

Rorden, C., & Brett, M. (2000). Stereotaxic display of brain lesions. *Behavioural Neurology, 12*, 191–200.

Sakurai, Y., Sakai, K., Sakuta, M., & Iwata, M. (1994). Naming difficulties in alexia with agraphia for Kanji after a left posterior inferior temporal lesion. *Journal of Neurology, Neurosurgery and Psychiatry, 57*, 609–613.

Schmolck, H., Kensinger, E. A., Corkin, S., & Squire, L. R. (2002). Semantic knowledge in patient H.M. and other patients with bilateral medial and lateral temporal lobe lesions. *Hippocampus, 12*, 520–533.

Tombaugh, T. N., & Humbley, A. M. (1997). The 60-item Boston Naming Test: Norms for cognitively intact adults aged 25 to 88 years. *Journal of Clinical and Experimental Neuropsychology, 19*(6), 922–932.

Vandenberghe, R., Price, C., Wise, R., Josephs, O., Frackowiak, R. S. J. (1996). Functional anatomy of a common semantic system for words and pictures. *Nature, 383*, 254–256.

Warrington, E. K., & Shallice, T. (1984). Category specific semantic impairments. *Brain, 110*, 829–854.

Whatmough, C., & Chertkow, W. (2002). Neuroanatomical aspects of naming. In A. E. Hillis (Ed.), *The handbook of adult language disorders: Integrating cognitive neuropsychology, neurology and rehabilitation* (pp. 143–161). New York: Psychology Press.

APHASIOLOGY, 2004, *18* (5/6/7), 555–565

Priming auditory comprehension in aphasia: Facilitation and interference effects

Heather Harris Wright

University of Kentucky, Lexington, KY, USA

Marilyn Newhoff

San Diego State University, CA, USA

Background: Researchers have shown that adults with aphasia often demonstrate better comprehension for discourse than for single sentences. Investigations have included presenting preceding linguistic context to facilitate comprehension of target sentences in adults with aphasia. Priming paradigms have also been used to investigate sentence and discourse processing in adults with aphasia. In priming studies, significantly faster reaction times to related lexical probes compared to unrelated probes indicate the information activated during processing. However, the possible influence of the lexical probe on participants' comprehension of target sentences is unknown. It has been suggested that linguistic context provides redundant information that may allow the limited processing resources available to adults with aphasia to be adequately distributed to meet task demands; possibly, a related lexical probe, as opposed to other probe types, serves a similar purpose.

Aims: The objective of the current study was to examine the influence of related, incorrect, and neutral lexical probes on comprehension of sentence pairs by participants with aphasia and neurologically intact participants (NI).

Methods & Procedures: A total of 40 adults (20 presented with aphasia, 20 NI) participated in a cross-modal task. Stimuli were sentence pairs that required revision of the interpretation of the first sentence for adequate comprehension to occur. Participants listened to sentence pairs and completed a lexical decision task following each sentence pair. Lexical decisions consisted of target words that represented either the intended (revised) interpretation, initial (incorrect) interpretation, a neutral word (unrelated to the sentence pair's meaning), or a nonword. Following each sentence pair, participants answered four yes/no questions pertaining to the respective sentence pair.

Outcomes & Results: Results indicated that adults with aphasia and NI participants answered correctly significantly more questions when the lexical probe represented the intended interpretation of the sentence pair as compared to the baseline condition (neutral word). Also, participants missed significantly more questions when the lexical probe represented the initial (incorrect) interpretation as compared to the baseline.

Conclusions: Results of the study indicated that the type of probe presented influenced participants' comprehension of the sentence pairs. It is suggested that the presence of the inference revision target probe allowed participants to overcome limitations in working memory capacity or processing resources available to complete the task. Additionally, the initial inference target probe overextended participants' working memory capacity limits or available processing resources; thus, they did not perform as well during this condition.

Address correspondence to: Heather Harris Wright, The University of Kentucky, Division of Communication Disorders, CHS Building, 900 S. Limestone, Lexington, KY 40536-0200, USA. Email: hhwrig2@uky.edu

© 2004 by Taylor & Francis.

http://www.tandf.co.uk/journals/pp/02687038.html

DOI: 10.1080/02687030444000192

Discourse processing is an everyday skill involving extracting main ideas from sentences. For comprehension to occur, the extracted information must be integrated with context presented in preceding sentence(s). The extracted main idea or theme may consist of information inferred from the sentence, and not explicitly stated, yet representing the gist of the sentence (Kintsch, 1998). Adults with aphasia have demonstrated better comprehension for discourse than would be assumed by their single sentence comprehension performance (e.g., Brookshire & Nicholas, 1984), and it has been suggested that continuous presentation of related context facilitates their comprehension ability (Cannito, Hough, Vogel, & Pierce, 1996; Cannito, Jarecki, & Pierce, 1986; Hough, Pierce, & Cannito, 1989; Pierce, 1991).

Several researchers have found that comprehending target sentences in isolation is more difficult for adults with aphasia than comprehending target sentences preceded by a contextual paragraph (Boyle & Canter, 1986; Cannito et al., 1996; Cannito et al., 1986; Hough et al., 1989; Hough, Vogel, Cannito, & Pierce, 1997). Further, it has been shown that the *type* of context in the preceding paragraph does not matter. For example, both information that predicts the linguistic context (i.e., predicts the target information) and additional information that does not predict linguistic context, facilitate equally comprehension performance by adults with aphasia (Cannito et al., 1996; Hough et al., 1989). Several explanations for these findings have been suggested, such as, presentation of the preceding linguistic context facilitates processing of target information (Germani & Pierce, 1992), it limits the number of plausible events that can occur (Hough et al., 1989), and it provides redundancy of narrative information (Hough & Pierce, 1993; Pierce, 1991). Further, facilitating information processing, limiting the number of plausible events, and providing redundant information may allow for adequate distribution of the limited processing resources available to adults with aphasia so that task demands are met (McNeil, Odell, & Tseng, 1991; Miyake, Carpenter, & Just, 1994, 1995). This could account for their improved comprehension performance (Hough & Pierce, 1993; Hough et al., 1997; Pierce, 1991). It has been well documented that resource allocation deficits, whether they are due to a reduction in resource capacity or a reduction in ability to allocate the resources, negatively affect auditory comprehension abilities in adults with aphasia (McNeil, 1981; McNeil et al., 1991; Miyake et al., 1994, 1995). Thus, any strategy that may allow for the available resources to adequately meet task demands will likely result in improved task performance.

Priming paradigms have also been used in investigations of sentence and discourse processing in adults with and without aphasia. Results from these studies have shed additional light on the influence of context on comprehension. For example, with neurologically intact adults, several researchers have investigated activation of inferences generated during sentence processing (Long, Oppy, & Seely, 1994; Till, Mross, & Kintsch, 1988; Wright & Newhoff, 2002). Briefly, the priming paradigm used in these studies consisted of sentences presented visually or auditorily; following sentence presentation, a short pause (i.e., interstimulus interval [ISI]) occurred, then a letter string was presented. The letter string represented either the intended interpretation, a neutral word, or a nonword. Participants made a decision as to whether the letter string was an English word or nonword. Priming occurred when participants' reaction times were significantly faster for the target word (i.e., intended interpretation) than the neutral word. Results from these studies indicated that non-brain-damaged participants activated the intended interpretation following sentence presentation, thus supporting Kintsch's (1998) theory that the gist of a sentence is extracted and active for integration with future sentences.

Typically, in these priming studies, yes/no questions randomly follow sentence presentation. The questions may be fact-based or based on inferences generated. One of the purposes of including questions in sentence priming investigations is to ensure that participants are attending to the information presented in the sentence(s). In our earlier work (Wright & Newhoff 2002, in press), four question types followed each sentence pair—two based on facts and two based on inferences generated. Accuracy of responses was analysed and results indicated that neurologically intact participants performed at ceiling levels; not surprisingly, adults with aphasia missed significantly more questions than their non-brain-damaged counterparts. It is not surprising that the participants with and without aphasia missed significantly fewer questions based on facts than those based on inferences generated. As a result of these findings, in the present work we were interested in whether the type of lexical probe (i.e., intended, incorrect, or neutral) might influence how well comprehension occurs when it is measured by accurate responses to such questions. Further, we were interested in how participants responded to questions that could not be answered from explicitly presented information, but required the generation of an inference. Cognitive functions, including access to one's world knowledge and working memory, are required for generating an inference. Additional context, such as presentation of a related or unrelated lexical probe, could potentially influence participants' performance on the task by affecting the information they may access to process the sentences.

Based on results from investigations of contextual influences on comprehension, we expected that targets related to the sentences' intended meanings would positively influence response performance (comprehension). Hough et al. (1989) had suggested that presentation of preceding linguistic information limits the number of plausible events that may occur, thus facilitating comprehension of target sentences. Our thinking was that presentation of a lexical probe related to the sentence's intended meaning might result in the same outcome; that is, it might direct the individual to the intended meaning of the sentence thereby facilitating comprehension. Alternatively, presenting a lexical probe that represents an incorrect interpretation could negatively affect comprehension performance.

To test these hypotheses, we investigated the influence of probe type on inference comprehension performance in adults with and without aphasia. Stimuli consisted of sentence pairs requiring participants to revise their initial interpretation, generated from the first sentence, in order to comprehend the sentence pairs. Probes consisted of targets representing the intended (revised) interpretation, the incorrect (initial) interpretation, and neutral words that had no relation to the sentence pair meanings.

METHOD

Participants

A total of 40 adults participated in the study: 20 had unilateral left brain damage subsequent to cerebrovascular accident and 20 served as the control subjects without known neurological impairment (NI). Mean age was 65.8 (SD = 14.1) for the aphasia group and 64.3 (SD = 13.0) for the NI group. Mean years of education completed for each group were 15.1 (SD = 2.8) and 15.6 (SD = 3.0) for the aphasia and NI groups, respectively. Criteria for participants with aphasia included: (a) no more than one CVA, and that one CVA in the left hemisphere; (b) at least 6 months post onset of the stroke; (c) mild to moderate severity of aphasia; and (d) sufficient single word reading abilities. Adults with aphasia were excluded if their medical records documented evidence of bilateral lesions, multiple CVAs, or cognitively deteriorating conditions such as Alzheimer's or Parkinson's. Additionally, all participants met the following criteria: (a) demonstrated appropriate visual acuity to read stimuli presented on the computer; (b) aided or unaided hearing within normal limits for conversational purposes; and (c) sufficient dexterity control to make responses using an internal mouse.

Type and severity of aphasia were confirmed by performance on the Western Aphasia Battery (WAB: Kertesz, 1982). Aphasia quotients (AQ) were obtained for each participant (X = 82.8, SD = 5.6) and types of aphasia were as follows: anomic (N = 8), conduction (N = 2), Broca's (N = 3), and transcortical motor (N = 7). All participants responded with greater than 90% yes/no reliability on the WAB auditory verbal comprehension subtest, establishing that they were able to reliably respond to yes/no questions. The single word subtests from the Reading Comprehension Battery for Aphasia-2 (RCBA-2: LaPointe & Horner, 1998) were administered to confirm participants' reading ability at this level. The maximum raw score for the three subtests is 30; the cut-off raw score for study participants was 25/30. Participants also completed a lexical decision task (LDT), similar to the experimental LDT, to ensure their ability to adequately read stimuli presented on the computer and respond to whether the letter string represented a word or nonword. All participants responded with 85% or greater accuracy for making the lexical decisions.

The NI participants denied any previous neurological episodes or conditions, and scored 27 or higher on a cognitive screening assessment, the Mini Mental State Examination (MMSE: Folstein, Folstein, & McHugh, 1975) (M = 29.2; SD = 1.1). Table 1 shows demographic and clinical data for the groups.

TABLE 1
Summary of aphasia and NI groups'
demographic and clinical data

	Aphasia group	NI group
Age		
Mean (SD)	65.8 (14.1)	64.3 (13.0)
Range	38–86	42–84
Education		
Mean (SD)	15.1 (2.8)	15.6 (2.9)
Range	10–20	11–20
Months post onset		
Mean (SD)	72.3 (91.9)	
Range	6–341	
WAB AQ		
Mean (SD)	82.8 (5.6)	
Range	71–90	
MMSE		
Mean (SD)		29.2 (1.1)
Range		27–30

NI = neurologically intact; WAB AQ = Western Aphasia Battery Aphasia Quotient (Kertesz, 1982); MMSE = Mini Mental State Examination (Folstein, Folstein, & McHugh, 1975).

Tasks

A cross-modal task (CMT) was the format for sentence pair presentation. Participants listened to sentence pairs, then completed a visual lexical decision task (LDT) following each sentence pair. Sentence pairs consisted of the first sentence, leading the listener to make an initial inference; then a second sentence was presented. Based on the meaning of the second sentence, and in order to successfully comprehend the sentence pair, the listener was required to revise his/her initial inference. For example, in the following sentence pair:

> Bill bumped the car in front of him while going around the curve. At the end of the ride, Bill got out of the bumper car.

the inference initially generated by the listener is that Bill was in a car accident; however, after listening to the second sentence, the listener revises his/her initial interpretation and concludes that Bill was not in an accident, he was on a county fair ride.

Stimuli were the same as in Wright and Newhoff (2002, in press) and consisted of 120 sentence pairs; 80 were sentence pairs requiring an inference revision and 40 were filler sentence pairs. The LDT occurred 750 ms after the sentence pair and possible letter strings included inference revision targets (e.g., *fair*), initial inference targets (e.g., *accident)*, neutral words (e.g., *substantial*), and nonwords (e.g., *akimet*). Participants had 20 opportunities for responding to each of the following: inference revision targets, initial inference targets, and neutral words. Nonwords, equal to the total number of English words, were constructed to follow phonological rules of English.

Following each sentence pair, participants answered four yes/no questions, two factual and two inferencing. In Wright and Newhoff (in press) participants with and without aphasia performed significantly better on the fact questions than inferencing questions. The fact questions were based on explicitly stated information and did not require participants to draw inferences to answer them correctly (e.g., *Was Bill in a bumper car?*). For the present study, we were interested in how participants responded to questions that required generation of an inference. Thus, results are reported for participants' performance on the inferencing questions only. The inferencing questions consisted of one question related to the initial inference (e.g., *Was Bill in an accident?*), and one question related to the inference revision (e.g., *Was Bill at a county fair?*).

Experimental procedures

Participants heard the sentences projected from the speakers of a computer at a volume they confirmed was comfortable. LDT words and nonwords appeared in the centre of the computer screen in lowercase letters. The questions were presented via live voice and participants responded verbally either *yes* or *no* to each question. Participants were given as much time as necessary to answer the questions before the next sentence pair was presented. Order of questions following each sentence pair was randomised across participants.

Participants with aphasia attended two sessions. In their first session, informed consent was obtained and the WAB and RCBA-2 were administered. In the second session, the practice LDT, then practice items that were identical to the experimental task, were completed. The practice stimuli consisted of four inference revision sentence pairs and four questions following each pair. Participants were encouraged to repeat the practice items as many times as necessary until they were comfortable with the task. Following administration of the practice stimuli, three blocks containing 40 sentence pairs each of the CMT were administered. The NI participants completed all their testing in one session. Order of presentation of the three blocks was randomised across participants. Additionally, order of presentation of the questions was randomised following each sentence pair and across participants.

For the CMT, participants were instructed to listen carefully to each sentence pair, and when a letter string appeared on the computer screen, to quickly press the *yes* button if the letter string was an English word, or the *no* button if it was a nonword. The response buttons were the left (*yes*) and right (*no*) buttons of the internal computer mouse, centrally positioned below the keyboard. Participants responded with their dominant hands, or in the case of some of the participants with aphasia, their strongest hand, using a single finger. After each response, participants returned their finger to the same position, which was equidistant from the two response buttons. Participants' accuracy for making the lexical decisions ranged from 9% to 22% items missed (i.e., 1.8–4.4 items missed) for the aphasia group and 3% to 13% items missed (i.e., 0.6–2.6 items missed) for the NI group.

RESULTS

Auditory comprehension: Facilitation

A facilitation effect for auditory comprehension would be assumed to occur if participants answered correctly significantly more questions during the inference revision target condition as compared to the neutral condition. A mixed analysis of variance (ANOVA) of group (NI, aphasia) by question type (initial inference, revised inference) by target condition (inference revision, neutral) was performed. Results indicated significant main effects for group, $F(1, 38) = 24.2$, $p < .0001$, question type, $F(1, 38) = 4.2$, $p < .05$, and target condition, $F(1, 38) = 11.3$, $p < .01$. The group by question type interaction was also significant, $F(1, 38) = 8.0$, $p < .01$. The NI group missed fewer questions than the aphasia group.

Both groups performed better during the inference revision target condition compared to the neutral condition, and these results indicate a facilitation effect for auditory comprehension. Post-hoc analysis of the simple effects indicated that the aphasia group performed better on the initial inferencing questions than the revised inferencing questions, whereas there was no significant difference between response performance on question types for the NI group. Group performances are reported in Table 2.

Auditory comprehension: Interference

An interference effect for comprehending the sentence pairs would be assumed if participants made more errors responding to questions about sentences in the initial inference target condition as compared to the neutral condition. A mixed ANOVA of group by question type by target condition (initial inference, neutral) was performed. Results indicated significant main effects for group, $F(1, 38) = 24.0$, $p < .0001$, and target condition, $F(1, 38) = 10.4$, $p < .01$, as well as significant interactions for group by question type, $F(1, 38) = 8.6$, $p < .01$, and question type by target condition, $F(1, 38) = 7.4$, $p < .01$. The NI group missed fewer questions compared to the aphasia group. Inspection of the target condition main effect indicated that more questions were missed during the initial inference target condition compared to the neutral target condition, demonstrating that the initial inference target interfered with participants' comprehension of the sentence pairs. Post hoc analysis of the simple effects indicated that the aphasia group performed

TABLE 2
Interference revision and neutral conditions

Question types	Aphasia group		NI group	
	Inference revision	Neutral	Inference revision	Neutral
Initial inference				
Mean	16.0	14.9	18.1	17.1
SD	2.4	2.6	1.5	2.3
Inference revision				
Mean	13.7	13.2	18.2	17.7
SD	4.1	3.8	1.8	1.9

Means and standard deviations for correct responses during the inference revision and neutral conditions for the questions related to the initial inference and inference revision for the aphasia and NI groups.
NI = neurologically intact.

TABLE 3
Initial inference and neutral conditions

Question types	Aphasia group		NI group	
	Initial revision	Neutral	Initial revision	Neutral
Initial inference				
Mean	13.7	14.9	15.1	17.1
SD	2.0	2.6	2.8	2.3
Inference revision				
Mean	12.8	13.2	17.3	17.7
SD	3.8	3.8	2.1	1.9

Means and standard deviations for correct responses during the initial inference and neutral conditions for the questions related to the initial inference and inference revision for the aphasia and NI groups.
NI = neurologically intact.

better on the initial inference questions, and there was no significant difference in response performance for the NI group. Group performances are reported in Table 3.

DISCUSSION

The objective of this study was to examine the possible influence of probe placement on comprehension of sentences by individuals who were either aphasic or NI. Specifically, using a cross-modal task, we measured participants' response performance to questions pertaining to initial (incorrect), and revised (correct) inferences as presented in a series of sentence pairs. When the lexical probe represented the revised (intended) interpretation of the sentence pair, participants performed significantly better on the questions as compared to their performance during the neutral condition. Also, participants missed significantly more questions when the lexical probe represented the initial (incorrect) interpretation. We believe these findings are attributable to limitations in allocation of resources and/or reduced working memory capacity.

It is clear from the data that when the lexical probe represented the intended interpretation of a sentence pair, it served as a contextual cue. It has been suggested that linguistic context increases the redundancy of information presented (Hough & Pierce, 1993; Pierce, 1991) and limits the number of plausible outcomes that the listener may derive (Hough et al., 1989). This, in turn, allows for the processing resources available to be adequately distributed to meet the task demands, thereby resulting in better performance. Since adults with aphasia present with reduced processing resources (McNeil, 1981; McNeil et al., 1991), any strategy that may limit the demands on the resources available should result in improved task performance. Generating an initial interpretation then revising it to comprehend the meaning of sentence pairs may have required more processing resources than were available for our participants. However, the contextual cue did function to direct participants to the intended meaning, thus reducing the amount of processing resources needed to generate the correct interpretation; again, resulting in better performance on the comprehension task.

Conversely, during the initial inference condition participants were presented with a lexical probe that represented an incorrect interpretation of the sentence pairs' meanings. Consequently, more questions were missed during this condition. Presenting an alternative choice increased the number of interpretations that the listener generated and it eliminated the opportunity for redundancy of information. Increasing the possible outcome choices and not confirming the interpretation likely increased the demand on the processing resources available. One possibility for the decreased performance during the initial inference condition, then, may be that presentation of the incorrect interpretation required additional processing resources to address it as an outcome, thus overextending the resources available to process and comprehend the sentence pairs.

An alternative, but related, explanation for the results of the study is that processing these sentence pairs exceeded participants' working memory capacity. Researchers have suggested that adults with aphasia present with an impairment in working memory capacity (Caspari, Parkinson, LaPointe, & Katz, 1998; Procter, Wilson, Sanchez, & Wesley, 2000; Ronnberg, Larsson, Fogelsjoo, Nilsson, Lindberg, & Angquist, 1996; Tompkins, Bloise, Timko, & Baumgaertner, 1994). Further, Hough et al. (1997) found differences in performance between older and younger participants with aphasia on a picture-pointing task measuring comprehension of active and passive sentences. These authors attributed the difference to "an age-related impairment in working memory capacity that was overlaid upon their aphasic language deficit" (p. 244). They suggested that their older participants with aphasia evinced an "immediacy effect"; that is, since processing the sentences exceeded their working memory capacity limits, they identified with the last noun heard as the agent of the sentence and performed better on the passive than active sentences.

Possibly our participants experienced an "immediacy effect" as well, although it was not age-dependent. They performed best during the inference revision condition and poorest during the initial inference condition. When the inference revision or initial inference target word was presented, participants identified with it as representing the intended meaning of the sentence pairs. Thus, the lexical probe did not reduce the burden on the participants' working memory capacity for processing the sentence pairs; instead it served as a means for determining the sentence pairs' outcome in spite of the impairment.

Individual participant performance

From our results it does appear that the lexical probes did influence participants' performance on the inferencing questions; however, our participants presented with mild comprehension impairments and performed well on the task during the neutral condition, too. One might argue that the participants did not make large gains in performance as a result of the contextual cue because they were already successful when completing the task during the neutral condition. In past investigations of contextual influences on comprehension performance, NI groups have not been included and the adults with aphasia have presented with more severe comprehension deficits than those in the present study (e.g., Cannito et al., 1986; Hough et al., 1989, 1997). In these earlier works, the influence of linguistic context on comprehension of reversible passive sentences in participants with aphasia has been investigated. It had been shown that adults with aphasia with high comprehension scores do not benefit from prior linguistic context when comprehending these sentence types (Pierce & Beekman, 1985; Pierce & Wagner, 1985). In our study, both the participants with and without aphasia performed similarly on the task. Our findings suggest that participants with aphasia with mild comprehension deficits, as well as the NI participants, benefited from presentation of contextual cues for confirming inferences generated during sentence pair presentation, even when their baseline performance on the task was relatively good.

It might also be argued that, although our results were statistically significant, they do not demonstrate significant gains in performance from a clinical standpoint. When inspecting group means, the adults with and without aphasia responded correctly to approximately one question more during the revised (intended) inference condition and missed approximately one more question during the initial (incorrect) inference condition when compared to the neutral condition; and these results are similar to those found in previous investigations (Boyle & Canter, 1986; Cannito et al., 1986; Hough et al., 1997). The difference, however, still appeared small; so we inspected the data to see how participants performed on the task. Fourteen participants with aphasia responded correctly to more questions during the inference revision condition than the neutral condition; one had an equal number of correct responses in both conditions, and five had more correct responses during the neutral condition. Participants who responded better answered between one and nine more questions correctly during the inference revision condition, whereas those who did better during the neutral condition answered only one to three questions correctly. The NI participants performed as follows: eleven with better performances during the inference revision condition, four with no difference between conditions, and five with better performances during the neutral condition.

When inspecting individual performance during the initial inference condition, ten participants with aphasia missed more of these questions than during the neutral condition, three performed the same in both conditions, and seven performed better during the neutral condition. Although there was greater variability in aphasic individual performances when comparing these conditions, the difference in response performance was not as variable. That is, larger differences were found for those who responded better during the neutral condition than those who responded better during the initial inference condition. The NI participants performed as follows: fifteen performed better during the neutral condition, four performed equally during the initial inference and neutral conditions, and only one performed better during the initial inference condition.

Inspection of the individual data further demonstrates that the intended interpretation did benefit participants' performance on the task; and the initial (incorrect) interpretation hindered their performance on the task. Boyle and Canter (1986) found that their participants, who included individuals with nonfluent and fluent aphasia with good and poor comprehension abilities, performed significantly better when linguistic context preceded the target sentence than when the target sentence was in isolation. However, only 19 of their 36 participants demonstrated better performance during the contextual condition. From our results, it appears that adults presenting with mild-to-moderate aphasia do respond well to lexical probes; future investigations are warranted to determine if adults with more severe aphasia presentations benefit from this type of contextual cue for generating inferences during sentence and discourse processing.

Conclusion and clinical implications

In summary, the results of our study indicate that the type of probe presented influences comprehension performance by adults with and without aphasia. Possibly, the presence of the inference revision target probe allowed participants to overcome limitations in working memory capacity or processing resources available to complete the task; whereas the initial inference target probe overextended participants' working memory capacity limits or available processing resources. However, our conclusions should be interpreted cautiously because we did not include a measure of participants' working memory capacity. Future studies might further investigate the effect of resource allocation and working memory capacity deficits on discourse processing to determine their influence or role in language abilities of adults with aphasia. Thus, future investigations should include a measure of participants' working memory capacity. In terms of clinical applicability, Cannito et al. (1996) suggested using narrative contexts as a clinical tool for facilitating comprehension abilities of individuals with aphasia. Providing participants with lexical contextual cues, such as words related to the intended meaning or gist of a sentence or narrative, may also serve as a clinical tool to facilitate comprehension at sentence and discourse levels.

REFERENCES

Boyle, M., & Canter, G. J. (1986). Verbal context and comprehension of difficult sentences by aphasic adults: A methodological problem. *Clinical Aphasiology: Proceedings of the Conference, 16*, 38–44.

Brookshire, R. H., & Nicholas, L. E. (1984). Comprehension of directly and indirectly stated main ideas and details in discourse by brain-damaged and non-brain-damaged listeners. *Brain and Language, 21*, 21–36.

Cannito, M. P., Hough, M., Vogel, D., & Pierce, R. S. (1996). Contextual influences on auditory comprehension of reversible passive sentences in aphasia. *Aphasiology, 10*(3), 235–251.

Cannito, M. P., Jarecki, J. M., & Pierce, R. S. (1986). Effects of thematic structure on syntactic comprehension in aphasia. *Brain and Language, 27*, 38–49.

Caspari, I., Parkinson, S. R., LaPointe, L. L., & Katz, R. C. (1998). Working memory and aphasia. *Brain and Cognition, 37*, 205–223.

Folstein, J. A., Folstein, S. E., & McHugh, P. R. (1975). ''Mini-Mental State'': A practical method for grading the mental state for the clinician. *Journal of Psychiatric Research, 12*, 189–198.

Germani, M. J., & Pierce, R. S. (1992). Contextual influences in reading comprehension in aphasia. *Brain and Language, 42*, 308–319.

Hough, M. S., & Pierce, R. S. (1993). Contextual and thematic influences on narrative comprehension of left and right hemisphere brain-damaged adults. In H. Brownell & Y. Joanette (Eds.), *Narrative discourse in normal aging and neurologically-impaired adults* (pp. 213–238). San Diego, CA: Singular Publishing Group.

Hough, M. S., Pierce, R. S., & Cannito, M. P. (1989). Contextual influences in aphasia: Effects of predictive versus nonpredictive narratives. *Brain and Language, 36*, 325–334.

Hough, M. S., Vogel, D., Cannito, M. P., & Pierce, R. S. (1997). Influence of prior pictorial context on sentence comprehension in older versus younger aphasic subjects. *Aphasiology, 11*(3), 235–247.

Kertesz, A. (1982). *Western Aphasia Battery.* New York: Grune & Stratton.

Kintsch, W. (1998). *Comprehension: A paradigm for cognition.* New York: Cambridge University Press.

LaPointe, L. L., & Horner, J. (1998). *Reading Comprehension Battery for Aphasia-2.* Austin, TX: Pro-Ed.

Long, D. L., Oppy, B. J., & Seely, M. R. (1994). Individual differences in the time course of inferential processing. *Journal of Experimental Psychology: Learning, Memory, and Cognition, 20*(6), 1456–1470.

McNeil, M .R. (1981). Auditory comprehension in aphasia: A language deficit or reduced efficiency of processing supporting language? *Clinical Aphasiology, 10*, 342–345.

McNeil, M. R., Odell, K., & Tseng, C. H. (1991). Toward the integration of resource allocation into a general theory of aphasia. *Clinical Aphasiology, 20*, 21–39.

Miyake, A., Carpenter, P. A., & Just, M. A. (1994). A capacity approach to syntactic comprehension disorders: Making normal adults perform like aphasic patients. *Cognitive Neuropsychology, 11*, 671–717.

Miyake, A., Carpenter, P. A., & Just, M. A. (1995). Reduced resources and specific impairments in normal and aphasic sentence comprehension. *Cognitive Neuropsychology, 12*, 651–679.

Pierce, R. S. (1991). Contextual influences during comprehension in aphasia. *Aphasiology, 5*(4–5), 379–381.

Pierce, R. S., & Beekman, L. (1985). Effects of linguistic and extralinguistic context on semantic and syntactic processing in aphasia. *Journal of Speech and Hearing Research, 28*, 250–254.

Pierce, R. S., & Wagner, C. (1985). The role of context in facilitating syntactic decoding in aphasia. *Journal of Communication Disorders, 18*, 203–214.

Procter, A., Wilson, B., Sanchez, C., & Wesley, E. (2000). Evaluation of attention process training and brain injury education in persons with acquired brain injury. *Brain Injury, 14*(7), 633–647.

Ronnberg, J., Larsson, C., Fogelsjoo, A., Nilsson, L., Lindberg, M., & Angquist, K. (1996). Memory dysfunction in mild aphasics. *Scandinavian Journal of Psychology, 37*, 46–61.

Till, R. E., Mross, E. F., & Kintsch, W. (1988). Time course of priming for associate and inference words in a discourse context. *Memory and Cognition, 4*, 283–298.

Tompkins, C. A., Bloise, C. G. R., Timko, M. L., & Baumgaertner, A. (1994). Working memory and inference revision in brain-damaged and normally aging adults. *Journal of Speech and Hearing Research, 37*, 896–912.

Wright, H. H., & Newhoff, M. (in press). Inference revision processing in adults with and without aphasia. *Brain and Language.*

Wright, H. H., & Newhoff, M. (2002). Age-related differences in inference revision processing. *Brain and Language, 80*, 226–239.

APHASIOLOGY, 2004, *18* (5/6/7), 567–579

Confrontation naming and semantic relatedness judgements in Spanish/English bilinguals

Lisa A. Edmonds and Swathi Kiran

University of Texas at Austin, USA

Background: The results of many current studies on naming in bilingualism have provided converging evidence for a semantic representation common to both languages within a bilingual individual. However, the interaction between lexical access and semantic representation in bilinguals is relatively unclear.

Aims: To further understand this relationship in normal bilingual individuals, we asked the following questions: (1) Is there homogeneity in naming accuracy for both languages across subjects? We predicted that naming accuracy would differ across subjects based on their proficiency levels in each language. (2) After separating subjects into groups based on their proficiency levels (balanced, Spanish dominant, English dominant), is there a difference in their mean ratings of the semantic similarity of word pairs across proficiency groups? According to the mixed model (De Groot, Dannenburg, & van Hell, 1994), it was predicted that similar mean ratings would be observed across all groups.

Methods & Procedures: A total of 23 Spanish/English bilinguals (average age = 35.5 years) completed a confrontation naming task and a semantic relatedness questionnaire in both languages. The same set of stimuli, controlled for various factors, was used for each task in both languages and counterbalanced by language across two sessions. Based on naming performances, participants were assigned to the balanced bilingual (N = 10), English dominant (N = 10), or Spanish dominant (N = 3) group (Kohnert, Hernandez, & Bates, 1998).

Outcomes & Results: Overall English mean correct was 94.29%; Spanish was 88.19%. Significant differences in naming were seen between groups, $F(2, 85)$ = 4.3, p = .01, and within the language dominant groups across subjects ($p < .05$) and items ($p < .05$). On the semantic relatedness task, no significant difference was observed between the ratings of word pairs in each language across participants or items in any group.

Conclusions: Despite differences in lexical access, participants in all proficiency groups rated word pairs similarly, indicating a shared semantic representation for both languages. The mixed model (de Groot et al., 1994) can explain the findings for all groups. Results of this study have clinical implications for bilingual aphasic patients. It is imperative to ascertain a patient's pre-morbid language use prior to brain damage in order to gauge pre-morbid proficiencies. Treatment should consider proficiency levels in both languages, with consideration that the strength of connections between each lexicon and from each lexicon to semantic memory may differ.

As the number of Spanish/English bilinguals in the United States increases, it is imperative that research be focused on the fundamental aspects of cognition and language in bilingualism. This information is necessary to assess and treat acquired disorders of language and cognition in bilingual adults, especially among the elderly Hispanic

---

Address correspondence to: Lisa A. Edmonds, Department of Communication Sciences and Disorders, Jones Communication Building, CMA A2.200, Mail Code A1100, The University of Texas at Austin, Austin, TX 78712-1094, USA. Email: lisaedmonds@mail.utexas.edu

http://www.tandf.co.uk/journals/pp/02687038.html   DOI:10.1080/02687030444000057

population, which is the fastest growing ethnic minority in the United States (ASHA, 1989, 1991). Naming deficits are the most common characteristic in all types of aphasia (Goodglass, 1998), and they are often the first language deficit detected in early Alzheimer's disease. In order to assess and treat naming deficits, it is crucial to understand the organisation, relationship, and processing within and between the lexicons of bilingual adults.

Evidence from numerous experimental sources reveals that the two languages of a bilingual individual access a common semantic network (Francis, 1999). Semantic comparisons between words of different languages have been shown to take *no longer* than comparisons between words in the same language, suggesting integration of semantic information between languages (Dufour & Kroll, 1995; Potter, So, vonEckardt, & Fedlman, 1984). Similarly, cross-language categorisation experiments have found that bilinguals show no difference in reaction times within and across language conditions (Caramazza & Brones, 1980; Potter et al., 1984). It has also been demonstrated through picture–word interference studies that words in the non-target language are active during production of words in the target language (Herman, Bongarts, De Bot, & Schreuder, 1998).

In addition to behavioural studies, neuroimaging studies utilising various semantic processing paradigms have demonstrated similar cortical localisation of activation for L1 and L2 languages (e.g., Chee, Tan, & Thiel, 1999; Hernandez, Dapretto, Mazziotta, & Bookheimer, 2001; Illes et al., 1999; Klein, Milner, Zatorre, Meyer, & Evans, 1995; Perani et al., 1996; Wartenburger, Heekeren, Abutalebi, Cappa, Villringer, & Perani, D., 2003).

While there appears to be converging evidence for a semantic representation that is common to both languages in a bilingual individual, the mechanism of phonological access of lexical items across two languages appears less evident (but see Roelofs, 2003, for a detailed investigation of phonological planning in Dutch/English unbalanced bilingual adults, and Pallier, Colomé, & Sebastián-Gallés, 2001, for a discussion of the influence of native-language phonology on lexical access in highly fluent Catalan/ Spanish bilinguals).

A few studies have investigated lexical access in bilingual adults using naming tasks. Roberts and Deslauriers (1999) investigated naming of cognates and noncognates in French/English normal and aphasic bilinguals, with the hypothesis that phonetic similarity of cognates would facilitate naming across languages. However, in general, they did not find significantly higher naming of cognates over noncognates. Kohnert, Bates, and Hernandez (1999) conducted timed naming tasks on Spanish/English bilinguals from age 5 through college. All subjects had learned English as a second language at school between ages 4 and 6. Based on accuracy and reaction times in naming, they found a gradual dominance shift to English culminating by college age. Kohnert et al. (1998) also tested 100 young, educated Mexican-American Spanish/English bilingual adults who learned both languages before age 8 on the Boston Naming Test (BNT) (Kaplan, Goodglass, & Weintraub, 1983). They found that 75% of their participants named fewer pictures in Spanish than in English, and the progression of difficultly on the BNT normally seen in English monolinguals was not evident in Spanish. In both of these studies, the authors argue that age of acquisition is less important a factor in proficiency than use, and that the critical period theories for language learning may be over-simplified. In an attempt to evaluate the performance of other bilingual groups on the BNT, Roberts, Garcia, Desrochers, and Hernandez (2002) tested English monolingual, Spanish/English bilingual, and French/English bilingual groups. The English group served as a control group that the Kohnert et al. (1998) study did not have. They found that the bilingual groups scored significantly lower than the monolingual group in English.

Most naming studies with bilingual adults aim to establish normative data (e.g., Kohnert et al., 1998; Kremin et al., 2003; Roberts et al., 2002), and they are not directed at answering theoretical questions about naming. Further, interpretation of the data is occasionally difficult based on what authors have reported. For example, Roberts et al. (2002) did not report within-group differences in naming across languages. Roberts and Deslauriers (1999), unlike Kohnert et al. (1998), did not separate the bilingual groups into categories of dominance, as the authors assumed a certain degree of equal proficiency based on questionnaires given to the participants regarding language use. Further, the authors did not report how each bilingual group performed across languages, and they only tested two semantic categories of words.

Numerous models have been proposed to explain semantic representation and access of lexical items between two languages (L1 and L2). The word association model, first described by Potter et al. (1984), assumes that second language words (L2) gain access to concepts only through first language mediation (L1). This model predicts that translation from L1 to L2 will be faster than picture naming in L2, because translation from L1 to L2 relies on the lexical links and can thus bypass conceptual access. In contrast, the concept mediation model (Potter et al., 1984) proposes that second language words directly access concepts, and predicts that translation from L1 to L2 and picture naming in L2 should be similar because both require conceptual access prior to the retrieval of L2 lexical items. Potter et al. (1984) investigated translation and picture naming in a group of fluent Chinese/English bilinguals and found that the times to translate from L1 to L2 and to name pictures in L2 were very similar, thus providing support for the concept mediation model. However, application of these models to groups of bilingual adults depends on respective proficiency in each language. For instance, Kroll and Curley (1988) performed a similar task as Potter et al. (1984) with bilinguals with low and high L2 proficiency, and they observed evidence for the word association model in the low-proficiency bilinguals as well as evidence for the concept mediation model in the high-proficiency bilinguals.

The revised hierarchical model proposed by Kroll and Stewart (1990, 1994) includes connections between both L1 and L2 and the central concept. However, the links differ in their strengths as a function of proficiency in L1 relative to L2. Therefore, L1 presumably has a larger lexicon than L2, and lexical associations from L2 to L1 are assumed to be stronger than those from L1 to L2. Further, the links between words and concepts are assumed to be stronger for L1 than for L2. Kroll and Stewart provide support for the revised hierarchical model from observations of increased latencies when translating from L1 to L2 than vice versa, and shorter latencies when translating categorised lists versus randomised lists from L1 to L2. They infer from the data that a longer latency implies that the translation is being moderated by conceptual memory, whereas shorter latencies imply a direct translation between lexicons.

Finally, de Groot (1992) proposed the mixed model, which combines the word association and concept mediation models. This model argues that the lexicons of a bilingual are directly connected to each other as well as indirectly connected by way of a shared semantic representation. However, de Groot (1992) based her theory on forward translation (L1 to L2) only in L1 dominant subjects. Therefore, in a follow-up study De Groot et al. (1994) examined forward and backward translation with six predictor variables (imageability, context availability, definition accuracy, familiarity, word frequency, and length) in two Dutch/English bilingual groups that differed in L2 proficiency. Results revealed a significant effect of imageability on forward translation, implying semantic mediation, and a smaller effect of imageability on backward translation. Therefore, while de Groot et al. (1994) agree that the data support a weak version of the asymmetrical model (direct and strong L2 to L1 link in backward translation without concept mediation), they argue for the mixed model since this model predicts concept mediated backward translation, but with less "strength" in the link from L2 to conceptual memory than L1 to conceptual memory.

In order to further understand the relationship between lexical access and semantic representation in bilingual adults, the present study investigated the relationship between oral confrontation naming and semantic representation in bilingual adults by using the same set of stimuli for both tasks. Semantic representation was evaluated by semantic relatedness ratings of pairs of words in English and Spanish in order to discern if there are differences in how bilinguals "conceptualise" word pairs in each of their respective languages. This task was chosen because we believed that there would be a ceiling effect in a semantic categorisation task and because a semantic relatedness judgement task would require the subjects to extract features from pairs of items being compared. Although both experiments were untimed, we predicted the results to be accounted for by the general predictions of de Groot's mixed model (de Groot et al., 1994). Further, the results of our experiment were expected to provide a theoretical basis to guide treatment methods for bilingual individuals with aphasia.

All of the participants learned both languages before age 10 and described themselves as functionally bilingual. However, due to the existing nature of variability within bilinguals, we categorised our participants into three dominance groups based on their naming performance in each language using the methods of Kohnert et al. (1998). We then examined the relationship between lexical access (through oral naming) and semantic processing (through semantic relatedness ratings) across the three groups. The following were our research questions and predictions.

1. Is there homogeneity in naming accuracy for both languages across subjects? We predicted that naming accuracy would not be homogeneous between subjects based on their proficiency levels in each language. Based on their naming accuracy in both languages, subjects would be assigned to one of three groups: balanced bilingual, English dominant, or Spanish dominant (Kohnert et al., 1998).

2. Is there a difference in semantic relatedness judgements across languages as measured by mean ratings of word pairs in English and Spanish in any of the proficiency groups? According to the mixed model, it was predicted that similar mean ratings on word pairs would be observed across all groups since L1 and L2 both have links to a shared conceptual memory. However, if differences between word pair ratings are observed, we would predict these differences to occur in the language dominant groups, since the strengths of the links between L1 and conceptual memory and L2 and conceptual memory would theoretically be different in these groups. Any significant differences in mean ratings of word pairs across languages for the dominant groups would have to be reconciled by alternative bilingual language processing models, such as the asymmetrical model (Kroll & Stewart, 1990, 1994).

METHOD

Participants

A total of 23 Spanish/English normal bilingual individuals ranging in age from 22 to 71 years (average = 35.5; SD = 14.2) participated in the study. All participants had normal or corrected to normal vision and normal hearing. They all had at least a high-school degree with a mean education of 15.6 years (SD = 2.01). Exclusionary criteria included neurological disorders such as stroke, transient ischaemic attacks, Parkinson's disease, Alzheimer's disease, psychological illness, learning disability/dyslexia, seizures, and attention deficit disorder. All participants learned English ($Mean$ = 3.3 years; SD = 3.3) and Spanish ($Mean$ = 0.6; SD = 1.7) before the age of 10 years and described themselves as "functionally bilingual". In order to characterise language use and proficiency further, participants filled out a language usage questionnaire (Muñoz, Marquardt, & Copeland, 1999) during their first session that asked questions about usage and self-evaluation of their language skills. See Table 1 for further description of participants.

Stimuli

Oral naming and semantic relatedness judgement tasks were developed for this experiment. We expected the participants to perform at near 100% accuracy levels on a semantic processing task such as semantic matching, which would make it difficult to discern differences in semantic processing within the different proficiency groups.

TABLE 1
Participant information

Subject	Gender	Age	Years ed	Age learned English	Age learned Spanish	Eng-S	Eng-C	Span-S	Span-C
1	F	22	15	0	0	7	7	6	6
2	F	23	17	0	0	7	7	6	7
3	F	33	15	3	0	7	7	7	7
4	F	46	16	4	0	7	7	6	6
5	F	38	16	0	0	7	7	7	7
6	F	24	15	6	0	7	7	7	7
7	F	24	18	3	0	7	7	6	7
8	M	29	12	0	5	7	7	6	6
9	F	37	14	3	0	7	7	6	7
10	F	59	12	4	0	7	7	7	7
11	M	35	16	8	0	5	6	7	7
12	F	23	17	10	0	7	7	6	7
13	F	22	16	5.5	0	7	7	7	7
14	F	71	16	8.5	0	7	7	7	7
15	F	50	18	0	0	7	7	7	7
16	F	23	17	9	0	6	6	7	7
17	F	49	16	0	5	7	7	7	7
18	F	21	14	5	0	6	7	5	6
19	M	58	12	0	5	7	7	7	7
20	F	23	17	0	0	5	5	7	7
21	F	42	20	0	0	7	7	6	7
22	M	35	14	0	0	7	7	7	7
23	F	30	17	6	0	5	5	7	7
	Average	35.52	15.65	3.26	0.65	6.65	6.74	6.56	6.83
	SD	14.17	2.01	3.35	1.68	0.71	0.62	0.59	0.39

Eng-S = Self-ratings of English speaking in informal situations. Eng-C = Self-ratings of English comprehension in informal situations. Span-S = Self-ratings of Spanish speaking in informal situations. Span-C = Self-ratings of comprehension of Spanish informal situations.

Further, we wanted the subjects to engage in a task that involved extracting semantic information and using it to make semantic decisions. Finally, the results of our experiment were expected to provide a theoretical basis to guide treatment methods for bilingual individuals with aphasia. Therefore, we administered a semantic relatedness judgement task in each language to investigate the degree to which participants rated the similarity in meaning of two related items.

From an original corpus of 200 words that varied across semantic categories, 150 were selected based on the following criteria. Cognates (e.g., *elephant* and *elefante*) and words with at least 50% phonetic similarity (e.g., *cat* and *gato*) were eliminated from the set to avoid facilitation of naming across languages. Words between one and four syllables (English average = 1.53; Spanish = 2.58) were then chosen. Finally, high to moderate frequency words were selected in each language (English = 5 or higher, Spanish = 3 or higher; Frances & Kučera, 1982; Juilland & Chang-Rodriguez, 1964; respectively) such that the average frequency for both languages (English = 53.86, SD = 107.35; Spanish = 58.50, SD = 126.47) was matched as determined by a paired t-test (t = 0.707; p = .480). Colour pictures were chosen from Art Explosion Software® (NOVA Inc), modified to equal approximately 4 × 6 inches, and centred on 8 × 11 inch white paper. Two sets of stimuli were prepared, one for each language, and placed in a binder with the pictures in a pseudorandomised order controlled to avoid more than two consecutive examples from the same category (e.g., *table* could not follow *chair*).

The semantic relatedness task employed the same stimuli as the oral naming task. Each of the 150 words was paired with another word from the same list. The word pairs were either category coordinates (e.g., *apple* and *orange*) or word associations (e.g., *soap* and *razor*), so were intended to be similar in meaning. In order to create more semantic variation in pairs, some words were used more than once, resulting in 157 pairs of words. All word pairs were typed onto a sheet and a 4-point rating scale where "1" (indicating "very similar") and "4" (indicating "not similar") was typed beneath each word pair. The questionnaire was 11 pages long with approximately 1.5 spaces between each pair of words.

Procedures

Both the naming and the semantic relatedness tasks were conducted across two sessions that were at least 1 day apart, with the order of language counterbalanced across participants. First the naming task was conducted. Participants were required to name each picture with no feedback provided. After naming the pictures, each participant completed a semantic relatedness questionnaire in the same language as the naming task to avoid cross-linguistic interference. For this task, participants were required to rate how similar they considered the meanings of pairs of words on a scale of 1 ("very similar") to 4 ("not similar") by circling the appropriate number. The directions written on the top of the first page were as follows: "*For this task, you need to make decisions about pairs of words. Please look at each pair of words and decide how similar the words are in meaning. If you do not know a word, cross it out and do not do anything else with that pair of words.*" The Spanish version had a translation of these directions. The directions were also provided verbally with an example, and participants were instructed to ask questions if they did not understand the task.

Scoring

For the naming task, the total number of pictures named correctly in each language was calculated. Responses were considered incorrect if they could not be found in an English or a Spanish dictionary with an appropriate definition or in a bilingual dictionary with an appropriate translation. Further, alternative responses reflecting dialectal or acceptable lexical variations in Spanish were credited (e.g., *cerillas* and *fósforos* were both accepted for *matches*). For the semantic relatedness task, only word pairs that were rated were calculated.

RESULTS

Grouping of participants

Based on their naming performances, participants were divided into three groups: balanced bilingual ($N = 10$), English dominant ($N = 10$), and Spanish dominant ($N = 3$). Dominance for each subject was calculated by comparing the difference between their naming performance in both languages against the mean difference in naming for all of the participants (*Mean* = 6.1) (Kohnert et al., 1998). Participants more than one standard deviation from the mean were deemed dominant in the language with the higher naming score. For example, participant 13 was deemed English dominant because she achieved 98% accuracy in English and 90.6% accuracy in Spanish, a difference of 7.4. See Table 2 for groupings and scores.

Naming accuracy

A 3×2 ANOVA on the naming accuracy revealed a significant main effect only for group, $F(2, 85) = 4.3$, $p = .01$. A Bonferroni post-hoc analysis across groups revealed a significant difference between the balanced bilingual and the Spanish dominant group ($p < .001$) and the English dominant and Spanish dominant group ($p < .001$). These results were expected, since groups were composed based on the naming performance of the participants. Interaction effects were not pursued because the interaction between the groups was not the point of this study.

Data for the groups were then separated and analysed with paired t-tests to determine if there were differences in naming across participants and items (subject and item analyses). No significant difference was found between English and Spanish naming on the subject analysis in the balanced bilingual group ($t = 1.60$; $p = .130$), but there was a significant difference between English and Spanish naming in the English dominant ($t = 5.69$; $p < .001$) and Spanish dominant groups ($t = 4.74$; $p = .009$, see Figure 1a). Next, paired t-tests were performed on each group to see if there were any differences in naming across items for both languages. The results showed that naming accuracy across both languages was significantly different across items for the English dominant, $t(149) = 8.13$, $p < .05$, and Spanish dominant groups, $t(149) = 5.64$, $p < .05$. These results are consistent with the naming across participants results for each group. There was also a significant difference across items for the balanced bilingual group, $t(149) = 2.59$, $p < .05$. Given that the overall means for naming accuracy were close (English *Mean* = 96.25; $SD = 9.19$, Spanish *Mean* = 94.14, $SD = 11.36$), this inconsistent finding appears to be due to a few items consistently named incorrectly in Spanish.

Semantic relatedness judgements

Participants were instructed to avoid rating word pairs for which they did not recognise one or both words, resulting in elimination of less than .1% of the word pairs from the data set. A 3×2 ANOVA on the remaining ratings indicated an overall significant main effect only for group, $F(2, 892) = 8.00$, $p = .0001$. A Bonferroni post hoc analysis

TABLE 2
Naming accuracy for all three groups

Balanced bilingual group				English dominant group				Spanish dominant group			
Subject #	English naming %	Spanish naming %	/E/-/S/	Subject #	English naming %	Spanish naming %	/E/-/S/	Subject #	English naming %	Spanish naming %	/E/-/S/
5	98.6	98.6	0	1	98	63.3	34.7	11	76	90.6	14.6
6	92.6	90	2.6	2	96.6	70.6	26	20	82	96.6	14.6
9	98.6	96.6	2	3	98.6	84.6	14	23	83.3	95.3	12
12	96	90	6	4	99.3	91.3	8				
14	91.3	90	1.3	7	95.3	80	15.3				
15	98.6	97.3	1.3	8	93.3	75.3	18				
16	94	93.3	0.7	10	96	86.6	9.4				
17	98.6	96	2.6	13	98	90.6	7.4				
19	96.6	94	2.6	18	96	81.3	14.7				
22	95.3	93.3	2	21	98	83.3	14.7				
Average	96.02	93.91	2.11	Average	96.91	80.69	16.22	Average	80.43	94.17	13.73
SD	2.70	3.19	0.49	SD	1.81	8.83	7.02	SD	3.89	3.16	0.74

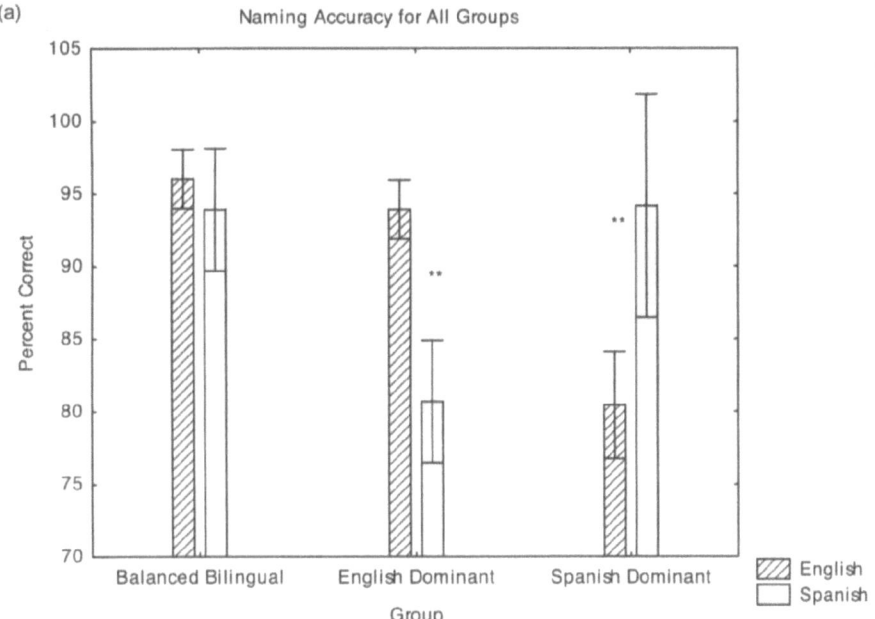

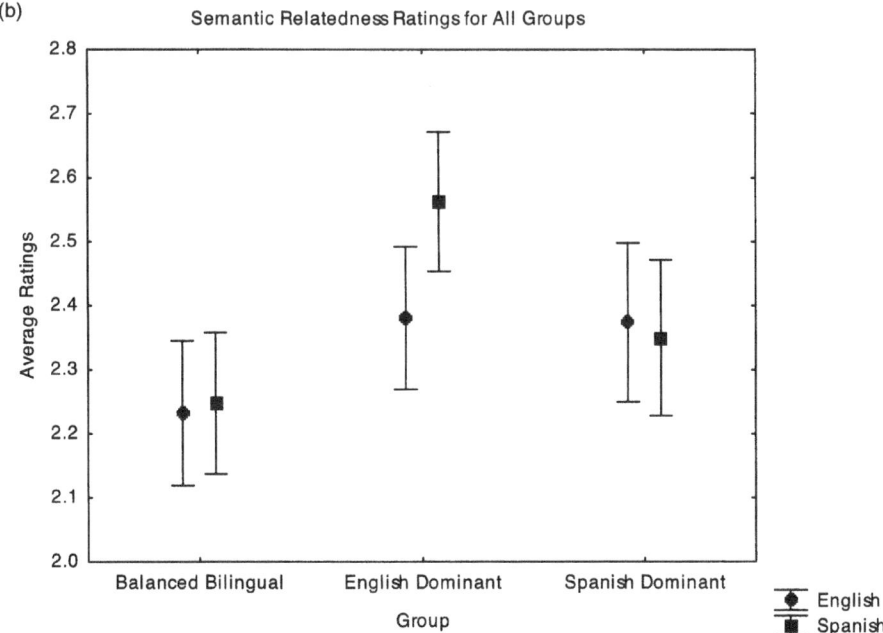

Figure 1. (a) Naming accuracy for all groups across participants. ** indicates $p < .0001$ significance. (b) Semantic relatedness judgements across items for all groups.

revealed that there was a significant difference in rating between the balanced bilingual group and the English dominant (p = .00421) and balanced bilingual group and Spanish dominant group (p < .001). In other words, the balanced bilingual group rated word pairs in English and Spanish significantly lower (more alike) than both the English and Spanish dominant groups. Implications for these findings will be explored in the Discussion.

Data for the three groups were then separated and analysed with a paired t-test to determine if there was a difference in ratings between languages across participants and items (subject and item analysis). The results showed that there was no significant difference between languages on the subject analysis in any group—balanced bilingual: $t(9)$ = 0.48, p = .64; English dominant: $t(9)$ = 0.39, p = .71; Spanish dominant: $t(2)$ = 1.57, p = .26. Further, on the item analysis, no significant difference between English and Spanish semantic ratings was noted within any group—balanced bilingual: $t(138)$ = 0.77, p = .44; English dominant: $t(123)$ = 0.65, p = .51; Spanish dominant: $t(136)$ = 0.85, p = .39; see Figure 1b. Assuming that the semantic relatedness judgements are a reflection of semantic representation (albeit a less sensitive measure than online measures), non-significant differences in ratings across participants within each group seem to indicate that semantic representation of both languages is shared across participants.

Self-rating across groups

The self-rating scores that the participants gave themselves on their speaking and comprehension abilities in both languages were also analysed. Two 3×2 ANOVAs across groups revealed overall significant main effects for group differences in self-ratings for production, $F(4, 38)$ = 19.13, p < .001, and comprehension, $F(4, 38)$ = 15.21, p < .001. A Bonferroni post-hoc analysis for both production and comprehension revealed a significant difference in ratings between the balanced bilingual and Spanish dominant group (p < .001) and the English dominant and Spanish dominant group (p < .001). Thus, the subjects' self-ratings reflected their naming abilities in both languages. This appears to indicate that naming tasks may be a good indicator of overall language proficiency, and also that bilingual adults provide accurate information regarding their linguistic abilities in both languages.

DISCUSSION

The present experiment investigated the relationship between oral picture naming and semantic relatedness judgements on the same set of stimuli across two languages in normal bilingual adults. Based on naming performance, three groups with significantly different proficiency profiles emerged: balanced bilingual, English dominant, and Spanish dominant. Overall, the balanced bilingual group showed no difference in naming across languages. However, the English dominant group named better in English than in Spanish, and the Spanish dominant group named better in Spanish than in English.

On the semantic rating task, there was a significant difference in ratings between the balanced bilingual group and both other groups, with the balanced bilingual group rating word pairs as more alike in both English and Spanish as compared to the English and Spanish dominant groups. A notable finding was that, unlike the naming results within each group, no significant differences were observed between English and Spanish word-pair ratings for any group across participants or items. These results are particularly striking because they seem to indicate that the participants conceptualised the items in both languages similarly. Assuming that the semantic relatedness judgement task measures semantic representation, since participants were forced to extract semantic information about the two words that they were instructed to compare, then the results seem to indicate that there is a shared semantic representation for both languages for all groups *despite* differences in naming abilities (lexical access) and proficiency in each language. Further, the self-rating scores that the participants gave themselves on their English and Spanish speaking abilities revealed a significant difference in ratings between the three groups. These differences reflected the dissimilarity observed in naming abilities across groups. Thus, self-rating questionnaires may provide useful information related to proficiency.

To summarise, findings from this study indicate that despite differential access for naming of L1 and L2 across languages, semantic representation (concepts) is the same in English and Spanish for normal adult bilinguals. Specifically, we found that the English dominant group demonstrated superior naming in English compared to Spanish, while the Spanish dominant group demonstrated superior naming in Spanish compared to English. However, despite these differences, we found no significant difference in rating the semantic relatedness of word pairs within any group. Therefore, it can be surmised that even though there may be a wide variation in proficiency within bilinguals who learn both languages before age 10, this variation does not seem to affect a shared semantic representation between their two lexicons.

As hypothesised in the introduction, the findings of this experiment can be explained by de Groot's mixed model (1994). This model predicts that each lexicon is connected directly to a shared representation in conceptual memory as well as by a direct connection between the two lexicons. Further, the model predicts that the strength of the weight from L2 to conceptual memory is weaker than that from L1. This premise would explain both the findings of the current study—namely (a) lexical access or naming is weaker in L2 than in L1 and (b) semantic representations from a shared conceptual memory (as measured by semantic feature extraction and similarity ratings for word pairs) are similar between L2 and L1 for all bilingual groups. Further, the model would also account for the non-significant but notable differences in the mean ratings between English (*Mean* = 2.38) and Spanish (*Mean* = 2.56) in the English dominant group. In other words, the English dominant group rated word pairs more similarly in their dominant language (L1) than in L2, suggesting a "stronger" connection between L1 to conceptual memory than from L2 to conceptual memory.

An alternative explanation for the results can be provided by the asymmetrical model proposed by Kroll and Stewart (1994). This model argues for a stronger link from L2 to L1 and a weak connection between L2 and the shared conceptual system, and thus would predict that semantic relatedness judgements would be mediated by L1 for both languages. This premise would account for the similar semantic judgements in the dominant groups but may imply that participants in the dominant groups translated the word pairs in the weaker language into their stronger language in order to make judgements (since the link from L2 to L1 is stronger than that between L2 and conceptual memory in this model). However, this model cannot satisfactorily explain the findings of the balanced bilingual group, where mean semantic ratings for English (*Mean* = 2.23) and Spanish (*Mean* = 2.24) were almost identical.

A more parsimonious explanation for all three subject groups can be obtained from de Groot's mixed model (1992, 1994), since this model would suggest the weighted connection between L2 and conceptual memory falls along a continuum determined by L2 proficiency. Therefore, in balanced bilingual individuals, L2 and L1 connections to conceptual memory are equally weighted, whereas in L1 dominant groups, the L2 connections to conceptual memory can be weighted lesser than the L1 connections to conceptual memory.

The data in the current study provide further empirical support for the increasing notion that the frequency of usage, and not age of acquisition, more accurately describes bilingual proficiency. For example, the three Spanish dominant participants in the present study were born in Spanish-speaking countries and spoke Spanish at home, but learned English in school and used English in addition to Spanish on a fairly regular basis. These participants are currently students and have been in the United States for 2–3 years. This profile is distinctly different from the subjects in the English dominant group, who were primarily born and educated in the United States, so their English usage has been much higher than their Spanish usage despite using Spanish at home as children. The majority of the participants in the balanced bilingual group, by contrast, were professional translators and bilingual teachers whose work involves switching between both languages simultaneously on a regular basis. Therefore, it seems that language proficiencies are clearly on a continuum and are not static, and one of the strongest factors influencing proficiency is language usage. Support for this premise also comes from Kohnert et al. (1998, 1999) who propose that continued language use may be more important for L1 and L2 proficiency than factors such as age of acquisition, which is often of main concern in critical period theories of second language learning.

Further investigation is needed on other groups of bilingual adults, including proficient bilinguals that learned L2 after age 10. In addition, the present study was restricted to high- to mid-frequency concrete words. Less frequent and abstract words also need to be evaluated in order to have a more complete picture of the relationship between lexical access and semantic representation. Finally, other measures of semantic representation, including online measures, are needed to replicate the present findings.

Results of the present study have clear clinical implications for bilingual patients with aphasia. First, during the case history it is imperative to ascertain a patient's amount of usage in each language *immediately prior* to brain damage in order to gauge pre-morbid proficiency in each language. In addition, interpretation of test results should account for prior proficiency so that a lower score in one language is not necessarily interpreted as a deficit due to brain damage. Further, treatment should take into account proficiency level in both languages, with consideration that both lexicons most likely share a semantic representation but the strengths of the connections between each lexicon and semantic representation may differ based on proficiency. Therefore, a semantic approach to naming may improve the target in both languages if it were only remediated in one, assuming that the strength of the connection between semantic memory and the untreated language is strong enough to support the generalisation. If not, direct translation treatment may be needed in order to mediate through the dominant language. We recognise that this method is not the most efficient, and are currently investigating the most efficient manner in which to treat naming deficits in bilingual people with aphasia.

REFERENCES

American Speech-Language-Hearing Association. (1989). *Office of minority concerns newsletter, 10*(1). Rockville, MD: American Speech-Language-Hearing Association.

American Speech-Language-Hearing Association. (1991). Cultural diversity in the elderly population. *ASHA, 33. 66.10* (1). Rockville, MD: American Speech-Language-Hearing Association.

Caramazza, A., & Brones, I. (1980). Semantic classification by bilinguals. *Canadian Journal of Psychology, 34,* 77–81.

Chee, M. W. L., Tan, E. W. L., & Thiel, T. (1999). Mandarin and English single word processing studied with functional magnetic resonance imaging. *The Journal of Neuroscience, 19*, 3050–3056.

De Groot, A. M. B. (1992). Determinants of word translation. *Journal of Experimental Psychology: Learning, Memory and Cognition, 18*, 1001–1018.

De Groot, A. M. B., Dannenburg, L., & van Hell, J. G. (1994). Forward and backward word translation by bilinguals. *Journal of Memory and Language, 33*, 600–629.

Dufour, R., & Kroll, J. (1995). Matching words to concepts in two languages: A test of the concept mediation model of bilingual representation. *Memory and Cognition, 23*(2), 166–180.

Frances, N., & Kučera, J. (1982). *Frequency analysis of English usage*. Boston: Houghton Mifflin & Company.

Francis, W. S. (1999). Cognitive integration of language and memory in bilinguals: Semantic representation. *Psychological Bulletin, 125*, 193–222.

Goodglass, H. (1998). Stages of lexical retrieval. *Aphasiology, 12*(4), 287–298.

Herman, D., Bongarts, T., De Bot, K., & Schreuder, R. (1998). Producing words in a foreign language: Can speakers prevent interference from their first language? *Bilingualism: Language and Cognition, 1*, 213–229.

Hernandez, A., Dapretto, M., Mazziotta, J., & Bookheimer, S. (2001). Language switching and language representation in Spanish-English bilinguals: An fMRI study. *NeuroImage, 14*, 510–520.

Illes, J., Francis, W. S., Desmond, J. E., Gabriele, J. D., Glover, G. H., Poldrack, R. et al. (1999). Convergent cortical representation of semantic processing in bilinguals. *Brain and Language, 70*(3), 347–363.

Juilland, A., & Chang-Rodriguez, E. (1964). *Frequency dictionary of Spanish words*. London: Mouton & Co.

Kaplan, E., Goodglass, H., & Weintraub, S. (1983). *Boston Naming Test*. Philadelphia: Lea & Febiger.

Klein, D., Milner B., Zatorre, R., Meyer, E., & Evans, A. (1995). The neural substrates underlying word generation: A bilingual function-imaging study. *Proceedings of the National Academy of Sciences USA, 92*, 2899–2903.

Kohnert, K. J., Bates, E., & Hernandez, A. E. (1999). Balancing bilinguals: Lexical-semantic production and cognitive processing in children learning Spanish and English. *Journal of Speech, Language, and Hearing Research, 42*, 1400–1413.

Kohnert, K. J., Hernandez, A. E., & Bates, E. (1998). Bilingual performance on the Boston Naming Test: Preliminary norms in Spanish and English. *Brain and Language, 65*(3), 422–440.

Kremin, H., Akhutina, T., Basso, A., Davidoff, J., De Wilde, M., Kitzing, P. et al. (2003). A cross-linguistic data bank for oral picture naming in Dutch, English, German, French, Italian, Russian, Spanish, and Swedish (PEDOI). *Brain and Cognition, 53*, 243–246.

Kroll, J. F., & Curley, J. (1988). Lexical memory in novice bilinguals: The role of concepts in retrieving second language words. In M. Gruneberg, P. Morris, & R. Sykes (Eds.), *Practical aspects of memory* (Vol. 2, pp. 389–395). London: John Wiley & Sons.

Kroll, J. F., & Stewart, E. (1990). *Concept mediation in bilingual translation*. 31st Annual Meeting of the Psychonomic Society, New Orleans.

Kroll, J. F., & Stewart, E. (1994). Category interference in translation and picture naming: Evidence for asymmetric connections between bilingual memory representations. *Journal of Memory and Language, 33*, 149–174.

Muñoz, M., Marquardt, T., & Copeland, G. (1999). A comparison of the codeswitching patterns of aphasic and neurologically normal bilingual speakers of English and Spanish. *Brain and Language, 66*, 249–274.

Pallier, C., Colomé, A., & Sebastián-Gallés, N. (2001). The influence of native-language phonology on lexical access: Exemplar-based versus abstract lexical entries. *Psychological Science, 12*(6), 445–449.

Perani, D., Dehaene, S., Grassi, F., Cohen, L., Cappa, S., Dupoux, E. et al. (1996). Brain processing of native and foreign languages. *NeuroReport, 7*, 2439–2444.

Potter, M., So, K., vonEckardt, B., & Fedlman, L. (1984). Lexical and conceptual representation in beginning and proficient bilinguals. *Journal of Verbal Learning and Verbal Behavior, 23*, 23–381.

Roberts, P. M., & Deslauriers, L. (1999). Picture naming of cognate and non-cognate nouns in bilingual aphasia. *Journal of Communication Disorders, 32*, 1–23.

Roberts, P. M., Garcia, L. J., Desrochers, A., & Hernandez, D. (2002). English performance of proficient bilingual adults on the Boston Naming Test. *Aphasiology, 16*(4–6), 635–645.

Roelofs, A. (2003). Shared phonological encoding processes and representations of languages in bilingual speakers. *Language and Cognitive Processes, 18*(2), 175–204.

Wartenburger, I., Heekeren, H. R., Abutalebi, J., Cappa, S. F., Villringer, A., & Perani, D. (2003). Early setting of grammatical processing in the bilingual brain. *Neuron, 37*, 159–170.

APHASIOLOGY, 2004, *18* (5/6/7), 581–588

Generative word fluency skills in adults with Parkinson's disease

Monica Strauss Hough

East Carolina University, Greenville, NC, USA

Background: Studies addressing cognitive function of adults with Parkinson's disease (PD) have revealed inconsistencies relative to language disturbances. Whereas some researchers have observed no evidence to support language dysfunction on semantic/generative naming tasks, others have found that adults with PD display decreased performance on these tasks. Generative naming may be problematic for adults with PD but its usefulness as a predictor for identifying cognitive impairment in this population is unclear.

Aims: The purpose of the investigation was to examine performance of a group of 20 PD individuals and an age-, education-, and gender-matched control group of 20 individuals on generative naming tasks for nouns, verbs, and adjectives. The primary hypothesis was that the adults with PD would demonstrate a deficit in verb generation.

Methods & Procedures: All participants with PD had a diagnosis based on the presence of two of three classic PD signs, bradykinesia, resting tremor, and rigidity, as determined by a neurologist. All participants were native English speakers, had normal or corrected vision, passed a hearing screening, and had no history of developmental disabilities, head injury, or substance abuse. There were no significant differences between groups on premorbid Full Scale IQ or cognitive functioning as measured by the MMSE. The experimental procedure consisted of noun, verb, and adjective fluency tasks. Participants were instructed to name as many exemplars as possible in 60 seconds for each part of speech. Scores were based on total number and percentage of accurate responses.

Outcomes & Results: Both groups produced significantly more nouns than verbs and adjectives. Percentage of accuracy data revealed that: (1) the control group was significantly more accurate than the Parkinson's group; (2) the Parkinson's group was significantly less accurate than controls on adjective generation; and (3) significantly higher accuracy was observed for nouns and verbs than adjectives across groups. Overall word retrieval performance as measured by the Test of Adolescent/Adult Word Finding was significantly related to adjective generation only.

Conclusions: The group with PD exhibited an impairment in adjective generation as compared to controls. Mental representations for adjectives appear to be more multifaceted than representations for nouns and verbs. The increased complexity of semantic networks for adjectives may be vulnerable to the effects of brain damage associated with PD.

Parkinson's disease (PD) is a progressive and degenerative neurological disorder characterised by brainstem degeneration, reduction of dopamine secondary to gradual degeneration of cells in the substantia nigra, and possible frontal lobe degeneration

Address correspondence to: Monica Strauss Hough, East Carolina University, Communication Sciences & Disorders, Greenville, North Carolina 27858, USA. Email: HoughM@Mail.ecu.edu

The author would like to thank Eastern North Carolina Parkinson's Support Groups, and especially the Pitt County-Greenville group, for their participation and support in this project. The author also would like to thank Ann Cralidis for her assistance in collecting reliability data.

http://www.tandf.co.uk/journals/pp/02687038.html   DOI:10.1080/02687030444000101

associated with depletion of dopamine in the striatum (Duffy, 1995; Freed, 2000; Roseberry-McKibbin & Hegde, 2000). Concomitant linguistic and non-linguistic deficits that may accompany the disease, coupled with the possible onset of dementia often confound a perspective of the patient's cognitive abilities (Savage, 1997; Yorkston & Garrett, 1997). Studies addressing language and cognitive function in adults with PD have revealed some inconsistencies relative to specific disturbances (Barbosa, Limongi, & Cummings, 1997; Bayles, Tomoeda, Wood, Cruz, Azuma, & Montgomery, 1997; Lubinski, 1997). Few studies address the effects that PD may have on language functioning, and reported findings have often been inconsistent. Whereas Beatty and Monson (1989) found no evidence to support language dysfunction in individuals with PD on semantic or generative naming tasks, Bayles et al. (1997) observed that adults with PD accompanied by mild and questionable dementia displayed decreased performance on these types of tasks. Thus, tasks such as generative naming may be problematic for adults with PD; however, the usefulness of these tasks as predictors for identifying cognitive impairment or dementia in this population is unclear.

Several studies have revealed that brain changes secondary to PD are variable across different samples of individuals with PD relative to particular linguistic tasks (Azuma, Bayles, Cruz, Tomoeda, Wood, & McGeagh, 1997; Bayles, Trosset, Tomoeda, Montgomery, & Wilson, 1993; Beatty & Monson, 1989; Piatt, Fields, Paolo, Koller, & Troster, 1999). In addition, specific cognitive and linguistic impairments in individuals with PD appear to vary secondary to an overlap in deficits associated with both cortical and subcortical dementia, as well as other clinical manifestations associated with PD (Barrett, Crucian, Schwartz, & Heilman, 2000; Colcher & Simuni, 1999). Raskin, Sliwinski, and Borod (1992) examined generative naming for semantic and letter categories in a group of PD patients without dementia and a group of normal controls. The PD participants produced fewer items than the controls for semantic retrieval but there were no significant between-group differences on letter fluency. Using similar tasks, Bayles et al. (1993) studied the performance of PD adults with and without dementia and normal controls, among other populations. In contrast to Raskin et al.'s (1992) findings, letter naming was more difficult than semantic retrieval for both PD groups. PD participants without dementia (as measured by the MMSE) performed more poorly than the normal controls for both tasks. In a similar study, Azuma et al. (1997) examined PD adults with and without dementia and normal controls on letter, noun, and semantic category fluency. Consistent with Bayles et al.'s (1993) results, the PD participants without dementia produced fewer responses for the letter than the semantic fluency tasks. The control group performed equally well on all three tasks, suggesting that the performance of the PD patients without dementia may reflect a specific lexical processing deficit secondary to PD. Furthermore, these findings indicate that verbal fluency skills in adults with PD may be influenced by the nature of the individual categories or specific fluency task; some fluency tasks may be differentially sensitive to the linguistic abilities of PD adults.

Piatt et al. (1999) examined lexical, semantic, and action (verb) word fluency abilities in adults with PD with and without dementia and normal elderly adults. The PD participants with dementia performed significantly worse than the other groups on all tasks, but especially on action fluency. The PD participants without dementia did not show any significant differences in performance from the controls except for a trend towards significantly poorer performance on action fluency. Piatt et al. hypothesised that performance on action fluency may be an indicator of the progressive fronto-subcortical degeneration noted in PD, as opposed to the occurrence or severity of cognitive deficits in general. Thus, the results of this study suggest a notable relationship between PD, neuroanatomical site, and cognitive-linguistic impairment; however, the exact nature of this relationship remains unclear. The utility of action fluency as a predictor for early dementia in PD associated with fronto-subcortical impairment requires further investigation. Because of the subtlety of this possible deficit and the contradictory findings in letter and semantic categories, the investigation of other grammatical word class categories is warranted. In the present investigation, performance on generative naming tasks for nouns, verbs, and adjectives was examined in a group of individuals with PD and a non-brain-damaged control group. Relationships between generative word production and word retrieval skills were also investigated.

METHOD

A total of 20 adults with PD and 20 normal elderly control participants (NC) were included in the study as participants. The two groups were participant-matched for age, education, and gender (12 males, 8 females). All participants with PD were diagnosed by a neurologist based on the presence of two of three classic PD signs: bradykinesia, resting tremor, and rigidity. All NC participants reported no history of any neurological disorder or medications that may impair cognitive function, via questionnaire.

In addition, all participants met the following inclusionary criteria: (1) Native speakers of English; (2) No self-report of history of or dependence on drugs or alcohol, or other substance abuse, no diagnosis of mental illness; (3) No self-report of developmental disabilities; (4) No self-report of significant head injury with loss of consciousness; (5) Hearing sufficient to pass a modified hearing screening for older adults (ASHA, 1992); (6) Normal or corrected vision, screened using an eye chart placed at 20 feet from the participant. Criteria 2–4 were examined via questionnaire.

The regression equation from the Demographically Based Index of Premorbid Intelligence (Barona, Reynolds, & Chastain, 1984), which uses demographic information to appraise intelligence, was used to estimate Verbal, Performance, and Full Scale IQ (FSIQ) for all participants. An independent t-test conducted on the FSIQ data revealed no significant difference between groups. The Mini-Mental State Examination (MMSE: Folstein, Folstein, & McHugh, 1975) was given to evaluate the cognitive status of all participants. Only two participants (PD group) scored below 25 on this measure (22, 23). An independent t-test conducted on the overall MMSE scores revealed no significant difference between groups. All participants also administered the Test of Adolescent/Adult Word Finding (TAWF: German, 1990) to examine the relationship between performance on convergent word retrieval and generative naming. An independent t-test conducted on the TAWF standard scores revealed a trend towards significance ($t = 3.274$; $p = .054$). Means, standard deviations, and ranges for age, education, estimated FSIQ, MMSE, and TAWF are presented in Table 1.

The experimental procedure consisted of noun, verb, and adjective fluency tasks administered to all participants to evaluate generative naming. Participants were instructed to name as many exemplars as possible in a 60-second timeframe for each of the three parts of speech. Prior to the task, all individuals were provided with descriptions and examples of nouns, verbs, and adjectives. Several sentences highlighting each part of speech were presented to each participant and any questions regarding the task procedure were also addressed. Scores for all three tasks were based on the total number of items produced as well as the percentage of correct items produced during the 60-second period. The order of the three generative naming tasks was randomised across participants. The examiner wrote down all responses during the administration task. The three

TABLE 1

Means, standard deviations, and ranges for participant characteristics and pre-experimental test scores

	PD			NC		
	Mean	SD	Range	Mean	SD	Range
Age	72.8	6.6	55–81	73.2	8.3	57–91
Education	15.6	2.8	9–21	15.6	3.0	12–19
FSIQ*	109	8.5	87–119	110	4.4	101–114
MMSE**	27.6	.51	22–30	29.5	.15	28–30
TAWF***	105.4	3.5	76–135	122.5	3.9	91–157

* Full Scale Intelligence Quotient (Barona et al., 1984).
** Mini-Mental State Examination (Folstein et al., 1975); maximum score = 30.
*** Test of Adolescent/Adult Word Funding (German, 1990) standard scores.

tasks also were audio-taped on a Marantz Professional PMD201 audio-cassette recording attached to a Shure SM58 Vocal Microphone for additional verification.

Intra-examiner reliability for percentage of accuracy was determined by having the author re-score the three fluency tasks for each participant approximately 2 weeks after the initial scoring of the set of tasks. Percentage of agreement for noun, verb, and adjective generation was 100%, 99%, and 99%, respectively. Inter-examiner reliability for percentage of accuracy was determined by having an experienced, certified speech-language pathologist randomly score one of the three fluency tasks for each participant. Percentage of agreement for noun, verb, and adjective generation was 100%, 100%, and 98%, respectively.

RESULTS

Means and standard deviations (SD) for the total number of responses for both groups on the three generative naming tasks are presented in Table 2. A mixed repeated measures Analysis of Variance (ANOVA) with one between-subjects (group) and one within-subjects (grammatical category) variable conducted on these data revealed a significant main effect of grammatical category only, $F(2, 76) = 58.184; p < .001$. There were no other significant findings.

Means, SDs, and ranges for the significant grammatical category finding are as follows: (1) nouns: 22.95, 1.24, 20.45–25.45; (2) verbs: 14.78, .87, 13.02–16.53; (3) adjectives: 13.68, 1.12, 11.40–15.95. Bonferroni pairwise comparisons conducted on the

TABLE 2

Means and standard deviation for the total number of responses on nouns, verbs, and adjectives for both groups

	PD		NC	
	Mean	SD	Mean	SD
Nouns	21.4	8.2	24.5	7.4
Verbs	13.6	5.2	16.0	5.8
Adjectives	11.4	5.9	16.0	8.1

TABLE 3
Means and standard deviation for the percentage of accurate
responses on nouns, verbs, and adjectives for both groups

	PC		NC	
	Mean	SD	Mean	SD
Nouns	97.5	4.1	99.3	1.5
Verbs	94.1	8.8	96.4	4.8
Adjectives	67.8	39.5	91.2	14.7

significant main effect revealed a significant difference between the total number of nouns and adjectives ($p < .01$) and between nouns and verbs ($p < .01$), regardless of group. There was no significant difference between adjectives and verbs.

Means and standard deviations for the percentage of accurate responses for both groups on the three generative naming tasks are presented in Table 3. A mixed repeated measures ANOVA with one between-subjects (group) and one within-subjects (grammatical category) variable conducted on these data revealed significant main effects for group, $F(1, 38) = 7.776$; $p < .01$, and grammatical category, $F(2, 76) = 13.177$; $p < .001$, and a significant group × grammatical category interaction, $F(2, 76) = 4.928$; $p < .02$. Overall, the NC group showed a significantly higher percentage of accuracy than the group with PD. A significantly higher percentage of accurate responses were produced for both nouns and verbs than adjectives across groups.

Post hoc analyses, in the form of Tukey's Least Significant Difference (LSD) test, were conducted on the mean differences of the significant group × grammatical category interaction. There were no significant differences relative to the percentage of accuracy between each of the grammatical categories for the control group; however, the group with PD had a significantly lower percentage of accuracy for adjectives than both nouns ($p < .05$) and verbs ($p < .05$), with no difference between verbs and nouns. Scheffe tests conducted on the between-group means for each grammatical category revealed that the group with PD performed significantly worse than the NC group on adjective generation ($p < .01$); there were no significant differences between the groups for either verbs or nouns.

Pearson Product Moment Correlations were conducted between the percentage of accuracy for each of the grammatical categories and (1) TAWF standard scores; (2) estimated FSIQ based on the Barona et al. (1984) index; and (3) MMSE score. Scores were collapsed across groups and then correlated. Results revealed significant positive correlations between percentage of accuracy for adjectives and all three clinical test scores: TAWF standard score ($r = .51$; $p < .01$), MMSE score ($r = .55$; $p < .01$), and FSIQ ($r = .49$; $p < .01$). There were no other significant findings.

DISCUSSION AND CONCLUSIONS

The results revealed that the group with PD appeared to exhibit an impairment in the generation of adjectives as compared to the control group, when temporally constrained. Although both groups produced significantly fewer adjectives than nouns, there was no significant difference between the groups on the number of adjectives produced. It was only the PD group that displayed significantly less accuracy in their adjective than noun and verb generation. Furthermore, although both groups produced significantly fewer verbs than nouns, percentage of accuracy was not significantly different for these two grammatical categories for either group. Overall word retrieval performance, as measured by the TAWF, was found to be significantly related to adjective generation only.

A few researchers have shown that generative naming tasks are sensitive to the subtle linguistic changes that may accompany Parkinson's disease (Piatt et al., 1999; Raskin et al., 1992). However, it appears that this observation has been more prevalent with PD participants who have confirmed dementia (Azuma et al., 1997; Bayles et al., 1993, 1997; Piatt et al., 1999). As mentioned, in the current cohort, only two participants scored below the normal cognitive functioning cut-off on the MMSE; these two individuals were in the questionable range of functioning. However, upon inspection of their individual performance, it was found that these two participants performed similarly to the normal control group. Thus, the observed reduction in percentage of accuracy for adjective generation in the group with PD is a noteworthy finding.

It is interesting to note that the initial hypothesis relative to investigation outcome was that the participants with PD would demonstrate a deficit in verb rather than adjective generation. The development of this hypothesis was related to the nature of brain damage associated with PD, specifically the possible prevalence of frontal lobe degeneration as the result of depletion of dopamine in the striatum. Research has revealed that aphasic patients with anterior left hemisphere damage and traumatic-brain-injured adults (motor vehicle accidents) with similar areas of damage have frequently been observed to exhibit selective impairments of verb retrieval/naming (Goodglass, Klein, Carey, & Jones, 1966; Kim & Thompson, 2000; Miceli, Silveri, Villia, & Caramazza, 1984). Several investigators have suggested strong connections between neuroanatomical structure/site and representation of particular lexical categories: anterior/frontal left hemisphere regions associated with verb/action representation, posterior regions with noun representation (Miceli, Silveri, Nocentini, & Caramazza, 1988; Zingeser & Berndt, 1990). Piatt et al.'s (1999) research with adults with PD explored a similar hypothesis with remarkable results; however, their tasks did not include adjective generation. Thus, it was speculated that PD may disrupt the representation, access to, and/or generation of verbs.

Consequently, instead, the issues to explore are: (1) the uniqueness of adjectives and (2) the finding that participants with PD with normal cognitive functioning have more difficulty in accurately generating adjectives. Although nouns and verbs can have more than one meaning, a difference in meaning is usually accompanied by a change in the word's part of speech. That is, when a noun has a different meaning, this different meaning makes the word a verb or possibly an adjective. For example, the noun "record" in "Let's make a *record*" becomes a verb in "*Record* the statement". Or the noun "stable" in "*stable* of horses" becomes an adjective in "The table is *stable*". This observation is not the same for adjectives; many adjectives are homographs. These words elicit more than one distinct meaning, yet are represented by only one spelling. Furthermore, not only do adjectives frequently have more than one meaning; these different meanings are also adjectives. For example, the adjective "warm" can refer to temperature ("*warm* milk") or kindness ("He is a *warm* person") but still remains an adjective. Thus, adjectives are often ambiguous by nature and require reliance on contextual information (linguistic, extralinguistic, or paralinguistic) for their appropriate interpretation (Pierce, 1984; Rubenstein, Lewis, & Rubenstein, 1971; Simpson, 1981). Consequently, mental representations for adjectives may be more multifaceted than representations for nouns and verbs. This increased complexity of semantic networks for adjectives may be more vulnerable to the effects of brain damage associated with PD. This speculation, however, requires further investigation as it relates to PD and other neurological disorders. Additionally, the large standard deviation associated with the mean accuracy percentage on adjectives for the group with PD suggests that problems with adjectives may be observed only in a subgroup of individuals with PD. The characteristics of such a subgroup require delineation.

The significant relationship between overall word retrieval as measured by the TAWF and adjective generation is a surprising observation, particularly because of the nature of theTAWF. Although the TAWF is more multifaceted than most word retrieval tests because it examines retrieval of both nouns and verbs, it does not include any subtests involving adjective generation. Thus, it appears that, regardless of naming task, one's ability to generate adjectives may be related to overall retrieval of words (including nouns and verbs), at least for this sample of older adults. Additionally, the significant relationships between MMSE scores and adjective generation as well as between FSIQ and adjective generation suggest that generative naming, and adjective fluency in particular, may be a useful and sensitive predictor of early cognitive decline in PD patients. Additional research regarding the utility of generative naming as a tool in identifying cognitive and linguistic deficits associated with PD is in order. Furthermore, continued research on the nature of adjectives, strategies used to generate adjectives, and their mental representation and organisation is certainly warranted.

REFERENCES

ASHA Ad Hoc Committee on Hearing Screenings in Adults. (1992). Consideration in screening adults/older persons for handicapping hearing impairments. *ASHA, 34*, 81–87.

Azuma, T., Bayles, K. A., Cruz, R. F., Tomoeda, C. K., Wood, J. A., & McGeagh, A. (1997). Comparing the difficulty of letter, semantic, and name fluency tasks for normal elderly and patients with Parkinson's disease. *Neuropsychology, 11*(4), 488–497.

Barbosa, E. R., Limongi, J. C., & Cummings, J. L. (1997). Parkinson's disease. *Psychiatric Clinics of North America, 20*(4), 769–790.

Barona, A., Reynolds, C. R., & Chastain, R. (1984). A demographically-based index of premorbid intelligence for the WAIS-R. *Journal of Consulting and Clinical Psychology, 52*(5), 885–887.

Barrett, A. M., Crucian, G. P., Schwartz, R. L., & Heilman, K. L. (2000). Testing memory for self-generated items in dementia. *Neurology, 54*(6), 1258–1264.

Bayles, K. A., Tomoeda, C. K., Wood, J. A., Cruz, R. F., Azuma, T., & Montgomery, E. B. (1997). The effect of Parkinson's disease on language. *Journal of Medical Speech-Language Pathology, 5*(3), 157–166.

Bayles, K. A., Trosset, M. W., Tomoeda, C. K., Montgomery, E. B., & Wilson, J. (1993). Generative naming in Parkinson's disease patients. *Journal of Clinical and Experimental Neuropsychology, 15*, 547–562.

Beatty, W. W., & Monson, N. (1989). Lexical processing in Parkinson's disease and multiple sclerosis. *Journal of Geriatric Psychiatry and Neurology, 2*(3), 145–152.

Colcher, A., & Simuni, T. (1999). Parkinson's disease and Parkinsonian syndromes: Clinical manifestations of Parkinson's disease. *Medical Clinics of North America, 83*(2), 327–347.

Duffy, J. (1995). *Motor speech disorders: Substrates, differential diagnosis, and management.* St Louis, MO: Mosby Year Book, Inc.

Folstein, M. F., Folstein, S. E., & McHugh, P. R. (1975). Mini-Mental State: A practical method for grading the cognitive state of patients for the clinician. *Journal of Psychiatric Research, 12*, 189–198.

Freed, D. (2000). *Motor speech disorders: Diagnosis and treatment.* San Diego,CA: Singular Publishing Group.

German, D. J. (1990). *Test of Adolescent and Adult Word Finding.* Austin, TX: Pro-Ed Publishers.

Goodglass, H., Klein, B., Carey, P., & Jones, K. (1966). Specific semantic word categories in aphasia. *Cortex, 2*, 74–89.

Kim, M., & Thompson, C. (2000). Patterns of comprehension and production of nouns and verbs in agrammatism: Implications for lexical organization. *Brain and Language, 74*(1), 1–25.

Lubinski, R. (1997). Perspectives on aging and communication. In R. Lubinski & D. J. Higginbotham (Eds.), *Communication technologies for the elderly: Vision, hearing, and speech* (pp. 1–21). San Diego, CA: Singular Publishing Group.

Miceli, G., Silveri, M. C., Nocentini, U., & Caramazza, A. (1988). Patterns of dissociation in comprehension and production of nouns and verbs. *Aphasiology, 2*, 351–358.

Miceli, G., Silveri, M. C., Villa, G., & Caramazza, A. (1984). On the basis for the agrammatic's difficulty in producing main verbs. *Cortex, 20,* 207–220.

Piatt, A. L., Fields, J. A., Paolo, A. M., Koller, W. C., & Troster, A. I. (1999). Lexical, semantic, and action verbal fluency in Parkinson's disease with and without dementia. *Journal of Clinical and Experimental Neuropsychology, 21*(4), 435–443.

Pierce, R. S. (1984). Comprehending homographs in aphasia. *Brain and Language, 22,* 339–349.

Raskin, S. A., Sliwinski, M., & Borod, J. C. (1992). Clustering strategies on tasks of verbal fluency in Parkinson's disease. *Neuropsychologia, 30*(1), 95–99.

Roseberry-McKibbin, C., & Hegde, M. N. (2000). *Neurologically based communication disorders and dysphagia. An advanced review of speech-language pathology: Preparation for NESPA and comprehensive examination* (pp. 411–483). Austin, TX: Pro-Ed.

Rubenstein, H., Lewis, S., & Rubenstein, M. (1971). Homographic entries in the internal lexicon: Effects of systematicity and relative frequency of meanings. *Journal of Verbal Learning and Verbal Behavior, 10,* 57–62.

Savage, C. R. (1997). Neuropsychology of subcortical dementias. *Psychiatric Clinics of North America, 20*(4), 911–931.

Simpson, G. (1981). Meaning dominance and semantic context in the processing of lexical ambiguity. *Journal of Verbal Learning and Verbal Behavior, 20,* 121–136.

Yorkston, K. M., & Garrett, K. L. (1997). Assistive communication technology for elders with motor speech disability. In R. Lubinski & D.J. Higginbotham (Eds.), *Communication technologies for the elderly: Vision, hearing, and speech* (pp. 235–261). San Diego, CA: Singular Publishing Group.

Zingeser, L. B., & Berndt, R. S. (1990). Retrieval of nouns and verbs in agrammatism and anomia. *Brain and Language, 39*(1), 14–32.

APHASIOLOGY, 2004, *18* (5/6/7), 589–597

Naming and category concept generation in older adults with and without dementia

Monica Strauss Hough

East Carolina University, Greenville, NC, USA

Background: An intact semantic memory system is vital for accurate naming of objects; naming failures exhibited by individuals with dementia have been a means of identifying the nature of the semantic memory impairment. However, naming impairment has also been reported in healthy older adults. Categorisation is a process of concept formation within semantic memory. Category type influences ability to synthesise category concepts. Studies investigating categorisation skills in adults with dementia have revealed deterioration in conceptual knowledge as compared to age-matched healthy cohorts.
Aims: It is hypothesised that normal older adults are impaired at the lexical access stage of word retrieval; those with dementia have deficits in the earlier concept identification stages of word retrieval and lexical access difficulties.
Methods & Procedures: A group of adults with dementia of the Alzheimer's type (DAT) and a group of normal elderly adults were examined on naming and category concept generation tasks relative to accuracy and error types. Participants were 15 adults with DAT and 15 age-, education-, and gender-matched neurologically intact adults. MMSE results supported division of two groups. All participants were native English speakers, literate, with normal hearing. Experimental tasks were the Test of Adolescent/Adult Word Finding (TAWF) and a category concept generation task (CCGT). For the CCGT, participants were presented with four category examples for common and goal-directed categories and instructed to provide a category label. Context vignettes accompanied category examples for half the categories.
Outcomes & Results: For the TAWF, there were no significant group differences for standard scores. Further analysis revealed that: (1) the control group performed significantly poorer on picture naming: nouns than any other subtest; (2) normal controls performed better than the DAT group on all subtests except picture naming: nouns; and (3) the DAT group performed significantly worse on category naming than all other subtests. Analysis of CCGT revealed that: (1) normal controls performed better than the DAT participants on goal-directed categories with context but not without context; (2) performance was higher for goal-directed categories with context for controls only; and (3) performance was higher on common than goal-directed categories without context for controls.
Conclusions: The results indicate that normal older adults are impaired in lexical access; those with DAT have deficits in the earlier conceptual stages of word retrieval in addition to lexical access difficulties. DAT participants especially had difficulty with category naming. The DAT adults showed minimal differences in performance from a no-context to context condition. The findings support previous research that adults with DAT display semantic memory impairments.

Address correspondence to: Monica Strauss Hough, East Carolina University, Communication Sciences & Disorders, Greenville, North Carolina 27858, USA. Email: HoughM@Mail.ecu.edu

© 2004 by Taylor & Francis.
http://www.tandf.co.uk/journals/pp/02687038.html   DOI:10.1080/02687030444000110

The semantic memory system is a hierarchically organised network of conceptual knowledge that contains the permanent representation of the knowledge of objects, facts, and concepts as well as knowledge of words, their meanings, and their relationships. Semantic memory is the highest faculty in the cognitive system and the point in the information processing chain where information from the perceptual system is inter-related and synthesised with factual information (Au & Bowles, 1991; Bayles, Kaszniak, & Tomoeda, 1987; Tulving, 1983). An intact semantic memory system is vital for accurate identification and naming of objects as well as the understanding and production of written and spoken words (Au & Bowles, 1991; Bayles et al., 1987; Bowles & Poon, 1985; Herlitz & Viitanen, 1991; Nicholas, Obler, Au, & Albert, 1996).

Difficulty in naming or word retrieval has been observed to be the most obvious early symptom of dementia, regardless of cause, and has been found to occur before other language changes associated with the syndrome are measurable (Bayles, Tomoeda, Kaszniak, & Trosset, 1991; Bayles, Tomoeda, & Trosset, 1990; Chan, Butters, Paulsen, Salmon, Swenson, & Maloney, 1993; Emery & Breslau, 1989; Hodges, Salmon, & Butter, 1992; Huff, Corkin, & Growden, 1986; Shuttleworth & Huber, 1988; Sommers & Pierce, 1990). Naming has been considered a meaningful representation of the integrity of the semantic memory system; naming failures exhibited by individuals with dementia have been examined as a means of identifying the nature of the semantic memory impairment. However, naming is truly a measure of lexical memory. Furthermore, an impairment in naming ability has also been reported in healthy older adults (Albert, Heller, & Milberg, 1988; Au & Bowles, 1991; Bowles, Obler, & Albert, 1987; Carr, McCauley, Sperber, & Parmelee, 1982; Goulet, Ska, & Kahn, 1994; Nicholas, Obler, Albert, & Goodglass, 1985; Nicholas et al., 1996); thus, the exact nature of the naming deficit in individuals with dementia and healthy older adults is difficult to differentiate.

Categorisation, in which an individual decides whether something belongs to a par-ticular class, has been identified as a process of concept formation within semantic memory (Medin & Smith, 1984; Mervis & Rosch, 1981). Research on categorisation has been a major source of information on an individual's knowledge of concepts (Hough, 1989, 1993) and has revealed that the type of category influences an individual's ability to synthesise the category's concept. Common categories are groups of natural object concepts, such as "vegetables" and "clothing", that are well established in memory (Rosch, 1975; Rosch & Mervis, 1975). Goal-directed categories are concepts that are instrumental in achieving the goals of daily living, such as "things to take on a picnic" (Barsalou, 1982, 1983; Hough, 1989). In research with non-brain-damaged young adults, Barsalou (1983) found that goal-directed categories are dependent on context for their conceptualisation whereas common categories are context-independent. That is, concepts for common categories were as available without the presence of context as with lin-guistic context because their exemplar-to-concept associations are more established in memory than those for goal-directed categories. On the other hand, relevant contexts were found to prime goal-directed categories; goal-directed category labels were as obvious as common category labels when category examples were primed by linguistic contexts indicating current goals. Thus, goal-directed category concepts appear to require synthesis of additional sources of information for their realisation that is not needed to generate common category concepts (Hough, 1989, 1993).

Studies investigating categorisation skills in adults with dementia have revealed that these individuals show significant deterioration in the structure and/or contents of semantic and conceptual knowledge as compared to their age-matched healthy cohorts (Bayles et al., 1990; Binetti, Magni, Cappa, Padovani, Bianchetti, & Trabucchi, 1995;

Chan et al., 1993; Hough, 1998; Hough, May, & Givens, 1992; Sommers & Pierce, 1990). However, the nature and extent of the differences between individuals with dementia and normal elderly adults have not been clear. Furthermore, despite an extensive body of research on the effects of dementia on semantic memory, there continues to be a lack of agreement regarding whether dementia results in a loss of conceptual knowledge, remarkable difficulty in accessing this conceptual knowledge, or both types of deficits.

The present hypothesis is that normal older adults are impaired at the lexical access stage of word retrieval, whereas those with dementia have deficits in the earlier concept identification stages of word retrieval in addition to lexical access difficulties. Examination of word retrieval performance of healthy older adults and those with dementia on tasks of both naming and category conception may provide additional insight into identifying and understanding the nature of the deficits as well as assessing and treating these deficits more effectively. Thus, the purpose of the current investigation is to examine performance of a group of adults with dementia of the Alzheimer's type (DAT) and a group of normal elderly adults on naming and category concept generation tasks relative to accuracy and types of errors produced.

METHOD

Participants

A total of 15 adults presenting with a diagnosis of probable dementia of the Alzheimer's type (DAT) and 15 neurologically intact adults participated in the investigation. The DAT and control groups were participant-matched for age, education level, and gender (8 males, 7 females). All DAT participants had been medically and clinically diagnosed as having probable dementia of the Alzheimer's type (DAT) and who met the NINCSD-ADRDA criteria for DAT (McKhann, Drachman, Folstein, Katzman, Price, & Stadlan, 1984). All participants were administered the Mini-Mental State Examination (MMSE: Folstein, Folstein, & McHugh, 1975), with results supporting the division of two groups, those with and those without dementia. An independent t-test conducted on the MMSE scores revealed a significant difference between groups ($t = 5.763$; $p < .05$). The DAT group included mostly mild and some moderately impaired individuals based on scores from the MMSE. All participants were native speakers of English and were literate. All participants passed a modified pure-tone hearing screening for older adults (screening at 40 dB through the speech frequencies) (ASHA, 1992; Ventry & Weinstein, 1983, 1992). In addition, all participants were administered the Peabody Picture Vocabulary Test-III (PPVT-III: Dunn & Dunn, 1997). An independent t-test conducted on the PPVT-III standard score data revealed no significant difference between groups ($p > .05$). Premorbid IQ was estimated for all participants using the Barona, Reynolds, and Chastain (1984) regression equation from the Demographically Based Index of Premorbid Intelligence. An independent t-test conducted on the estimated Full Scale IQ (FSIQ) data revealed no significant differences between groups ($p > .05$). Means and standard deviations for age, education, PPVT-III standard scores, premorbid FSIQ, and MMSE are presented in Table 1.

Procedure

The experimental tasks involved administration of the Test of Adolescent/Adult Word Finding (TAWF: German, 1990) and a category concept generation task (CCGT) (Hough,

TABLE 1
Means and standard deviations for participant characteristics
and pre-experimental test scores

	Controls	DAT
Age (yrs.)	68.8	70.1
	(5.7)	(6.2)
Education (yrs.)	12.9	13.3
	(2.4)	(2.9)
Premorbid IQ*	98.4	101.2
	(7.9)	(11.1)
PPVT-III standard score**	100.8	96.8
	(8.8)	(17.1)
MMSE***	28.4	18.1
	(2.3)	(4.6)

Standard deviations are in parentheses.
* Based on Barona et al. (1984) demographic quotient.
** Peabody Picture Vocabulary Test-III; normal range 85–115.
*** Mini-Mental State Examination, maximum score = 30.

1988, 1989, 1993) developed and originally normed on both younger and older normal adults by the author. The TAWF assesses naming in five contexts/subtests. These five subtests include: Picture naming: nouns; Sentence completion; Descriptive naming/ naming to definition; Picture naming: verbs; and Category naming. Analysis and comparison between groups included: (a) TAWF standard score, (b) percentage of accuracy per TAWF subtest, and (c) error type. For the CCGT, the participant was auditorially/ visually presented with four examples (two highly and two moderately typical examples) of a particular category and was instructed to provide a category label. The categories were 8 common categories (fruits, sports, etc.) for which Rosch (1975) has developed typicality norms, and 16 goal-directed categories (things to take on a picnic, things that can be folded, etc.) for which Hough (1988) has developed norms with adults. For half of the categories, a context vignette was presented with the four category examples. Each context vignette described a character engaged in a goal-directed activity and primed the subsequent respective category label. Sample paragraphs with category examples for both the common and goal-directed categories are presented in Table 2. Performance accuracy and error type were examined relative to: (a) category type (common, e.g., fruits, sports, etc.; goal-directed, e.g., things to take on a picnic, things that can be folded, etc.); and (b) presence of prior context: half of the stimulus sets were preceded by the two-sentence context vignette. Contextual influences were of interest, particularly for the goal-directed categories that are context-dependent and almost always require the listener/reader to rely on linguistic context for accurate identification of the category label.

RESULTS

Means and standard deviations for TAWF standard scores and subtest percentages for both groups are presented in Table 3. An independent t-test conducted on the TAWF standard score data revealed no significant differences between groups ($p < .05$). A mixed repeated measures Analysis of Variance (ANOVA) conducted on the TAWF subtest

TABLE 2
Sample paragraphs and exemplars for the common and goal-directed categories

Common category: "Clothing"

Sarah loved to go shopping. She always looked forward to the end of the season because most items were on sale.

boots
shirt
stockings
suit

Goal-directed category: "Things to take on a camping trip"

Paul wanted to spend the weekend at a state park in the mountains. He packed up everything he would need for a few days of sleeping under the stars.

backpack
flashlight
tarp
air mattress

accuracy percentages with one between-subjects (group) and one within-subjects (subtest) variable revealed:

- a significant main effect for group, $F(1, 28) = 10.55$; $p < .05$;
- a significant main effect for subtest, $F(4, 112) = 12.61$; $p < .05$;
- a significant group × subtest interaction, $F(4, 112) = 13.07$; $p < .05$.

Overall, the control group performed significantly better than the DAT group and there was significantly less accuracy on the Picture naming: nouns subtest of the TAWF than any other subtest.

TABLE 3
Test of Adolescent/Adult Word Finding (TAWF) standard score and subtest percentage means and standard deviations for both groups

	Controls	DAT
TAWF standard scores*	91.5	86.3
	(11.6)	(14.3)
TAWF Subtest Percentages		
Picture naming: nouns	58.5	53.2
	(9.7)	(10.6)
Sentence completion	84.6	59.2
	(7.1)	(9.2)
Descriptive naming	88.6	61.4
	(10.2)	(9.8)
Picture naming: verbs	78.5	44.2
	(8.3)	(12.3)
Category naming	80.4	30.7
	(5.2)	(13.3)

Standard deviations are in parentheses.
* TAWF Standard Score normal range = 85–115.

Post hoc analyses in the form of the Tukey's Honestly Significant Difference (HSD) Test conducted on the significant interaction revealed the following:

1) The control group performed significantly poorer on Picture naming: nouns than any other subtest ($p < .01$).
2) There were significant differences between groups for all subtests ($p < .05$) except Picture naming: nouns. That is, the normal controls performed significantly better than the DAT group on all subtests except for Picture naming: nouns.
3) The DAT group performed significantly worse on Category naming than all other subtests ($p < .05$) and significantly worse on Picture naming: verbs ($p < .05$) than Picture naming: nouns, Sentence completion, and Descriptive naming.

Error types were analysed according to the error categories from the TAWF. Although not statistically analysed, the control group produced a similar percentage of semantic (42%) and visual (38%) errors (i.e., "horse" for "statue"), whereas the DAT group produced very few visual errors (3%), with similar percentages of no response (29%), nonspecific (28%) (i.e., "that thing"), and semantic (26%) errors. Most of the semantic errors produced by the control group were coordinate class errors (providing name of related item in the same category; "cane" for "crutch") (82%); most of the semantic errors produced by the DAT group were unrelated to the target ("table" for "crutch") (80%). These latter errors are still considered a semantic error on the TAWF (unrelated).

Means and standard deviations for percentage of accuracy for each of the category conditions on the CCGT for both groups are presented in Table 4. A mixed repeated measures ANOVA with one between-subjects (group) and two within-subjects (category type, presence of context) variables conducted on the accuracy percentage data revealed:

- a significant main effect of group, $F(1, 28) = 22.68$; $p < .01$;
- a significant main effect of category type, $F(1, 28) = 11.32$; $p < .05$;
- a significant group × category type interaction, $F(1, 28) = 12.76$; $p < .05$;
- a significant group × context interaction, $F(1, 28) = 9.83$; $p < .05$;
- a significant category × context interaction, $F(1, 28) = 10.72$; $p < .05$;
- a significant group × category type × context interaction, $F(1, 28) = 14.02$; $p < .05$.

TABLE 4
Means and standard deviations for percentage accuracy on the category concept generation task for both groups

Category type	Control	DAT
Common w/out context	92.7 (6.4)	66.8 (10.1)
Common with context	94.2 (5.7)	70.5 (9.7)
Goal-derived w/out context	64.4 (10.2)	58.3 (12.7)
Goal-derived with context	88.1 (10.2)	62.3 (9.8)

Standard deviations are in parentheses.

The control group performed significantly better than the DAT group overall for both common and goal-derived categories. The control group performed significantly better on common than goal-derived categories; the DAT group showed no significant difference in performance between the two category types. Furthermore, the control group performed significantly better in the presence of context than the DAT group and significantly better than in no-context conditions; the DAT group exhibited no significant differences between context and no-context conditions.

Post hoc analyses using Tukey's HSD test on the significant three-way interaction revealed the following:

1) There was a significant difference between groups for goal-directed categories with context but not without context: the normal controls performed significantly better than the DAT participants for generating category labels for the goal-directed categories when context was presented ($p < .05$).

2) Performance was significantly higher for goal-directed categories in the presence of context (versus no context) for controls only ($p < .05$).

3) Performance was significantly higher on common than goal-directed categories without context for only the control group ($p < .05$).

Although error types were not statistically analysed for the CCGT, it was evident that a high percentage of errors produced by the control group were semantically related to the target category label (Common: 97%; Goal-derived: 84%); for the DAT group, errors were primarily no response (Common: 39%; Goal-derived: 44%) or semantically unrelated to the target label (Common: 35%; Goal-derived: 32%).

DISCUSSION AND CONCLUSIONS

The results support the hypothesis that normal older adults are impaired in lexical access, particularly for retrieving object names or pictureable nouns. Individuals with dementia, and particularly DAT, appear to have deficits in the earlier conceptual stages of word retrieval in addition to lexical access difficulties. The access problems observed in DAT appear to minimally involve pictureable nouns and verbs, which were examined in the current investigation. The DAT participants especially had difficulty with category naming; this finding was observed on both experimental tasks. Category label generation appears to be dependent on somewhat intact knowledge of the semantic or referential field of a particular concept (Binetti et al., 1995; Hough, 1989, 1993). Even minimal loss of a category's referential field, as may be observed in the early stages of DAT, might result in difficulty in integrating perceptual and factual information adequately to generate category concepts.

It is interesting to note that on both tasks the participants with DAT had noticeably more no-response errors than the controls and a similar occurrence of this error type to the other error types committed. It appears that this observation may be consistent with deterioration in the contents of lexical and conceptual knowledge; that is, these individuals may frequently be unable to access any information, because the information is basically unavailable. The frequent occurrence of no-response errors on both naming and category concept generation tasks may be another representation of the significant disruption in both lexical and semantic memory, respectively.

As mentioned previously, adults with dementia have been observed to display significant deterioration in the structure and contents of semantic/conceptual knowledge as compared to their age-matched healthy cohorts (Bayles et al., 1990, 1991; Binetti et al., 1995; Chan et al., 1993; Hough et al., 1992). Furthermore, it has been indicated that the ability to generate concepts for different types of categories, particularly goal-directed categories, is influenced by the presence of context (Barsalou, 1982, 1983). In the current investigation, this ability to utilise context to enable concept generation was not observed for the DAT adults. They showed minimal differences in performance from a no-context to context condition for either category type, and especially for the goal-directed categories for which it was imperative that they utilise context to generate the appropriate category label. Thus, it appears that adults with DAT, even in mild and moderate stages of the disease, display a semantic memory impairment. This deficit is characterised by difficulty in consistently integrating all available information for accurate identification and generation of concepts, as well as basic word retrieval ability.

The TAWF appears to be a useful tool in identifying the distinctive patterns of lexical performance observed with normal ageing and in those individuals with mild and moderate impairments as a result of dementia. As was observed, the normal older adults had noticeable difficulty in retrieving lexical referents for pictureable object nouns as compared to other nouns or verbs on the TAWF. This naming pattern was also found in another group of older adults on the TAWF (Hough, 1998) as well as in other studies using similar stimuli (Au & Bowles, 1991; Bowles et al., 1987). Although the DAT group also exhibited deficits in the naming of pictureable nouns, they especially had difficulty with category naming on the TAWF. In fact, category labelling appeared to be a very difficult endeavour for the DAT participants on the category concept generation task as well. Thus, because of the varied naming demands on the TAWF, it may be a valuable tool for distinguishing patterns of lexical retrieval abilities in normally ageing adults and the DAT population as well as other cognitive and linguistically impaired groups.

REFERENCES

Albert, M. L., Heller, H. S., & Milberg, W. (1988). Changes in naming ability with age. *Psychology and Aging*, *3*(2), 173–178.

ASHA Ad Hoc Committee on Hearing Screenings in Adults. (1992). Consideration in screening adults/older persons for handicapping hearing impairments. *ASHA*, *34*, 81–87.

Au, R., & Bowles, N. (1991). Memory influences on language in normal aging. In D. Ripich (Ed.), *Handbook of geriatric communication disorders* (pp. 293–305). Austin, TX: Pro-Ed, Inc.

Barona, A., Reynolds, C. R., & Chastain, R. (1984). A demographically-based index of premorbid intelligence for the WAIS-R. *Journal of Consulting and Clinical Psychology*, *52*(5), 885–887.

Barsalou, L. W. (1982). Context-independent and context-dependent information in concepts. *Memory and Cognition*, *10*(1), 82–93.

Barsalou, L. W. (1983). Ad hoc categories. *Memory and Cognition*, *8*, 211–227.

Bayles, K., Kaszniak, A. W., & Tomoeda, C. K. (1987). *Communication and cognition in normal aging and dementia*. Austin, TX: Pro-Ed, Inc.

Bayles, K., Tomoeda, C. K., Kaszniak, A. W., & Trosset, M. W. (1991). Alzheimer's disease effects on semantic memory: Loss of structure or impaired processing? *Journal of Cognitive Neuroscience*, *3*(2), 166–182.

Bayles, K. A., Tomoeda, C. K., & Trosset, M. W. (1990). Naming and categorical knowledge in Alzheimer's disease: The process of semantic memory deterioration. *Brain and Language*, *39*, 498–510.

Binetti, G., Magni, E., Cappa, S. F., Padovani, A., Bianchetti, A., & Trabucchi, M. (1995). Semantic memory in Alzheimer's disease: An analysis of category fluency. *Journal of Clinical and Experimental Neuropsychology*, *17*, 82–89.

Bowles, N. L., Obler, L. K., & Albert, M. L. (1987). Naming errors in healthy aging and dementia of the Alzheimer type. *Cortex*, *23*, 519–524.

Bowles, N., & Poon, L. W. (1985). Aging and retrieval of words in semantic memory. *Journal of Gerontology*, *40*(1), 71–77.

Carr, T. H., McCauley, C., Sperber, R. D., & Parmelee, C. M. (1982). Words, pictures, and priming: On semantic activation, conscious identification, and the automaticity of information processing. *Journal of Experimental Psychology: Human Perception and Performance, 8,* 757–777.

Chan, A. S., Butters, N., Paulsen, J. S., Dalmon, D. P., Swenson, M. R., & Maloney, L. T. (1993). An assessment of the semantic network in patients with Alzheimer's disease. *Journal of Cognitive Neuroscience, 5,* 254–261.

Dunn, L. M., & Dunn, L. M. (1997). *Peabody Picture Vocabulary Test-III.* Circle Pines, MN: American Guidance Services.

Emery, O. B., & Breslau, L. D. (1989). The problems of naming in SDAT: A relative deficit. *Experimental Aging Research, 14*(4), 181–193.

Folstein, M. F., Folstein, S. E., & McHugh, I. (1975). Mini-Mental State: A practical method for grading the cognitive state of patients for the clinician. *Journal of Psychiatric Research, 12,* 189–198.

German, D. (1990). *Test of Adolescent/Adult Word Finding.* Allen, TX: DLM Teaching Resources.

Goulet, P., Ska, B., & Kahn, H.J. (1994). Is there a decline in picture naming with advancing age? *Journal of Speech and Hearing Research, 37,* 629–644.

Herlitz, A., & Viitanen, M. (1991). Semantic organization and verbal episodic memory in patients with mild and moderate Alzheimer's disease. *Journal of Clinical and Experimental Neuropsychology, 13*(4), 559–574.

Hodges, J. R., Salmon, D. P., & Butters, N. (1992). Semantic memory impairment in Alzheimer's disease: Failure of access or degraded knowledge? *Neuropsychologia, 30*(4), 301–314.

Hough, M. S. (1988). *Categorization in aphasia: Access and organization of ad hoc and common categories.* Unpublished doctoral dissertation, Kent State University, USA.

Hough, M. S. (1989). Category concept generation in aphasia: The influence of context. *Aphasiology, 3*(6), 553–568.

Hough, M. S. (1993). Categorization in aphasia: Access and organization of goal-derived and common categories. *Aphasiology, 7,* 335–357.

Hough, M. S. (1998). *Incidence of word finding deficits in normal aging.* Paper presented at the annual Clinical Aphasiology Conference, Asheville, NC, USA.

Hough, M. S., May, M. J., & Givens, G. D. (1992). *Exemplar generation for common and functional categories in Alzheimer's disease.* Paper presented at the NIH Quality of Life and Aging Conference, Washington, DC, USA.

Huff, F. J., Corkin, S., & Growden, J. H. (1986). Semantic impairment and anomia in Alzheimer's disease. *Brain and Language, 28,* 235–249.

McKhann, G., Drachman, D., Folstein, M., Katzman, R., Price, D., & Stadlan, E. (1984). Clinical diagnosis of Alzheimer's disease: Report of the NINCDS-ADRDA work group. *Neurology, 34,* 939–949.

Medin, D. L., & Smith, E. E. (1984). Concepts and concept formation. *Annual Review of Psychology, 35,* 113–138.

Mervis, C. B., & Rosch, E. (1981). Categorization of natural objects. *Annual Review of Psychology, 32,* 89–115.

Nicholas, M., Obler, L., Albert, M., & Goodglass, H. (1985). Lexical retrieval in healthy aging. *Cortex, 21,* 595–606.

Nicholas, M., Obler, L., Au, R., & Albert, M. (1996). On the nature of naming errors in aging and dementia: A study of semantic relatedness. *Brain and Language, 54,* 184–195.

Rosch, E. (1975). Cognitive representation of semantic categories. *Journal of Experimental Psychology: General, 104*(3), 192–233.

Rosch, E., & Mervis, C. B. (1975). Family resemblances: Studies in the internal structure of categories. *Cognitive Psychology, 7,* 573–605.

Shuttleworth, E. C., & Huber, S. J. (1988). The naming disorder of dementia of the Alzheimer's type. *Brain and Language, 34,* 222–234.

Sommers, L. M., & Pierce, R. S. (1990). Naming and semantic judgements in dementia of the Alzhemier's type. *Aphasiology, 4*(6), 573–586.

Tulving, E. (1983). *Elements of episodic memory.* Oxford: Oxford University Press.

Ventry, I., & Weinstein, B. (1983). Identification of elderly people with hearing problems. *ASHA, 25,* 37–42.

Ventry, I., & Weinstein, B. (1992). Considerations in screening adults/older persons for handicapping hearing impairments. *ASHA, 34,* 81–87.

APHASIOLOGY, 2004, *18* (5/6/7), 599–609

Inhibition and auditory comprehension in Wernicke's aphasia

Debra A. Wiener

Boston University School of Medicine, Boston, MA, USA

Lisa Tabor Connor

Washington University School of Medicine, St. Louis, MO, USA

Loraine K. Obler

Boston University School of Medicine, Boston, and City University of New York Graduate School and University Center, NY, USA

Background: While research findings support the presence of inefficiencies in allocation of attention in individuals with aphasia, the cognitive mechanisms behind these inefficiencies remain unclear. One mechanism that would affect resource allocation for selective processing is an impaired inhibitory mechanism which, when normally functioning, would actively suppress distracting information.

Aims: The purpose of this study was to investigate the cognitive process of inhibition, at the lexical-semantic level of language processing, and its relation to auditory comprehension in Wernicke's aphasia.

Methods & Procedures: The classic Stroop Colour-Word Test was adapted to be applicable for use with an aphasic population. We administered this computerised manual-response, numerical version of the Stroop test to five individuals with Wernicke's aphasia and twelve age- and education-matched non-brain-injured controls. Correlations with Stroop interference examined associations with auditory comprehension as measured by the Token Test and the Complex Ideational Material subtest of the Boston Diagnostic Aphasia Examination.

Outcomes & Results: Analysis of the Stroop reaction time and error percentage data indicated that the interference effect was significantly larger for the participants with Wernicke's aphasia than for the controls, without an accompanying increase in facilitation, reflecting an impairment of inhibition in Wernicke's aphasia. In addition, the magnitude of Stroop interference was significantly positively correlated with the clinical-behavioural symptom of severity of auditory comprehension deficits as measured by the Token Test.

Conclusions: Findings support an impairment in inhibition at the lexical-semantic level of language processing in Wernicke's aphasia, reflecting the inability to effectively ignore the automatically evoked, distracting stimulus. The significant correlation between the Stroop interference effect and the severity of auditory comprehension deficits suggests that at least part of the attentional difficulties contributing to the striking reductions in auditory comprehension in this population can be attributed to impaired inhibition. Our

Address correspondence to: Dr Debra Wiener, Harold Goodglass Aphasia Research Center, VA Medical Center (12A), 150 S. Huntington Avenue, Boston, MA 02130, USA. Email: WienerDobn@aol.com

This study was performed as part of a dissertation by the first author in partial fulfilment of the requirements for a PhD in Speech and Hearing Sciences at the City University of New York Graduate School and University Center. We thank Dr Errol Baker and Dr Avron Spiro III for their statistical guidance. This project was supported in part by the National Institutes of Health (NIDCD) and by the Medical Research Service of the Department of Veterans Affairs.

http://www.tandf.co.uk/journals/pp/02687038.html   DOI: 10.1080/02687030444000228

findings expand upon our understanding of resource allocation in aphasia and reinforce our need to clinically assess and treat reductions in attention for maximised rehabilitation outcome.

Increasingly, aphasiologists have been focusing on the role that attention plays in difficulties with auditory processing. While research findings support the presence of inefficient attention allocation in individuals with aphasia (e.g., McNeil, Odell, & Tseng, 1991; Murray, Holland, & Beeson, 1997; Tseng, McNeil, & Milenkovic, 1993), the cognitive mechanisms underlying these inefficiencies remain unclear. In theorising on the role of attentional control of language functions, McNeil et al. considered the interplay of controlled and automatic processing. One mechanism that would reduce the allocation of resources necessary for selective processing is an impaired inhibitory mechanism which, when normally functioning, would serve to limit the generation and maintenance of irrelevant information. The purpose of the present study was to investigate the cognitive process of inhibition at the lexical-semantic level of language processing and its impact on auditory comprehension in Wernicke's aphasia.

NEUROPSYCHOLOGICAL EVIDENCE

Theories of selective attention emphasise the role that the process of inhibition plays in suppressing irrelevant information for improved focus in such higher-level cognitive tasks as verbal working memory and language performance (e.g., Hasher & Zacks, 1988; Tipper, 1985). Traditionally, attention theories placed the emphasis on the target of selection. Unselected information was thought to passively decay (Broadbent, 1970). However, more recent theories of selective attention (e.g., Tipper, 1985) propose an active suppression or inhibition of distracting information during selection for increased efficiency of processing.

Support for inhibition theory comes from the negative priming paradigm (Tipper, 1985). A participant is asked to respond to a target item presented simultaneously with a similar distractor item. The critical manipulation occurs between consecutive trials. The participant responds to a target on the test trial that had been ignored on the previous trial. The negative priming effect is lengthened response time on experimental trials as compared with control trials, where the distractor is an item not seen before. The source of the slower response time to the repeated item is theorised to be the inhibition that has accrued to the current target during its role as an ignored item in the previous trial.

INHIBITORY FUNCTION IN WERNICKE'S APHASIA

Inhibitory function has been investigated in a variety of populations evidencing selection difficulties, including the elderly (e.g., Earles, Connor, Frieske, Park, Smith, & Zwahr, 1997; Hasher & Zacks, 1988), individuals with schizophrenia (e.g., Maher, 1983), and those with dementia of the Alzheimer type (e.g., Sullivan, Faust, & Balota, 1995). In addition, Milberg, Blumstein, Katz, Gershberg, and Brown (1995) investigated inhibitory function in the presence of aphasia.

Milberg et al. (1995) conducted experiments to examine the extent to which deficits in controlled or automatic processing could characterise lexical access deficits in Wernicke's and Broca's aphasia. They administered two auditory lexical decision priming experiments to seven participants with Wernicke's aphasia and ten with Broca's aphasia (mean age 68.3 and 59.6 years, respectively) and to young (college-aged) and older (mean age 63.8) non-brain-injured controls. In one experiment, they varied prime–target predictability. The expectation was that those with normal controlled processing would show slowed response times for unrelated prime–target pairs as compared with neutral pairs when the unrelated pairs had been preceded by an induction set consisting of a series of word pairs all semantically related. In the second experiment, they manipulated the prime–target interstimulus interval (ISI). At the 2000 ms ISI, both facilitation for related pairs and inhibition for unrelated pairs should be obtained. Of the four subject groups, neither the older control group nor the Wernicke's aphasics were affected by manipulations that were to have invoked controlled processes. That is, they did not demonstrate inhibition in the high-probability condition, nor did these two groups demonstrate inhibition at the 2000 ms ISI. Thus, while inhibitory function appears reduced in Wernicke's aphasia, it is unclear whether this reduction is due to the aphasia type or the impact of age. This distinction is an important one, as inhibitory control is thought to decrease with age (e.g., Balota, Black, & Cheney, 1992; Earles et al., 1997; Hasher & Zacks, 1988), and patients with Wernicke's aphasia are, on average, significantly older than individuals with Broca's aphasia (Obler, Albert, Goodglass, & Benson, 1978).

In the neuropsychological literature, a common tool used to measure inhibition in non-aphasic populations is the Stroop Colour-Word Test (Stroop, 1935). Although there are now many variations on this task, the basic design is such that a participant is asked to name the ink colour of a printed word and ignore the meaning of the word. Ink colour naming is slower when the ink colour and the word meaning are incompatible (e.g., *blue* written in red ink) than when they are compatible (e.g., *red* written in red ink) or when they are neutral (e.g., *XXX* written in red ink). The prevailing interpretation of this effect is that the word information is activated automatically, and the participant needs to inhibit this information during the slower process of colour naming (MacLeod, 1991). Greater interference on this task, as measured by the difference between reaction times to the incompatible versus neutral conditions, without an accompanying increase in facilitation (the difference between reaction times in the neutral and compatible conditions), has been interpreted as reflecting reduced inhibitory abilities.

This pattern of findings, a larger-than-normal interference effect accompanied by no-greater-than-normal facilitation effect, is an important way to distinguish the effects of reduced inhibitory control from generalised cognitive slowing. An example from the ageing literature demonstrates this issue quite effectively. Prior to 1998, 20 studies had been conducted comparing older adults to younger adults on variations of the Stroop task (see review by Verhaeghen & De Meersman, 1998). Nearly all had obtained findings of a larger interference effect in older adults than in younger adults. Nearly all of the authors of these studies concluded, on the basis of these findings, that older adults show poorer inhibitory control than younger adults. In every one of these studies, response latencies were much longer for older than for younger adults. Slowing across all conditions in the study not only produced larger interference effects for the old, but larger facilitation effects as well. Verhaeghen and De Meersman demonstrated through meta-analysis of these studies that generalised slowing of all cognitive processes was likely the cause of these larger than normal interference effects, rather than a deficit in inhibitory control *per se*.

The aphasia literature contains very few studies of the Stroop effect, probably due to the high verbal demands of the original task. The validity of measuring a cognitive function via a variably impaired verbal response is, obviously, questionable. In order to adapt the Stroop test for use with a Wernicke's aphasic population, a manual-response version appears necessary given the high frequency of verbal paraphasia associated with Wernicke's aphasia. MacLeod (1991) compiled an extensive review of studies investigating the Stroop effect since J. R. Stroop's classic 1935 article, concluding that although the interference effect may be reduced when response modality is switched from oral to manual, it remains robust. A number of researchers (e.g., Fox, Shor, & Steinman, 1971; Shor, 1971; Windes, 1968) have found that numbers also can produce significant interference effects. For example, the naming of an Arabic numeral is interfered with when it appears in incongruent quantities. Use of numerical stimuli appears warranted in an adaptation of the Stroop test for Wernicke's aphasia, as it allows for a manual, computer keyboard response. While such stimuli tap into the lexical-semantic level of language, they avoid the need for the participant's verbal response.

The present study involved administration of a computerised manual-response, numerical version of the Stroop test to individuals with Wernicke's aphasia and age- and education-matched non-brain-injured controls. In order to determine whether individuals with Wernicke's aphasia evidence impaired inhibition in processing lexical-semantic information, we compared them to age-matched controls to help disentangle effects of ageing from effects due to stroke. Moreover, to accept the hypothesis that individuals with Wernicke's aphasia have a specific deficit of inhibition and not generalised slowing due to stroke, our design required both that the size of the facilitation effect was equivalent in participants with aphasia and age-matched controls and that the size of the interference effect was significantly greater.

We suggest, further, that one possible behavioural manifestation of impaired inhibition may be reduced auditory comprehension. Correlating the severity of auditory comprehension deficits with the interference score obtained on the Stroop test permitted exploration of the relationship between inhibition and auditory comprehension.

METHOD

Participants

Five adult participants with chronic Wernicke's aphasia and twelve non-brain-injured controls were tested. Participants were recruited from the subject pool of the Harold Goodglass Aphasia Research Center, which consists of both individuals who have sustained aphasia and normal adults.

The five participants with Wernicke's aphasia were selected based on the following criteria: a single onset of a left posterior infarct post cerebral vascular accident; no history of dementia, prior neurological trauma, drug or alcohol abuse, or chronic psychiatric disorder; English as native and primary language; right-hand dominance; normal visual acuity, with or without correction; and normal hearing thresholds across the speech frequencies, with or without correction. The diagnosis of Wernicke's aphasia was based on clinical observation and language examination. Six subtests of the Neurosensory Center Comprehensive Examination for Aphasia (NCCEA: Spreen & Benton, 1969) were administered to each participant with aphasia: Visual Naming, Description of Use, Sentence Repetition, Word Fluency, Identification by Sentence (the Token Test), and Reading Names for Meaning (Pointing). In addition, the Complex Ideational Material subtest of the Boston Diagnostic Aphasia Examination (Goodglass & Kaplan, 1983) was administered. The "Speech" and "Understanding" subsets of the Functional Communication Profile (Sarno, 1969) also were rated for each participant with aphasia for purposes of a comprehensive participant profile. Table 1 summarises the relevant demographic and clinical characteristics of the aphasic participants. All of these parti-

TABLE 1
Demographic and clinical characteristics of the participants with Wernicke's aphasia

Subject	Age	Educ	Time post-onset	Aphasia severity	NCCEA range*	FCP speech**	FCP comp**
1	72 yrs	12 yrs	177 mos	moderate	20–88%	56%	57%
2	76 yrs	10 yrs	56 mos	mod-severe	20–61%	49%	55%
3	63 yrs	12 yrs	163 mos	moderate	13–88%	55%	58%
4	74 yrs	12 yrs	114 mos	severe	6–61%	50%	50%
5	75 yrs	11 yrs	102 mos	mod-severe	8–61%	49%	47%

Including: chronological age; level of formal education; time post-onset of CVA in months; overall aphasia severity rating; range of percentiles of subtests of the NCCEA (Spreen & Benton, 1969) administered; and percentiles of estimated function in "Speech" and "Understanding" subsets of the FCP (Sarno, 1969).

*Percentiles are based on an aphasic population.

**Percentile represents functional communicative effectiveness in this modality based on estimated premorbid language proficiency.

cipants were male. Their mean age was 72 years, with a range of 63–76 years. Their mean level of formal education was 11.4 years, with a range of 10–12 years.

The twelve non-clinical controls were selected using the same criteria as the participants with aphasia, with two additional requirements: no history of neurological trauma or disease and a score of 28 or greater on the Mini-Mental State Examination (Folstein, Folstein, & McHugh, 1975). They were matched to the aphasic participants by age (mean age of 71.5 years, range 62–77 years) and level of formal education (mean of 12.6 years, range 12–16 years). Six of the control participants were male (Participants 6–11) and six were female (Participants 12–17). All research participants were treated in accordance with the Human Studies Committees of Boston University School of Medicine, the VA Boston Healthcare System, and the City University of New York Graduate Center. Participants received a modest payment for their participation at the conclusion of the study.

In order to measure auditory comprehension, the Token Test and the Complex Ideational Material subtest of the BDAE were administered to all participants. The participants with Wernicke's aphasia obtained raw scores on the Token Test ranging from 73 to 104 out of a possible 163 correct, reflecting severe to moderate-severe deficits when plotted on the NCCEA aphasia profile. Their raw scores on the Complex Ideational Material subtest ranged from 5 to 9 of a possible 12 correct, reflecting moderate-severe to mild deficits when plotted on the BDAE aphasia summary profile. As expected, the non-brain-injured controls demonstrated only minimal reductions on these two tests, reflected by a mean score of 161 on the Token Test and 11.2 on the Complex Ideational Material subtest.

Materials

The variation of the Stroop test used was modelled after Salthouse and Meinz's (1995) version which lent itself to modifications for increased validity in a language-impaired population. In order to create a measure of facilitation and interference, three conditions were established. The compatible condition was represented by the Arabic numerals 1 to 4 presented in congruent quantities (e.g., 333), consisting of four stimuli. The neutral condition was represented by an "X" in its four possible quantities. The incompatible condition was represented by the Arabic numerals 1 to 4 presented in incongruent quantities (e.g., 33), consisting of 12 stimulus items. The three experimental conditions provide a measure of facilitation (compatible vs neutral condition) and interference (incompatible vs neutral condition).

The experimental task consisted of 216 items—72 items in each condition. For each condition to be equally represented, the stimuli in both the compatible and neutral conditions were tripled in quantity. Stimuli were presented in random order for each participant. Three filler items were presented at the beginning of the experiment but were not included in the analysis.

The experimental trials were preceded by 10 practice items presented in random order—3 compatible, 3 neutral, and 4 incompatible trials. The same set of practice items was administered to each participant in random order.

Procedure

Participants were seated at a comfortable distance in front of a Macintosh PowerBook 180 computer with a 10-inch black and white screen. On the attached keyboard, four keys were exposed labelled "1", "2", "3", and "4". Participants were instructed to press the key that corresponded to the quantity of items on the screen. They were told to respond as quickly as possible and directed to use their left hand only.

The stimuli were presented in black on a white background via the software package PsyScope (Cohen, MacWhinney, Flatt, & Provost, 1993). Practice items were given and repeated, when necessary, until comprehension of the task was demonstrated by three consecutive correct responses. The 216 experimental trials followed. A PsyScope button box was used to increase timing accuracy to 1 ± 4 ms. Responses and latencies were recorded. The stimulus remained on the screen until the participant depressed one of the four response keys. The inter-trial interval was 500 ms.

RESULTS

The data for each participant were screened for mistrials (response latencies greater than 5 seconds) and outliers. Outliers were defined as responses greater than three standard deviations from the mean of all remaining responses for that participant. The mean number of mistrials for participants with Wernicke's aphasia was 0.6%, and the mean number of outliers was 2%. For the non-brain-injured controls, the mean number of mistrials was 0.3%, and the average number of outliers was 1.4%.

Reaction time data

The mean reaction times of the Wernicke's aphasic group and the control group are displayed in Figure 1. A 2 (group) $\times$ 3 (condition) mixed factor ANOVA was conducted on reaction time. RTs were longer for the participants with aphasia, $F(1, 15) = 5.66$, $MSE = 67,710.77$, $p < .05$, there was a significant difference among the conditions, $F(2, 30) = 88.85$, $MSE = 582.83$, $p < .001$, and the condition by group interaction was significant, $F(2, 30) = 28.12$, $MSE = 582.83$, $p < .001$, indicating that the increase in response time across conditions was larger for the participants with Wernicke's aphasia than for the controls.

Each group was examined separately. Each group showed a significant difference among the conditions: Wernicke's aphasics, $F(2, 8) = 29.97$, $MSE = 1,492$, $p < .001$; controls, $F(2, 22) = 34.06$, $MSE = 252.22$, $p < .001$. Post-hoc Newman-Keuls t-tests were

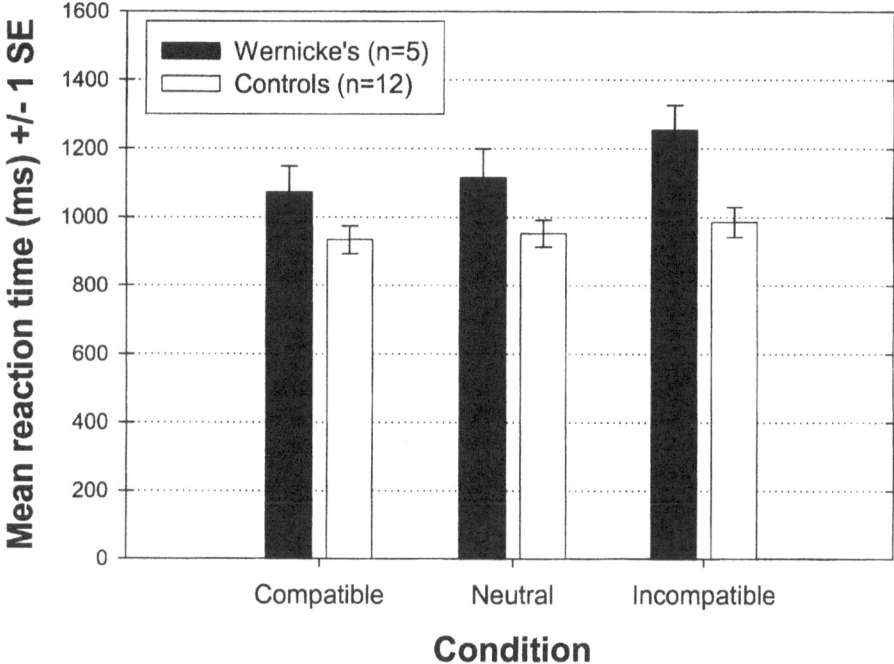

Figure 1. Stroop mean reaction times for the Wernicke's aphasic group and the non-brain-injured control group, by condition.

then performed. For each group, three paired comparisons were made: (1) the difference between the neutral and compatible conditions (the facilitation effect); (2) the difference between the incompatible and the neutral conditions (the interference effect); and (3) the difference between the facilitation effect and the interference effect. For the participants with Wernicke's aphasia, the facilitation effect was not significant, $t(8) = 2.50$, $p > .05$, although the interference effect, $t(8) = 7.99$, $p < .001$, and the difference between the facilitation and the interference effects, were significant, $t(8) = 10.48$, $p < .001$. For the controls, the facilitation effect, $t(22) = 4.18$, $p < .01$, the interference effect, $t(22) = 7.36$, $p < .001$, and the difference between the facilitation effect and the interference effect, $t(22) = 11.54$, $p < .001$, were all statistically significant.

The final step in the analysis of the reaction time data involved a comparison across groups, between the non-brain-injured controls and the participants with Wernicke's aphasia: the difference between the facilitation effect and the difference between the interference effect. The facilitation effect was no larger for the aphasic group ($M = 43$ ms) than for the controls ($M = 19$ ms), $t(15) = 1.91$, $p = .075$. However, the interference effect was significantly larger for the participants with Wernicke's aphasia ($M = 138$ ms) than for the controls ($M = 34$ ms), $t(15) = 4.35$, $p < .001$.

Error percentage data

The mean error percentages of the Wernicke's aphasic group and the control group, by condition, are displayed in Figure 2. Most participants made no errors in the compatible and neutral conditions, and error rate was very low in these conditions; however, for both

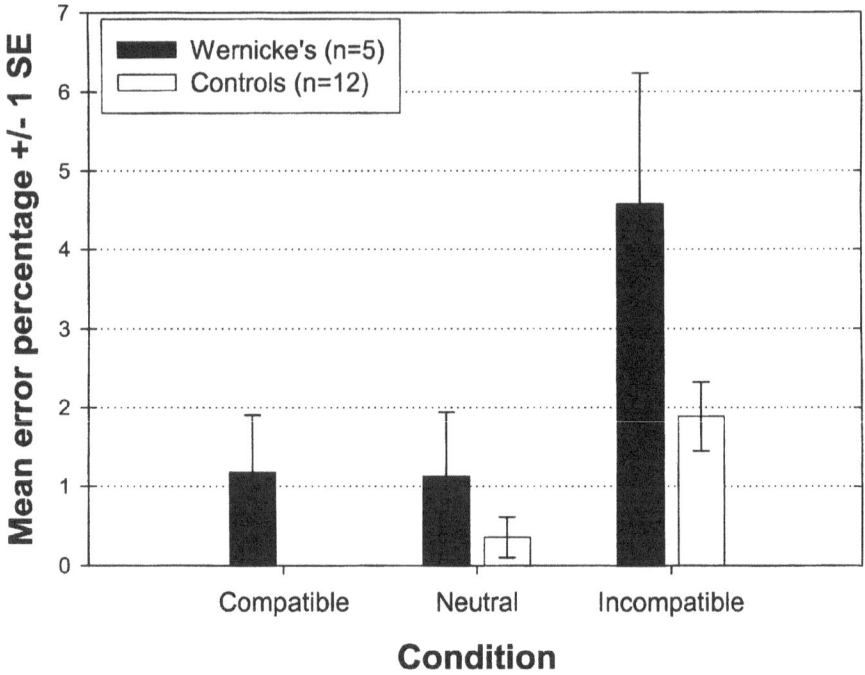

Figure 2. Stroop mean error percentages for the Wernicke's aphasic group and the non-brain-injured control group, by condition.

the aphasic group and the control group in the incompatible condition, the mean percentage of errors was significantly greater than zero, $t(4) = 2.77$, $p = .05$ and $t(11) = 4.30$, $p < .01$, respectively. The facilitation effect for errors (Wernicke's aphasics $M = -0.05$; controls $M = 0.35$) was not different between the groups, $t(15) = 0.637$, $p > .50$, whereas the interference effect for the aphasic group ($M = 3.45$) was significantly larger than for the controls ($M = 1.5$), $t(15) = 2.19$, $p < .05$.

Cross-measures comparisons

A Pearson correlation was performed to examine factors that may help to predict Stroop interference performance in Wernicke's aphasia, including the clinical-behavioural measures of auditory comprehension and the demographic factors of age, education, and time post-onset. Neither the Complex Ideational Material score nor the demographic factors examined were significantly correlated with Stroop performance, with all at $r < .77$, ns. However, a significant negative correlation was found between the Stroop error percentage interference effect and the Token Test score, $r(5) = -.91$, $p < .05$; that is, the greater the Stroop interference effect, the lower the Token Test score.

DISCUSSION

The goal of this study was to investigate inhibition at the lexical-semantic level of language processing in Wernicke's aphasia utilising the classic Stroop test, which we adapted to be applicable for an aphasic population. We expected that the participants with Wernicke's aphasia would show greater difficulty than the non-clinical controls in inhibiting the automatically activated word information, represented by the Arabic numeral, when attempting to respond to the quantity of items. We also examined whether there would be a significant association between the extent of inhibitory impairment and auditory comprehension deficit in Wernicke's aphasia.

Reaction time analyses indicated that the interference effect was significantly larger for the participants with Wernicke's aphasia than for the controls, without an accompanying increase in facilitation. Although the difference between the facilitation effect for these two groups might be considered as marginally significant, a post-hoc power analysis indicated that, with a difference of approximately 1 standard deviation between the mean reaction times of the Wernicke's aphasic group and the control group, we had nearly 90% power to detect it as significant (Cohen, 1988). Thus, the relatively small sample size ($n = 17$) was not an issue, and the facilitation effect was no larger for the aphasic group than for the controls. Likewise, not only were the error rates low, confirming that the reaction time data were not the result of a speed–accuracy trade-off, but these data, too, revealed significantly greater interference in the aphasic group than in the control group. Although the participants with Wernicke's aphasia were nearly 200 ms slower overall than their age-matched controls—a situation similar to that found in studies that compared Stroop performance between younger and older adults—there is no indication that generalised slowing could account for the results. That is, while the interference effect for the Wernicke's aphasic group was much larger than for the controls, the facilitation effects were equivalent for the two groups. Based on these findings, it appears that the individual with Wernicke's aphasia has a selective deficit of inhibitory control.

One might argue that our findings in this study reflect brain damage more generally, rather than damage resulting exclusively in Wernicke's aphasia. Recall, however, that Milberg et al. (1995) demonstrated relatively preserved inhibitory function in their 10 participants with Broca's aphasia. In the future, comparing the performance of individuals with Broca's aphasia on our version of the Stroop test with our data from Wernicke's participants will be useful to confirm these differences in inhibitory function between the aphasia types. Furthermore, examination of a group of individuals with Broca's aphasia with pure frontal lesions will increase our understanding of the interactions between frontal and posterior brain regions in the modulation of attention (e.g. Mesulam, 1981).

Additionally, the exploratory correlational analyses between inhibitory control deficits and impairment in auditory comprehension revealed a statistically significant association between the magnitude of Stroop interference and auditory comprehension as measured by the Token Test. Although the participants with Wernicke's aphasia were also impaired on auditory comprehension as measured by the Complex Ideational Material subtest of the BDAE, there was no correlation with the magnitude of Stroop interference. Of course it is difficult to support any particular argument for this pattern of results given the low statistical power. However, one may speculate that this pattern may be due to inhibitory control at different levels of the cognitive system for two measures of auditory comprehension. The large Stroop interference effect in the participants with Wernicke's aphasia corresponds to deficits at the lexical-semantic level of the language system, and the Token Test appears to be more heavily weighted towards proper inhibitory control at that lexical-semantic level (e.g., touch the large white circle and the small green square) than does Complex Ideational Material. If a participant has difficulty in inhibiting competing lexical information that has become activated (in the example above, both white and green, large and small, and circle and square are active), then comprehension performance will suffer. To perform successfully on Complex Ideational Material, lexical semantic inhibitory control does not seem as important as the ability to build a coherent structure for the narratives.

These findings expand on our understanding of resource allocation in aphasia. First, the relative dissociation between automatic and controlled processing in Wernicke's aphasia is further reinforced. Not only does automatic processing, regarding both lexical-semantic activation (e.g., Blumstein, Milberg, & Shrier, 1982) and deactivation (Wiener, 2000), appear to be preserved in Wernicke's aphasia, but our finding of a smaller facilitation effect than would be predicted based on the overall performance speed of the Wernicke's participants assures us that the greater interference evidenced was not a result of more potent automatic activation. Second, the results not only reinforce semantic impairments in this population when attentional resources are demanded at the level of controlled processing, but also direct us towards a faulty mechanism. The individual with Wernicke's aphasia cannot effectively ignore the automatically evoked, distracting stimulus. This deficit is not due to more potent automatic activation, but rather due to decreased inhibition. This faulty mechanism may result in a reduction in the ability to allocate attention, although it is premature to conclude that the inhibition effect is primary and causal, as the impaired inhibitory mechanism may itself be the result of inefficient resource allocation. Nonetheless, as the necessary interaction between the inhibitory mechanism and attention allocation is impaired, reduced effectiveness of auditory processing may result. Further research is clearly warranted to delineate the role of inhibitory function in auditory comprehension in aphasia.

REFERENCES

Balota, D. A., Black, S. R., & Cheney, M. (1992). Automatic and attentional priming in young and older adults: Reevaluation of the two-process model. *Journal of Experimental Psychology: Human Perception and Performance, 18*, 485–502.

Blumstein, S. E., Milberg, W., & Shrier, R. (1982). Semantic processing in aphasia: Evidence from an auditory lexical decision task. *Brain and Language, 17*, 301–315.

Broadbent, D. E. (1970). Stimulus set and response set. In D. I. Mortofsky (Ed.), *Attention: Contemporary theories and analysis.* New York: Appleton-Century-Crofts.

Cohen, J. (1988). *Statistical power analysis for the behavioral sciences, Second edition.* New York: Academic Press.

Cohen, J. D., MacWhinney, B., Flatt, M., & Provost, J. (1993). PsyScope: An interactive graphic system for designing and controlling experiments in the psychology laboratory using Macintosh computers. *Behavior Research Methods, Instruments and Computers, 25*, 257–271.

Earles, J. L., Connor, L. T., Frieske, D., Park, D. C., Smith, A. D., & Zwahr, M. (1997). Age differences in inhibition: Possible causes and consequences. *Aging, Neuropsychology, and Cognition, 4*, 45–57.

Folstein, M. F., Folstein, S. E., & McHugh, P. R. (1975). "Mini-Mental State": A practical method for grading the cognitive state of patients for the clinician. *Journal of Psychiatric Research, 12*, 189–198.

Fox, L. A., Shor, R. E., & Steinman, R. J. (1971). Semantic gradients and interference in naming color, spatial direction, and numerosity. *Journal of Experimental Psychology, 91*, 59–65.

Goodglass, H., & Kaplan, E. (1983). *The assessment of aphasia and related disorders, Second edition.* Philadelphia: Lea & Febiger.

Hasher, L., & Zacks, R. T. (1988). Working memory, comprehension, and aging: A review and a new view. In G. H. Bower (Ed.), *The psychology of learning and motivation, Vol. 22.* San Diego, CA: Academic Press.

MacLeod, C. M. (1991). Half a century of research on the Stroop effect: An integrative review. *Psychological Bulletin, 109*, 163–203.

Maher, B. A. (1983). A tentative theory of schizophrenic utterance. In B. A. Maher & W. B. Maher (Eds.), *Progress in experimental personality research, Vol. 12.* New York: Academic Press.

McNeil, M. R., Odell, K. & Tseng, C-H. (1991). Toward the integration of resource allocation into a general theory of aphasia. *Clinical Aphasiology, 20*, 21–39.

Mesulam, M. M. (1981). A cortical network for directed attention and unilateral neglect. *Annals of Neurology*, *10*, 309–325.

Milberg, W., Blumstein, S. E., Katz, D., Gershberg, F., & Brown, T. (1995). Semantic facilitation in aphasia: Effects of time and expectancy. *Journal of Cognitive Neuroscience*, *7*, 33–50.

Murray, L. L., Holland, A. L., & Beeson, P. M. (1997). Auditory processing in individuals with mild aphasia: A study of resource allocation. *Journal of Speech, Language, and Hearing Research*, *40*, 792–808.

Obler, L. K., Albert, M. L., Goodglass, H., & Benson, D. F. (1978). Aphasia type and aging. *Brain and Language*, *6*, 318–322.

Salthouse, T. A., & Meinz, E. J. (1995). Aging, inhibition, working memory, and speed. *Journal of Gerontology: Psychological Sciences*, *50B*, P297–P306.

Sarno, M. T. (1969). *The Functional Communication Profile*. New York: New York University Medical Center, Rusk Institute of Rehabilitation Medicine.

Shor, R. E. (1971). Symbol processing speed differences and symbol interference effects in a variety of concept domains. *The Journal of General Psychology*, *85*, 187–205.

Spreen, O., & Benton, A. L. (1969). *Neurosensory center comprehensive examination for aphasia*. Victoria, Canada: University of Victoria, Department of Psychology, Neuropsychology Laboratory.

Stroop, J. R. (1935). Studies of interference in serial verbal reactions. *Journal of Experimental Psychology*, *18*, 643–662.

Sullivan, M. P., Faust, M. E., & Balota, D. A. (1995). Identity negative priming in older adults and individuals with dementia of the Alzheimer type. *Neuropsychology*, *9*, 537–555.

Tipper, S. P. (1985). The negative priming effect: Inhibitory priming by ignored objects. *Quarterly Journal of Experimental Psychology*, *37*A, 571–590.

Tseng, C-H., McNeil, M. R., & Milenkovic, P. (1993). An investigation of attention allocation deficits in aphasia. *Brain and Language*, *45*, 276–296.

Verhaeghen, P., & De Meersman, L. (1998). Aging and the Stroop effect: A meta-analysis. *Psychology and Aging*, *13*, 120–126.

Wiener, D. A. (2000). *Mechanisms of inhibition in Wernicke's aphasia*. Unpublished doctoral dissertation, City University of New York, USA.

Windes, J. D. (1968). Reaction time for numerical coding and naming of numerals. *Journal of Experimental Psychology*, *78*, 318–322.

APHASIOLOGY, 2004, *18* (5/6/7), 611–623

Control and description of visual function in research on aphasia and related disorders

Brooke Hallowell

Ohio University, Athens, OH, USA

Natalie Douglas

Munroe Regional Medical Center, Ocala, FL, USA

Robert T. Wertz

Tennessee Valley Healthcare System and Vanderbilt University VA Medical Center, Nashville, TN, USA

Sunny Kim

Ohio University, Athens, OH, USA

Background: Most experimental and assessment tasks in studies of neurogenic language disorders rely on visual information processing. Failure to describe and/or control for visual function may lead to invalid data collection and interpretation.

Aims: An empirical study was initiated to describe current practice and needs for improvement in the description of and control for visual acuity, colour perception, visual fields, visual attention, and oculomotor functions.

Methods & Procedures: Data were collected from all articles ($N = 668$) on aphasia (subsequent to left hemisphere damage) and related language disorders (subsequent to TBI and right hemisphere damage) in adults published during a 10-year period in each of 17 journals.

Outcomes & Results: Few authors control for or describe even basic aspects of vision.

Conclusions: Specific needs and strategies for improvement are discussed. The need for improved continuing education concerning means of screening for various forms of visual function is highlighted. Researchers are encouraged to employ basic screenings corresponding to the visual functions implemented in their assessment and experimental tasks for a given study. Improved feedback to manuscript authors and those seeking grant funding regarding appropriate control for and description of visual function is advocated.

In a classic article in the aphasia literature, Brookshire (1983) describes the need for careful description and experimental control of numerous subject characteristics that may influence the results of research on persons with neurogenic language disorders: "Investigators who carry out experiments involving aphasic subjects should provide

Address correspondence to: Brooke Hallowell, School of Hearing, Speech and Language Sciences, Ohio University, W231 Grover Center, Athens, OH 45701, USA. Email: hallowel@ohiou.edu

This work was supported in part by grant number DC00153-01A1 from the National Institute on Deafness and Other Communication Disorders. The authors wish to thank Sojung Kim, Amy Reid, Leetal Cuperman, Lollie Vaughan, Stacey Commerford, Angie Evans, and Christine Jackson for assistance with data collection, and Dr Sherry Crawford for consultation and training on visual assessment and screening issues and methods.

http://www.tandf.co.uk/journals/pp/02687038.html   DOI: 10.1080/02687030444000084

reasonably detailed descriptions of those subjects in the published reports of their experiments'' (p. 343). Several other authors have emphasised that careful experimental control and participant description are essential to valid testing, experimentation, and interpretation of findings (e.g., Leonard & Orchard, 1996; Ska & Joanette, 1996; Skenes & McCauley, 1985; Wickstron, Goldstein, & Johnson, 1985). Brookshire's (1983) study of articles published over the course of approximately 10 years in four journals indicated that "many, if not most, investigators fail to provide this information" (p. 343).

To date, no published empirical studies, including Brookshire's, have addressed the need to describe and control for visual acuity (accuracy of near and far vision), colour perception (ability to discriminate some or all colours), visual fields (areas of the visual space in which corresponding physical stimulation is available to the visual system), visual attention (ability to allocate and sustain sufficient cognitive resources to process visual stimuli for a given behavioural task), and oculomotor functions (ability to move and control movements of the eyes and their component parts) in research involving patients with neurogenic language disorders. Brookshire (1983) did track the general rubric of "visual acuity" as a factor considered in a review of published studies on aphasia, but does not specifically mention issues related to vision and its potential impact on validity. A table in that article does convey that only a minute proportion of articles, 2% in four journals published over a 10-year period, address visual acuity in aphasia patient participant descriptions.

Failure to control for and/or describe visual function in patients with neurogenic disorders is problematic for two primary reasons. First, most experimental tasks in such research, as well as a great deal of material used in testing of the speech, language, and cognitive abilities of participants, rely heavily on the processing of visual information. Typical assessment and experimental tasks presented to adults with aphasia and related language disorders include, but are not limited to, picture naming, reading, multiple choice selection of pictures and/or written text, picture description, and various decision tasks related to pictorial and/or graphic displays. Second, most patients with neurological disorders have some visual dysfunction, and many have multiple visual problems (Fisk, Owsley, & Mennemeier, 2002; Lincoln, 1991; Lubinksi, Moscato, & Willer, 1997; Myers & Brookshire, 1996). Examples of visual function deficits that may co-occur with language disorders due to a common underlying neurogenic impairment include visual neglect, visual field deficits, and colour perception deficits (Denes, Semenza, Stoppa, & Lis, 1982; Edmans & Lincoln, 1987; Kinsella & Ford, 1985; Wilson & Wyper, 1992). Additionally, other visual function deficits may present concomitantly with neurogenic language disorders. These include visual acuity deficits, often exacerbated by ageing and/ or peripheral neuropathic complications of diabetes and related metabolic disorders (Whitbourne, 1996), and congenital acuity or colour perception defects (Chang, 1995; Erie, 1992). Failure to screen and/or test for vision in the patient population may lead to a lack of experimental control for important aspects of vision, and a lack of adequate participant description for valid interpretation of experimental results.

IMPORTANT ASPECTS OF VISUAL FUNCTION IN LIGHT OF COMMON RESEARCH TASKS

Aspects of visual function most likely to be of highest relevance to studies of aphasia and related disorders are described briefly below. Visual characteristics are presented within a framework of (1) those that may be evaluated as part of a case history process, and (2) those that may be directly assessed or screened for by experimenters or collaborating

Case history information

History of visual problems and illnesses that may lead to or be associated with visual problems. Case history information may provide important indicators of concerns regarding visual functioning that may be relevant to assessment and/or experimental tasks. In some cases, previous diagnoses found in medical records or reported by patients and significant others have lasting symptoms of which the patient may or may not be aware. Such cases may include a history of illness that may lead to or be associated with visual dysfunction, such as diabetes and other metabolic diseases, thyroid disease, cancer, collagen vascular disease, or renal insufficiency, all of which have commonly associated aspects of visual dysfunction (Chang, 1995; Erie, 1992). Such cases may also include a history of specific visual problems, such as dyslexia, visual agnosia, visuospatial disorders, strabismus, amblyopia, glaucoma, cataracts, retinal problems, visual hallucinations, or blind spots (Denes et al., 1982; Edmans & Lincoln, 1987; Kinsella & Ford, 1985; Wilson & Wyper, 1992). Whether or not patients complain of persisting effects of such problems, being informed of such history will help the investigator attend to potential deficits that may influence performance in the study. For example, a patient's spouse may report that the patient's physician determined that the patient experienced right visual neglect immediately following a left hemisphere cerebrovascular accident, but there may have been no recent report of testing or screening for neglect; knowing the history of neglect may sensitise the researcher to the importance of screening in this important aspect of visual attention.

Wearing of glasses or contact lenses. Another potentially important factor is the patient's history of using glasses or contact lenses, most commonly prescribed for visual acuity problems. Not all patients appear for participation with the appropriate amplification to compensate for visual acuity problems. Explicitly knowing whether such amplification has been prescribed helps the investigator to consider the appropriate use of amplification for the study at hand. Also, some experimental methods may not permit the wearing of visual amplification (e.g., some eye tracking and tachistoscopic procedures); consideration of the consequences of the patient's viewing of experimental materials without amplification will be important in determining whether the patient should be included in the study and/or whether results should be scrutinised in terms of the potential influence of visual acuity problems.

Some glasses and contact lenses are prescribed to address visual problems other than or in addition to visual acuity problems. For example spot-field awareness prisms are designed to redirect information from a patient's blind visual field to the seeing visual field; Fresnel prisms may be added to glasses to help limit double vision and assist with balance problems by slightly offsetting the visual field from left to right. As in the case of visual acuity prescriptions, the consequences of not using glasses or contact lenses for assessment and experimentation should be considered in light of a given research study.

Visual discomfort. Requesting information about any visual discomfort, such as eyestrain, eye pressure, or dry or burning eyes, may help the investigator to consider the potential influence of such symptoms on comfort and potential distraction during any visual tasks administered during the study.

Screening and/or assessment of visual function

Ideally, screening and/or assessment of visual function for a given study incorporates all aspects of visual performance to be tapped by any and all assessment or experimental tasks to be presented to patients in a given study. Visual function should be considered even if no visual dysfunction is reported by the patient or his or her significant others. If the investigator has access to recent assessment or screening reports from an ophthalmologist or optometrist, he or she may not need to incorporate specific visual screenings. It remains important, however, that the status of visual function be reported in the publication of the study, to assure readers that visual function and its relevance to the study's validity have been addressed in inclusion/exclusion criteria, participant descriptions, analysis of results, and/or interpretation of results.

Specific procedures to assess or screen for visual acuity, colour perception, visual fields, visual attention, oculomotor functions, and methods for adapting those procedures for adults with language disorders, are beyond the scope of the current article. The importance of attending to the relevance of those functions in research on neurogenic language disorders is highlighted here.

Observation of the eyes. The observation of eye symmetry, lesions, swelling, or drainage at the time of research participation is important in terms of determining the need for further screening or assessment (Chang, 1995). Swelling and drainage, most often attributed to infectious disease or allergic reaction (Erie, 1992), may indicate potential discomfort and/or distraction during visual tasks that may confound patient performance. These conditions may also indicate a general sense of illness that may influence a patient's performance during participation on a given day. Asymmetry in the eyelids, eye orbits, or pupils is frequently indicative of neuromuscular involvement and may signal difficulties that will have potential impacts on visual function.

Although less likely to be relevant to cognitive and linguistic tasks generally employed in research on neurogenic language disorders, observation of the pupils may alert the researcher to potentially confounding visual performance factors. Pupil size varies among individuals and also changes as a function of alertness, emotional state, degree of accommodation, ambient room light, and age (Chavis & Hoyt, 1995). Abnormalities in the pupils may indicate neurological disorders (especially lesions of the optic pathways), current or past infectious diseases, alterations due to surgery, effects of ocular or systemic medications, and benign individual variations.

Visual acuity. Visual acuity is perhaps the most familiar of visual functions among researchers, as it pertains to the accuracy of vision for viewing stimuli and the degree to which vision is impaired or within normal ranges, and is the basis for most prescriptions for visual amplification. One author (Brookshire, 1983) has reported the frequency of reference to visual acuity in published reports on aphasia. Reviewing 52 research reports in four journals published in a 10-year period, Brookshire indicated that only 2% of the reports included any mention of visual acuity in patient descriptions. Given the reliance on visual acuity for accurate responding to a large proportion of assessment and experimental tasks for aphasia and related disorders, that finding signalled an important need for further attention to this important patient characteristic and potentially confounding factor.

Age-related macular degeneration is the most common cause of declining visual acuity, followed by diabetic retinopathy, glaucoma, and cataracts (Segal, 1996). Unless an experimental task involves an unlikely requirement that participants rely only on peripheral viewing of visual stimuli, central rather than peripheral acuity is of primary importance in research on neurogenic language disorders. Near central visual acuity involves viewing of materials at an average distance of 16 inches (Newell, 1992), and is most often tapped in visual tasks in traditional aphasia assessment and cognitive-linguistic experimentation, including reading of text, word cards, and computer displays, and viewing of real objects, pictures, or graphic displays. Far central visual acuity involves viewing of materials at an average distance of 20 feet (Newell, 1992), and thus is less apt to be tapped in the area of research under consideration. It may be of relevance, though, for tasks in a given study, such as the reading of public signs in real-world contexts or the viewing of slides projected at a distance of more than three feet.

In cases where all experimental tasks can be accomplished with glasses or contact lenses, it is ideal to have patient participants use such amplification during all testing and experimentation, and to have researchers report acuity for corrected vision. Only in cases where participants are unwilling or unable to wear appropriate amplification is it highly relevant to report unaided visual acuity.

Colour perception.   Colour perception difficulties may be congenital or acquired. The most common colour vision abnormality is red-green "colour blindness," a congenital X-chromosome linked deficiency in a single type of retinal photoreceptor. It occurs in approximately 8% of males and only 0.8% of females (Chang, 1995). Varied problems of colour perception are common in cases of cerebrovascular accident and traumatic brain injury (Newell, 1992), and thus are especially important in any research involving the presentation of coloured visual stimuli to patients with neurological disorders, especially if discerning colour is important to the task at hand. Likewise, colour perception problems tend to increase with advancing age, with older adults becoming less able to discriminate colours in the green-blue-violet spectrum (Weale, 1963). Test items requiring colour word comprehension and/or colour naming are included in most published aphasia batteries; interpretation of responses to such items, as well as to coloured experimental items, should be made only in light of information regarding patient participants' colour perceptual abilities.

Visual fields.   Visual fields refer to components of the area of the visual space subtended by an individual's actual visual range when the individual's head is stable. Visual field deficits involve a loss of visual information from specific areas of the visual space. Cases of heteronymous hemianopsia or quantrantopsia (lack of vision in a hemispace or quadrant of the visual space, corresponding to a contralateral lesion of the optic tract, optic radiations, or primary visual area of the cortex), homogeneous hemianopsia (or tunnel vision, corresponding to lesions of the optic chiasm), or scotoma (areas of no vision within the visual field, corresponding to lesions of the optic nerve or macula) are common following stroke and traumatic brain injury. Patients are not necessarily aware of visual field deficits, as they are less obvious and the symptoms tend to be more difficult for patients to describe than visual acuity problems. Both central and peripheral visual fields may be noted in terms of their relevance to the tasks involved. Both, but especially central visual fields, are relied on for successful participation in most visually based language assessment tasks (Harrington & Drake, 1990).

Visual attention.   Visual attention deficits, or problems allocating and sustaining sufficient cognitive resources to process visual stimuli for a given behavioural task, are common sequelae of stroke and traumatic brain injury (Denes et al., 1982; Kinsella & Ford, 1985). Problems with visual attention may stem from general attentional resource deficits affecting cognitive processing of information in all modalities. Generalised problems of inattention are especially common in patients with right hemisphere damage and diffuse traumatic brain injury (Myers, 1998; Tompkins, 1995; Ylvisaker, 1992). Exploration of the role of various aspects of attention is beyond the scope of this article, but still an important consideration in as much as any aspect of attention may influence assessment and experimental results.

A primary example of a specifically *visual* attention deficit in many patients with aphasia and related disorders, especially during the first 1–6 months post-onset, is visual neglect (Riddoch, 1991). Visual neglect reflects a failure to attend to visual information; it is almost always associated with inattention to the hemispace contralateral to the site of lesion. It may occur with or without incidence of visual field deficits (Varney & Sivan, 1986). Visual neglect may confound language assessment involving visual materials, especially if the investigator is unaware of the neglect and does not account for it in language testing or experimental design. Varied forms of dyslexia, especially those associated with neglect and letter-by-letter reading, are also associated with problems of visual attention (cf. Riddoch, 1991).

Oculomotor functions.   Oculomotor functions include any of the neuromuscular abilities that contribute to movements of the eyes or their component parts. Problems of oculomotor control are associated with any of the muscles controlling eye movement, deficits in the cranial nerves that innervate those muscles, and cortical influences on the formulation or conveyance of motor commands to the cranial nerves (Liesegang & McPhee, 1992; Newell, 1992).

Assessment of pupillary reactions is useful in localising lesions of the optic pathways (Chavis & Hoyt, 1995). Consensual pupillary constriction is the constriction of the right and left pupils as they converge to focus on the same visual target (Newell, 1992). Near constriction is of particular interest in most assessment tasks common to language assessment and experimentation.

Nystagmus is characterised by repetitive, rhythmic, oscillatory movements of the eyes. It influences visual acuity because the eyes are unable to maintain a steady fixation, especially when nystagmus appears in jerk form (with a slow movement in one direction followed by a rapid return to the initial position) as opposed to pendular form (with eye movements of equal amplitude, speed, and duration in each direction) (Hamburger, 1992).

Strabismus is a condition of abnormal deviation of the eyes such that both eyes are not simultaneously directed towards the same object. It may influence performance in any visual task where ocular alignment is required or beneficial. It may also detract from visual acuity, and is frequently associated with diplopia, or double vision (Eggers, 1995; Hohberger, 1992).

Oculomotor apraxia is a deficit in motor programming for movement of the eyes. It is most frequently associated with traumatic brain injuries and lesions affecting the frontal lobes. Patients are rarely specifically aware of the condition prior to diagnosis, although they may sense some trouble with their eye movements. As in other forms of apraxia, oculomotor apraxia is notable during volitional—in contrast to spontaneous or auto-matic—tasks and, as such, influences intentional planned movements of the eyes (Liesegang & McPhee, 1992; Newell, 1992). It may be relevant to assessment or experimental tasks in which patients are asked to use eye movements to indicate inten-tional responses in behavioural tasks, so it may be especially important to consider in visual scanning and eye tracking studies.

The current study

In the present study, specific characteristics of visual function as described above are considered in light of visual screening or assessment tasks that yield information that may therefore should be implemented and described when appropriate for any given study. Careful consideration of visual function abilities pertinent to the tasks presented in a given study helps researchers to constructively enhance their inclusion/exclusion criteria, control methods, and patient descriptions. Reporting specific considerations of visual function in published research reports enables readers to better evaluate the results and implications of a given study, and also enhances the replicability of studies reported.

The primary goal of the current study was to examine and describe practices in the control for and description of visual functions in research on neurogenic language disorders. A thorough evaluation of such practices is an essential first step for developing follow-up strategies to address needs for improved experimental control and participant description.

METHOD

Data were collected from all journal articles pertaining to aphasia (subsequent to left hemisphere damage) and related language disorders (subsequent to TBI and/or right hemisphere damage) in adults published in 17 journals for the period of September 1991 to August 2001. Journals selected were those likely to include peer-reviewed publications reporting original empirical research relevant to adult neurogenic language disorders. The journals included are listed in Table 1. Articles not including empirical data were excluded, as were case studies in which no specific independent variables were controlled for or manipulated.

Each published test battery, subtest, and experimental task mentioned in each of the articles was considered thoroughly in terms of whether or not it involved the use of visual

TABLE 1
Number of qualifying articles on adult aphasia and related neurogenic language disorders found in 17 journals between September 1991 and August 2001

Journals	Number of articles
American Journal of Speech-Language Pathology	19
Annals of Neurology	4
Aphasiology	190
Archives of Neurology	11
Archives of Physical Medicine and Rehabilitation	5
Brain and Cognition	12
Brain and Language	213
Clinical Aphasiology	108*
International Journal of Language and Communication Disorders (1992–2001), British Journal of Disorders of Communication (1991), and European Journal of Disorders of Communication (1992–1997)	24
International Journal of Rehabilitation Research	2
Journal of Communication Disorders	14
Journal of Head Trauma and Rehabilitation	0
Journal of Medical Speech Language Pathology	16
Journal of Rehabilitation Research and Development	0
Journal of Speech and Hearing Research (1992–1995) and Journal of Speech, Language and Hearing Research (1996–2001)	31
Language and Cognitive Processes	3
Neurology	16
Total	668

materials as testing stimuli; each study was coded accordingly in a binary coding scheme. For example, if the study included visual materials, it would be coded as "1" (signifying "yes") for inclusion of visual materials. For studies involving the use of visual materials for assessment and/or experimentation, aspects of visual function required (reading, drawing, colour discrimination, or multiple-choice with objects or pictures) were coded in the same way. For example, if the study included one or more tasks involving colour discrimination, it was coded as "1" (signifying "yes") for requirement of colour discrimination. Data points were coded as missing when the nature of visual materials or tasks could not be determined, e.g., in cases of unpublished materials administered but not clearly described in the included article.

Also noted was whether or not the authors described or controlled for various aspects of visual function or status in their patient samples, and whether authors used such aspects to determine inclusion and/or exclusion criteria for participants. To ensure a conservative approach, thus capturing any attention at all to visual function within each article, mention of visual function in inclusion/exclusion criteria, pre-testing to ensure task performance ability, experimental control, patient description, statistical analysis, and/or interpretation of results was coded as a "yes" for controlling for and/or describing visual function.

Selection of the visual function information to be tracked was determined through an extensive review of the clinical visual assessment literature, with a focus on aspects that were likely to affect the validity of assessment results in patients with aphasia. The list of items tracked was scrutinised and edited in consultation with a practising neurophalmologist and a practising optometrist until both were in agreement with the final list. Any description of and control for each of the visual function items, including case history, observation, and screening or assessment items, was coded in a binary fashion. The items investigated are outlined in Table 2. All are described in the introduction to this article.

Data were collected by a team of four graduate and two undergraduate students in communication sciences and disorders after training by the first author regarding the nature of the study and specific coding methods and criteria. Training involved 3 hours of discussion about the rationale and design of the study, a minimum of 2 hours of hands-on training in the implementation of a visual case history and screening protocol including each of the items listed in Table 2, and supervised review and coding of a minimum of five articles for each student. Additionally, the following were provided for reference by the scorers during data collection: a review glossary to ensure mutual understanding of visual function, screening and assessment terms, a list of decision criteria for each item to be tracked, and examples of coding scenarios.

Reliability and reproducibility

Reliability and reproducibility data for the coding of research articles were obtained through repeat scoring of a random sample of 30% of the articles by independent scorers. Repeat scorers were among the scorers trained and involved in the original data collection. No scorer performed repeat scoring on articles he or she had previously scored. For any item within an article that was not coded identically by both scorers, the original scorer and the second scorer reviewed the article in person together, discussing each discrepancy until there was 100% resolution of disagreements. Reliability statistics were calculated for every visual function item tracked. Near visual acuity was the item chosen as a basis for calculating reproducibility of results, given the clear import of this basic

TABLE 2
Visual function characteristics examined for each research article

I. Case history information reported, described or controlled
    A. History of illness that may lead to or be associated with visual dysfunction (with any specific reference to vision)
    B. History of visual problems such as strabismus, amblyopia, glaucoma, cataracts, retinal problems, visual hallucinations, blind spots, etc.
    C. Wearing of glasses or contact lenses
    D. Visual discomfort, such as eyestrain, eye pressure, or dry or burning eyes

II. Screening and/or assessment aspects reported, described or controlled
    A. Observation of symmetry, lesions, swelling, or eye drainage
       • Observation of pupil size
    B. Visual acuity
       • Near central visual acuity (aided and unaided)
       • Far central visual acuity (aided and unaided)
    C. Colour perception
    D. Visual fields (general)
       • Central visual fields
       • Peripheral visual fields
    E. Visual attention deficits
    F. Oculomotor functions
       • Pupillary constriction
       • Near constriction of pupils
       • Nystagmus
       • Strabismus
       • Oculomotor apraxia

aspect of visual function for effective processing of visual information presented in typical testing and experimental tasks.

RESULTS

Article representation by journal

In total, 668 articles met inclusion criteria. No qualifying articles were found in the *Journal of Head Trauma and Rehabilitation* or the *Journal of Rehabilitation Research and Development*. Among the 15 journals that contained at least one relevant article, *Brain and Language*, *Aphasiology*, and *Clinical Aphasiology* were the three that published the largest number of relevant articles.

Reliability and reproducibility

Reliability of data collection was tested through repeated data extraction for a random sample of 30% of the articles by an independent scorer. Prior to 100% agreement achieved by both scorers reviewing each discrepancy together, initial inter-scorer agreement for the coding of the specific visual function variables ranged from 79% to 96%.

Using the re-scored data pertaining to the same 30% of articles in the study used for reliability testing, reproducibility for data extraction was calculated for the description of near central visual acuity, selected for its high degree of relevance to the majority of typical assessment tasks involving visual materials. Two independent observers agreed on 190 (96%) of 198 articles regarding the appraisal or lack of appraisal of near central visual acuity. The associated Cohen's kappa showed a substantial agreement (Kappa = 0.62). Again, all discrepancies in data recorded for original versus reliability extraction were discussed by two independent scorers, and resolved through their consensus upon re-examination of the articles in question.

For each item tacked in all of the research articles included in the study, 95% confidence intervals, presented in Table 3, were calculated. They demonstrate low variability in the frequency (across all articles) of authors addressing visual function items.

Description of and control for visual function

All but one qualifying article (99.85%) involved presentation of visual materials for testing of speech, language, and/or cognitive abilities, and/or for tasks involved in reported experimental protocols. Data pertaining to the number of articles that do include visual materials in patient evaluation and/or experimental testing are summarised in Table 3, according to specific aspects of visual function that may influence patient performance in responding to testing and experimental stimuli.

Case history

No more than 2.7% of studies included any type of case history information regarding visual function for inclusion or exclusion criteria, patient description, or experimental control: 97.3% of authors failed to mention any information regarding the history of

TABLE 3

Results among studies in which visual materials were presented to patients during reported evaluation and/or experimental tasks

Description	Total number of articles*	Articles including description	Percent of articles including description	95% Confidence interval (lower limit, upper limit)
History of illness associated with visual dysfunction	668	18	2.7	.01, .04
History of visual problems	668	8	1.2	.02, .06
Wearing of glasses, contact lenses	668	16	2.4	.01, .04
Visual discomfort	668	3	0.4	0, .03
Observation of symmetry, lesions, eye swelling, drainage	667	5	0.7	0.2, 1.7
Pupil size	667	3	0.4	0, 1.3
Central visual acuity	666	31	5	3, 7
Near visual acuity	666	31	5	3, 7
Far visual acuity	666	33	5	3, 7
Colour vision**	318	5	1.6	0.2, 2.9
Visual fields	667	60	9	7, 11
Central visual fields	667	2	0.3	0.4, 1.0
Peripheral visual fields	667	4	0.6	0.2, 1.5
Visual attention	667	60	9	7, 11
Pupillary constriction	667	2	0.3	0, 1.1
Strabismus	667	3	0.4	0, 1.3
Nystagmus	667	3	0.4	0, 1.3
Oculomotor apraxia	667	3	0.4	0, 1.3

*Numbers of articles vary because articles for which information was not clear for a given item were excluded from analyses for that item.

**Includes only articles involving the use of materials in color.

illness that may lead to or be associated with visual dysfunction (e.g., strabismus, amblyopia, glaucoma, cataracts, retinal problems, visual hallucinations, blind spots); 98.8% did not mention anything about patient history of visual problems; 97.6% did not mention whether patients wore glasses or contact lenses; and 99.6% failed to mention whether patients experienced visual discomfort (e.g., eyestrain, eye pressure, or dry or burning eyes).

Screening and/or assessment

No more than 0.7% of studies included any information related to observation of the eyes: 99.3% made no mention of symmetry, lesions, swelling, or eye drainage; and 99.6% did not comment on pupil size.

Only 9% or fewer of all articles included any type of visual screening and/or assessment information for participant inclusion or exclusion criteria, participant description, or experimental control. Only 5% mentioned near acuity and only 5% mentioned far acuity.

Articles not involving visual material in colour were excluded from analyses of whether colour vision abilities were mentioned. Of the 47.6% articles that entailed use of coloured visual materials, only 1.6% included any description of or control for colour vision abilities.

Aspects of visual attention and visual field status were the most commonly reported of all factors monitored in the study, but neither was reported in more than 9% of the articles. A total of 91% of articles failed to include information regarding any aspect of visual attention, including visual neglect; 9% included information about patients' visual fields, with only 0.3% including specific information about central fields and 0.6% including information about peripheral fields.

Few articles included any mention of patients' oculomotor functions, including pupillary constriction (0.3%), nystagmus (0.4%), strabismus (0.4%), or oculomotor apraxia (0.4%)

DISCUSSION

The seriousness of consequence of the failure to mention a specific aspect of visual status in terms of experimental control and/or interpretation of results depends largely on three main factors to be considered in the context of each individual study. First, as highlighted in the introduction, the relevance of any particular aspect of visual function is relative to the specific assessment and experimental tasks involved in a specific research study. For example, it would not be important to address far visual acuity in a study involving only near vision tasks. Second, the severity of relevant visual function deficits that patient participants possess must be considered in the light of each particular study. For example, if a patient has a near visual acuity problem even when wearing contact lenses or glasses, but performs a near vision task for which his or her near visual acuity is sufficient (such as in reading text in large font at a close viewing distance), then the mere presence of a visual acuity problem may not influence the validity of results. Still, screening for visual acuity at least would be essential for determining whether these factors might have influenced patients' performance, and thus the validity of results. Third, there is the possibility that visual abilities are being assessed by some researchers but that screening methods or results are not included in the published reports. With heightened awareness of the potential influence of visual functioning on the validity of assessment and experimental results, authors may better convince readers of the validity of their results and conclusions.

Given the importance of considering any individual study in light of these three principles, the amassed data regarding specific aspects of visual function do not necessarily capture the relative importance of screening for each specific factor in the context of any particular study, and thus do not convey the relative risk in not describing or controlling for that factor. Still, given the extremely high-frequency use of visual material in assessment and experimental tasks—all but 1 of the 668 articles published in a broad array of journals over 10 years—the lack of mention, description, or control for even very basic aspects of visual function clearly indicates a need for improvement among researchers in this area. At a minimum, screening for visual field deficits, visual attention, near visual acuity, and colour perception are critical to the valid interpretation of findings from most assessment batteries for aphasia and related language disorders

Given that only reports involving visual materials were included in the monitoring of whether visual function was addressed, the status of control and description of visual function in research on aphasia and related disorders is clearly grim. Especially in light of the fact that many patients with neurological disorders display one or multiple types of deficits in visual functioning (Fisk et al., 2002; Lubinksi et al., 1997; Myers & Brookshire, 1996), failure to take into account relevant visual deficits when assessment or experimental tasks involve visual information may lead to invalid test results, experimental results, and/or interpretation of experimental findings.

It is critical that investigators carefully screen for, describe, and control visual performance in patients with neurogenic communication disorders when performing research that entails the use of visual materials for testing or experimental tasks. A vision screening protocol of subject inclusion or exclusion should be designed with careful consideration of the potential effects of any visual function deficit on the validity of results in light of the task requirements for a given study.

As training in visual assessment is not central to the education of most researchers in neurogenic communication disorders, guidance is needed in the development and implementation of visual screening protocols. Also needed are continuing education opportunities regarding specific means of screening for oculomotor functioning and visual acuity, processing, and attention. Constructive feedback concerning appropriate participant control and description is important in the peer review process for research publication and funding.

REFERENCES

Brookshire, R. H. (1983). Subject description and the generality of results in experiments with aphasic adults. *Journal of Speech and Hearing Disorders, 48,* 342–346.

Chang, D. F. (1995). Ophthalmologic examination. In D. Vaughan, T. Asbury, & P. Riordan-Eva (Eds.), *General ophthalmology* (pp. 2–50). Norwalk, CT: Appleton & Lange.

Denes, G., Semenza, C., Stoppa, E., & Lis, A. (1982). Unilateral spatial neglect and recovery from hemiplegia: A follow-up study. *Brain, 105,* 542–552.

Edmans, J. A., & Lincoln, N. B. (1987). The frequency of perceptual deficits after stroke. *Clinical Rehabilitation, 1,* 273–281.

Eggers, H. M. (1995). Strabismus. In D. Vaughan, T. Asbury, & P. Riordan-Eva (Eds.), *General ophthalmology* (p. 208). Norwalk, CT: Appleton & Lange.

Erie, C. J. (1992). Ophthalmic history and examination. In G. B. Bartley & T. J. Liesegang (Eds.), *Essentials of ophthalmology* (pp. 4–182). Philadelphia: J. B. Lippincott Company.

Fisk, G. D., Owsley, C., & Mennemeier, M. (2002). Vision, attention, and self-reported driving behaviors in community-dwelling stroke survivors. *Archives of Physical Medicine and Rehabilitation, 83,* 469–477.

Harrington, D. O., & Drake, M. V. (1990). *The visual fields.* St. Louis: The C.V. Mosby Company.

Hohberger, G. G. (1992). Ocular motility, strabismus and amblyopia. In G. B. Bartley, T.J. Liesegang, & T. J. McPhee (Eds.), *Essentials of ophthalmology* (pp. 254–255). Philadelphia: J. B. Lippincott Company.

Liesegang, T. J., & McPhee, T. J. (1992). Neuro-ophthalmology. In G. B. Bartley & T. J. Liesegang (Eds.), *Essentials of ophthalmology* (pp. 4–182). Philadelphia: J. B. Lippincott Company.

Leonard, C. L., & Orchard, D. (1996). The problem of generalizing to a language population: A "random" controversy. *Journal of Speech and Hearing Research, 39*, 406–413.

Lincoln, N. B. (1991). The recognition and treatment of visual perceptual disorders. *Topics in Geriatric Rehabilitation, 7*(1), 25–34.

Lubinski, R., Moscato, B. S., & Willer, B. S. (1997). Prevalence of speaking and hearing disabilities among adults with traumatic brain injury from a national household survey. *Brain Injury, 11*(2), 103–114.

Myers, P. S. (1998). *Right hemisphere damage: Disorders of cognition and communication*. San Diego, CA: Singular Publishing Group.

Myers, P. S., & Brookshire, R. H. (1996). Effect of visual and inferential variables on scene descriptions by right-hemisphere-damaged, and non-brain-damaged adults: *Journal of Speech and Hearing Research, 39*, 870–880.

Newell, F. W. (1992). *Opthalmology principles and concepts* (pp. 143–515, 525–543). St. Louis, MO: Mosby Year Book.

Riddoch, M. J. (1991) Neglect and the peripheral dyslexias. In M. J. Riddoch (Ed.), *Neglect and the peripheral dyslexias* (pp. 369–390). Hove, UK: Lawrence Erlbaum Associates Ltd.

Ska, B., & Joanette, Y. (1996). Discourse in older adults: Influence of text, task, and participant characteristics. *American Journal of Speech-Language Pathology and Audiology, 20*(2), 101–107.

Segal, E.S. (1996). Common medical problems in geriatric patients. In L. L. Cartensen, B. A. Edelstein, & L. Dornbrans (Eds.), *The practical handbook of clinical gerontology* (pp. 3–35). Thousand Oaks, CA: Sage Publications.

Skenes, L. L., & McCauley, R. J. (1985). Psychometric review of nine aphasia tests. *Journal of Communication Disorders, 18*, 461–474.

Tompkins, C. (1995). *Right hemisphere communication disorders: Theory and management*. San Diego. CA: Singular Publishing.

Weale, R. A. (1963). *The aging eye*. London: H.K. Lewis.

Whitbourne, S. K. (1996). Psychological perspectives on the normal aging process. In L. L. Cartensen, B. A. Edelstein, & L. Dornbrans (Eds.), *The practical handbook of clinical gerontology* (pp. 3–35). Thousand Oaks, CA: Sage Publications.

Wickstron S., Goldstein H., & Johnson, L. (1985). On the subject of subjects: Suggestions for describing the subjects in language intervention studies. *Journal of Speech and Hearing Disorders, 50*, 282–286.

Wilson, J., & Wyper, D. (1992). Neuroimaging and neuropsychological functioning following closed head injury: CT, MRI and SPECT. *Journal of Head Trauma Rehabilitation, 7*, 29–30.

Ylvisaker, M. (1992). Communication outcome following traumatic brain injury. *Seminars in Speech and Language, 13*, 239–251.

APHASIOLOGY, 2004, *18* (5/6/7), 625–637

Effects of training volunteers to converse with nursing home residents with aphasia

Ellen M. Hickey

Dalhousie University, Halifax, Nova Scotia, Canada

Michelle S. Bourgeois

Florida State University, Tallahassee, FL, USA

Lesley B. Olswang

University of Washington, Seattle, WA, USA

Background: Nursing home residents with aphasia often experience social isolation. Providing trained conversation partners is one way to combat this problem, but evidence is needed for the effects of training conversation partners for persons with aphasia. The use of four college student volunteers was based on evidence for the benefits of intergenerational service-learning programmes.
Aims: The purpose of this study was to examine the effects of training four college student volunteers (SVs) to use multi-modality communication with two nursing home residents with Broca's aphasia (RAs).
Methods & Procedures: An ABA multiple baseline across subjects (SVs) and partners (RAs) design was used to examine the effects of the training programme in probe conversations. Each RA interacted with two SVs. Training consisted of five steps, with a criterion to move through each step of the programme, and to withdraw training. Thorough treatment fidelity procedures were used to ensure consistent training across subjects.
Outcomes & Results: The SVs demonstrated marked increases in multi-modality communication, with concomitant increases in RAs' comprehensibility. Sequential analyses revealed that multi-modality communication is more likely than speech only to elicit RAs' comprehensible responses, with a stronger effect after training. Social validity ratings demonstrated that the changes in the quality of the conversations were clinically significant.
Conclusions: This study revealed positive effects of training conversation partners of persons with aphasia to use multi-modality communication. Intergenerational service-learning programmes are one viable method to decrease social isolation and to increase opportunities for nursing home residents with aphasia to reveal their communicative competence.

Given the psychosocial ramifications of aphasia (Le Dorze & Brassard, 1995), creative solutions are needed to increase access to positive social interactions for persons with aphasia. A variety of conversation partners have been considered for persons with aphasia living in their own homes. For example, family members (Booth & Perkins, 1999; Hopper,

Address correspondence to: Ellen M. Hickey, School of Human Communication Disorders, 5599 Fenwick Street, Halifax, NS B3H 1R2, Canada. Email: ehickey@dal.ca

This study was funded by NIA Grant AG13008 to the Florida State University. The authors would like to thank all participants and nursing home staff who made this research possible. The advice of Kathryn Yorkston, Howard Goldstein, and S. Natasha Beretvas is appreciated.

http://www.tandf.co.uk/journals/pp/02687038.html   DOI: 10.1080/02687030444000093

Holland, & Rewega, 2002; Olswang, Hickey, Alarcon, & Rogers, 1998; Simmons, Kearns, & Potechin, 1987) and community volunteers (Kagan, Black, Duchan, Simmons-Mackie, & Square, 2001; Lyon et al., 1997) have been trained to support communication and social interactions for individuals with aphasia. Evidence supports the use of these trained volunteer conversation partners to increase societal participation for persons with aphasia.

The communication needs of nursing home residents with aphasia have not been addressed using this type of intervention. Providing trained conversation partners may increase their participation in social interaction as well. An intergenerational service-learning programme, which promotes elder–youth interaction and incorporates community service into higher education (Arkin, 1998; McGowan, 1994), is one possibility. The aim of this study was to train college student volunteers to be conversation partners for nursing home residents with aphasia.

Volunteers reportedly have difficulty discovering facilitative communication strategies on their own (Simmons-Mackie & Kagan, 1999). Further, research is not conclusive about specific helpful versus unhelpful behaviours, although multi-modality communication is often reported as a supportive strategy (Hickey, Alarcon, Rogers, & Olswang, 1998; Kagan et al., 2001).

Studies of conversation partner training have rarely examined the direct effects of the partner's trained behaviours on the communication behaviours of the individual with aphasia. Booth and Perkins (1999) used conversation analysis to measure pre- and post-intervention interactions, and to demonstrate the relationship between partner behaviours and participation of the individual with aphasia. No studies have used quantitative sequential analysis to examine this relationship. Finally, the lack of treatment fidelity measures and/or social validity measures in this research leaves many unanswered questions concerning the connection between partner training and corresponding changes in behaviours of individuals with aphasia.

The purpose of this study was to examine the effectiveness of a training programme to increase student volunteers' use of multi-modality communication during conversational interactions with nursing home residents with aphasia. The goal was to increase the residents' utterances that were comprehensible to their conversational partners. The following research questions were addressed: (1) Is multi-modality communication training effective in changing the proportion of student volunteers' use of multi-modality utterances during probe conversations? If so, how many sessions does it take for student volunteers to reach criterion for proportion of multi-modality utterances in probe conversations, and is this maintained when training is withdrawn? (2) Do the residents' proportions of comprehensible utterances increase after the student volunteers are trained to use multiple modalities? (3) Are the residents' comprehensible utterances more likely to follow the student volunteers' use of multi-modality communication than use of speech-only communication, and does this change after training? (4) Are changes in communication in the dyads clinically significant, as determined by observations and ratings of unfamiliar judges?

METHOD

Participants

Student volunteers. Four student volunteers (SVs) were recruited from all first semester majors in Communication Science and Disorders at a large university in the south-eastern USA. All SVs were Caucasian females, 20 to 25 years old, and had no prior experience with individuals with aphasia or coursework on aphasia. All students signed

Residents with aphasia.   Two nursing home residents with aphasia (RAs) participated (see Table 1 for demographic and aphasia information). The RAs met the following inclusion criteria: (1) primary diagnosis of single left hemisphere stroke
resulting in right hemiparesis, apraxia of speech, and Broca's aphasia, as determined
by the Western Aphasia Battery (WAB: Kertesz, 1982), with a maximum aphasia
quotient of 40/100; (2) minimum of 6 months post stroke; (3) hearing and vision
within functional limits (aided or unaided). Informed consent was first obtained by the
residents' family members (the person listed as primary contact in the resident's chart)
and then by the resident, using multi-modality communication to explain the study
procedures.

Setting and apparatus

The study took place in two mixed-population, privately owned nursing homes with
similar staffing, size, and structure. Participants sat at a table in a quiet room of the RA's
choice. Probe conversations were videotaped and audio taped, and timed with a stopwatch.

Multi-modality communication training

The SVs received training three times per week to increase their use of multi-modality
communication in conversations with the RAs. The experimenter (EH), a certified
speech-language pathologist, administered the training, using a manual and data collection sheets to keep the training consistent (Hickey, 2000a, 2000b). The training

TABLE 1
Demographic and aphasia characteristics for residents with aphasia (RA)

Characteristic	RA1	RA2
Time post-CVA	37 months	72 months
Age	72	77
Education	12	12
Marital status	Widower	Widow
Number of children	0	6
Frequency of visitors	1–2 × /year	1 × /week
Participates in activities	Yes	No
Eats meals in dining room	Yes	No
Length of time at nursing home	37 months	48 months
WAB Aphasia Quotient	27.8/100	15/100
WAB Aphasia Classification	Broca's	Broca's
RCPM	77th %ile	83rd %ile
Description of functional communication	primarily stereotypy: "Dovanday"; empty speech; gestures/pointing	head nods/shakes, facial expressions; rare speech; gestures/pointing

WAB = Western Aphasia Battery (Kertesz, 1982).
RCPM = Raven's Coloured Progressive Matrices (Raven, 1938, 1960).

included five steps: (1) general education; (2) identification of communication modalities in videotaped conversations of others (trained partners) interacting with the RAs; (3) SV self-evaluation of the use of multi-modality communication in videotape review of baseline conversations; (4) conversational practice of multi-modality communication with on-line feedback; and (5) conversational practice of multi-modality communication without on-line feedback. Progress through the training was determined using a criterion for each step in the programme. (The detailed training manual is available from the first author.) Each training session was followed by a probe conversation at the nursing home.

Stimuli

During all interactions, a variety of visual stimuli were available to support the conversations, but the actual stimulus sets were different for training versus probe conversations. Stimuli included two current newspaper headlines with pictures, pencil and paper, a small atlas of the USA, five personalised communication cards, and five categorical communication cards (e.g., cards with pictures and words related to entertainment, places, hobbies, sports, etc.).

Data collection and procedures

Conversation probes. The SVs and RAs participated in 10-minute probe conversations one to three times per week throughout the study, using the multiple probe technique, described below. The dyads were instructed to converse as follows: "You will have a conversation for 10 minutes. You can talk about anything you want, including your family, your hobbies, or your daily activities. You can also talk about these cards and newspaper clippings. I'm going to leave for 10 minutes. Keep talking until I come back." After the instructions were provided, the video and audio recording and stopwatch were started, and the examiner left the room for 10 minutes.

Transcription and scoring. The probe conversations were first transcribed verbatim from audiotape, then descriptions of all nonverbal behaviours were added while viewing the videotapes, using Systematic Analysis of Language Transcripts (SALT: Miller & Chapman, 1998). Coding consisted of three steps. SV utterances were coded for specific modality of communication, then for general modality. Next, RAs' utterances were coded for comprehensibility, using the following operational definitions.

1. *SV and RA specific modality*: (a) *Speaking*: minimal encouragers (e.g., "mhm"), words and sentences. (b) *Drawing*: a drawn picture or symbol. (c) *Gesturing*: upper extremity movement to convey meaning. (d) *Pointing*: to visual stimuli such as objects (e.g., TV, clock), newspaper articles, written materials, or communication cards. (e) *Writing*: written words or numbers.
2. *SV general modality*: (a) *Speech-only* utterances (i.e., no use of nonverbal modalities), or (b) *Multi-modality* utterances (i.e., use of a nonverbal modality at least once, such as gesturing, drawing, writing, or pointing), with or without speaking.
3. *RA comprehensibility*: (a) *Comprehensible utterances* were understood by the SV as determined by the SV's response, including intelligible speech, and unambiguous and meaningful nonverbal communication behaviours. (b) *Incomprehensible utterances* were not understood by the SV as determined by the SV's response, including unintelligible speech, and ambiguous, perseverative, or empty communication acts.

Experimental design

An ABA multiple baseline across subjects (SVs) and partners (RAs) design (Hersen & Barlow, 1976) was employed to measure the effectiveness and effects of training SVs to use multi-modality communication with RAs with aphasia. Three phases were included in the design: (1) baseline (A); 2) training of the SVs (B); and (3) post-training (A). During all phases, probe conversations were conducted. The primary dependent variables included SVs' communication modalities and RAs' comprehensibility in probe conversations.

Baselines began concurrently for all SV–RA dyads. The training phase was introduced sequentially across dyads. Movement from baseline to training phases was made after visual inspection of a minimum of three data points indicated a stable or decreasing trend in use of multi-modality communication. Movement from training to post-training phases was made after the SV reached criterion for all training steps, and for use of multi-modality communication during the probe conversations. The criterion for probe conversations was use of multi-modality communication in at least 70% of utterances in a minimum of three probe conversations. While this criterion is high, an utterance was coded as multi-modality even if only one nonverbal modality was used to convey one concept in the utterance (e.g., "Do you like bingo?" while pointing to bingo on the communication card). In addition, the criterion was set high in order to ensure training receipt. The post-training phase ended after a minimum of three data points were collected for SV4 (the last SV to be trained), with a stable or increasing trend for proportion of multi-modality utterances.

Given the possibility of extended baseline and post-training phases, the multiple probe technique was used to limit the number of data collection sessions. Probes were collected once a week during the baseline phase, until the last 1–2 weeks immediately preceding training, when probes were collected three times a week. Post-training sessions were conducted in similar fashion, with three probe conversations per week for at least 1 week immediately following post-training, and then one probe conversation session per week until the last dyad completed post-training.

Social validation measures

Social validation measures (Kazdin, 1982) were obtained from 15 unfamiliar judges (10 undergraduate and 5 doctoral students in speech and hearing sciences) in order to determine if multi-modality communication training with SVs produced clinically significant changes in conversations with RAs, as observed by persons unfamiliar with the participants and target behaviours. One baseline and one post-training probe conversation were randomly selected for each dyad. Three-minute segments (i.e., minutes three to five) were dubbed onto a master tape, with the two segments for each dyad dubbed consecutively in counterbalanced order. The judges viewed the videotape twice. Then they completed rating scales on six dimensions using 5-inch visual analogue scales, ranging from 0% to 100% of the time, to rate each conversational segment for: (1) comfort level of each participant, (2) amount of information conveyed by RAs, (3) effectiveness of SVs' communication behaviours, (4) equity of turn-taking, and (5) topic maintenance. The tape was stopped after each dyad while the judges marked the rating scales. The judges used one page per dyad, with ratings for each conversation marked in different colours.

Reliability

Trained assistants computed reliability measures for transcription and dependent measures on four randomly selected probe conversations for each dyad and phase (22% for each dyad). For transcription reliability, any disagreements were marked on the transcript by the assistants while they watched the videotaped probe conversation. Word agreement was 96.7% to 99.5% and utterance agreement was 97.3% to 100% for each transcript. The dependent measures were independently coded, and reliability was calculated using Cohen's Kappa (Kazdin, 1982). Measurement reliability values of .95 to .98 for modality coding and of .63 to .65 for comprehensibility coding were considered acceptable (Hollenbeck, 1978).

Adherence to treatment procedures was accomplished by use of a manual that described the steps of the programme and criterion behaviour for each step, a script for the general education programme, and data collection sheets for the dependent variables and training procedures (Moncher & Prinz, 1991). This ensured that each SV received the same information, instructions, and minimum number of trials (e.g., number of trials in videotape review). In addition, an independent, trained observer watched videotapes of one training session from each step of the training programme (25% of sessions), and tallied the opportunities for experimenter behaviours and the number of times the experimenter used the expected behaviour (e.g., prompts, models, reinforcement). Adherence to the protocol was calculated using the formula $(EA \times 100)/ET$, where EA = the experimenter behaviours actually used, and ET = the total opportunities for the experimenter behaviours (Billingsley, White, & Munson, 1980). Procedural reliability was 95% to 100% for each step.

Data analyses

Research questions 1 and 2 were addressed by visual inspection of the data across experimental phases (within and across participants) with regard to changes in level, slope, and trend (Hersen & Barlow, 1976; Kazdin, 1982). Data for question 1 are SVs' proportions of speech-only versus multi-modality utterances. Data for question 2 are RAs' proportions of comprehensible versus incomprehensible utterances. Research question 3 was addressed using sequential analysis methods, described below. Data for research question 4 were the unfamiliar judges' social validity ratings on all dimensions for each dyad, with means compared across baseline and post-training phases using two-tailed paired-sample t-tests.

Sequential analyses.   The likelihood of RAs' production of comprehensible utterances following the SVs' speech-only versus multi-modality utterances was examined using sequential analyses. Utterance codes for the SV's given behaviours (i.e., speech-only versus multi-modality), and the RA's target behaviours (i.e., comprehensible versus incomprehensible) were entered into a computer using Multiple Option Observation System for Experimental Studies software (MOOSES: Tapp, 1996). One pooled list for each dyad for each phase was analysed using a lag-1 sequential analysis to determine the sequential association, in terms of Yule's Q, for the observed frequency of a RA target behaviour (i.e., comprehensible utterance) following an SV's given behaviour (i.e., speech-only versus multi-modality). Yule's Q was computed as an index of sequential association between the student behaviours and the resident behaviours (Bakeman &

Gottman, 1997; Tapp, 1996). Yule's Q is the transformation of the odds ratio of the target sequences, and ranges from -1 to $+1$ (Bakeman & Gottman, 1997).

RESULTS

SVs' use of multi-modality communication

The proportion of SVs' multi-modality versus speech-only utterances in probe conversations during baseline, training, and post-training phases is displayed in Figure 1. All four SVs used primarily speech-only utterances to communicate in baseline conversations, with a tendency to produce at least 70% speech-only utterances. All four SVs demonstrated an immediate increase in use of multi-modality communication and decrease in use of speech-only communication after the first training session. All SVs had an immediate increase in the proportions of speech-only versus multi-modality utterances. All SVs achieved criterion for each of the five steps of training in one session. SV1, SV3, and SV4 also achieved criterion for probe conversations after five training sessions, and training was withdrawn. SV2 had borderline performance in the probe conversation after the fifth training session, so one additional session of step 5 was conducted, for a total of six training sessions. All four SVs maintained high proportions of multi-modality utterances in post-training, with stable levels around the criterion of 70%.

RAs' comprehensibility

The proportion of RAs' comprehensible versus incomprehensible utterances is displayed in Figure 2, with each dyad's graphs presented in the same order as in Figure 1. RA1 had approximately 40% to 70% comprehensible utterances during baseline with SV1 and SV4. In both dyads, RA1 increased the proportion of comprehensible utterances during the training phase to approximately 75–85%. Furthermore, RA1's increase in the level of comprehensible utterances did not occur in either dyad until the SV began training. RA1's comprehensibility was stable at approximately 70–75% during post-training with both SVs. RA2's proportion of comprehensible utterances was approximately 70–90% with SV2 and SV3 during baseline. Once the SVs were trained, RA2's proportion of comprehensible utterances increased to approximately 85–97%. Although this was not a substantial increase, her comprehensible utterances were also more stable than during baseline.

Sequential association of SV–RA behaviours

The likelihood of the RAs' comprehensible response following the SVs' speech-only or multi-modality utterance was examined using lag-1 sequential analyses for each dyad during each phase. Figure 3 displays the results in terms of Yule's Q values. The likelihood of a comprehensible response following a speech-only utterance for dyads 1 and 4 was always less than when it followed a multi-modality utterance. During baseline, Yule's Q was approximately .55 to .62 for speech-only utterance–comprehensible response sequences, and approximately .70 for multi-modality utterance–comprehensible response sequences. This difference becomes greater during training and post-training phases, with the likelihood of speech-only utterance–comprehensible response sequences decreasing across phases (.25 to .44), while the likelihood of multi-modality utterance–comprehensible response sequences increasing slightly across phases (.79 to .86).

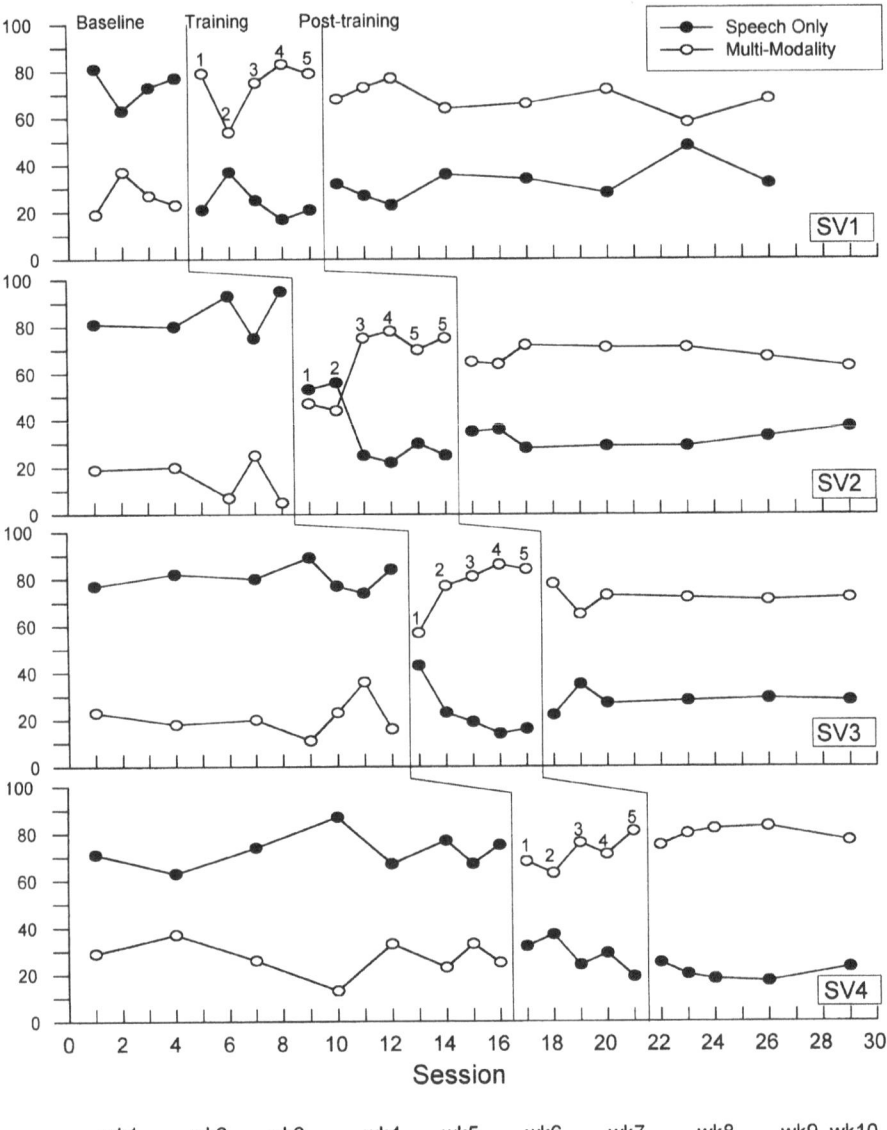

Figure 1. Proportion of student volunteers' (SVs) speech-only (black circles) versus multi-modality (white circles) utterances in 10-minute probe conversations with residents with aphasia (RAs). During the training phase, the numbers above the data points indicate the training step completed prior to each probe conversation.

The likelihood of comprehensible responses following speech-only versus multi-modality utterances for dyads 2 and 3 was about the same or slightly less during baseline, with values of approximately .41 to .46 for speech-only sequences, and .49 to .57 for multi-modality sequences. The likelihood of a comprehensible response following speech-only utterances decreased to chance levels (around zero) during training and post-training. However, the likelihood of comprehensible responses following multi-modality utterances increased for dyads 2 and 3 during training and post-training (up to .75).

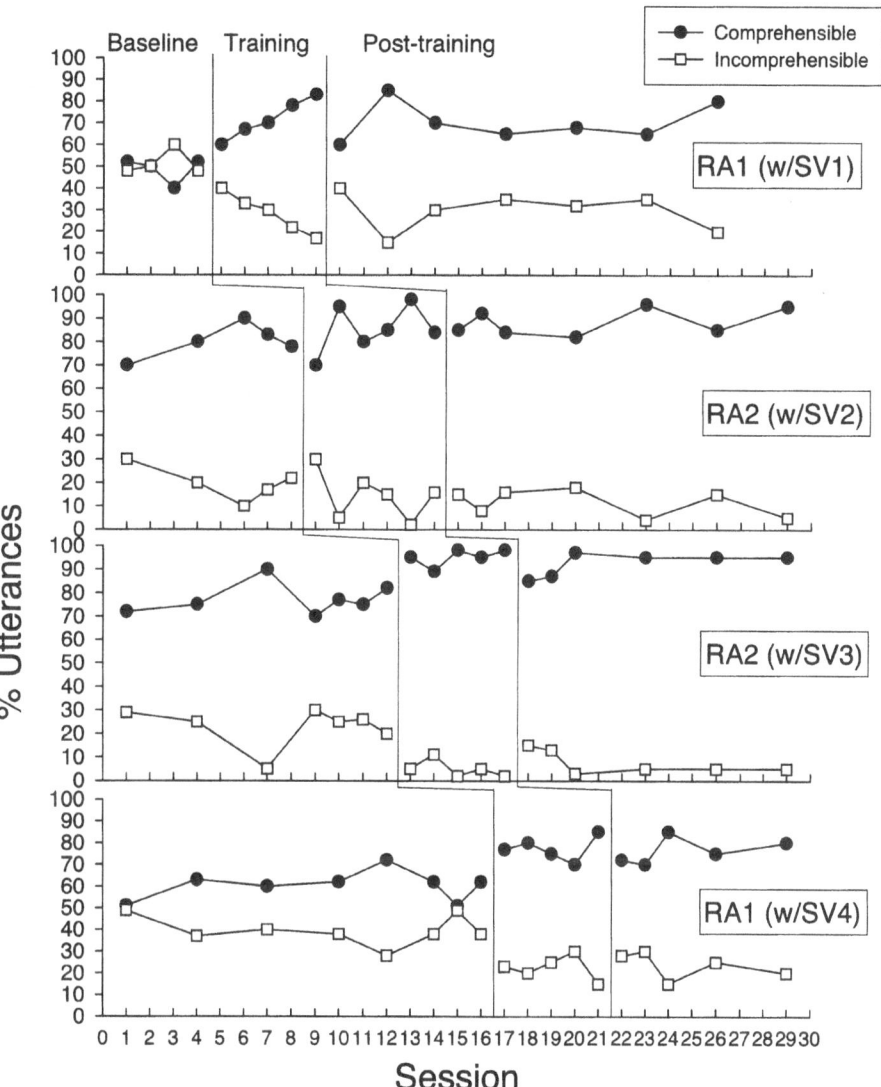

Figure 2. Proportion of residents' production of comprehensible (black circles) versus incomprehensible (grey squares) utterances during 10-minute probe conversations with student volunteers.

Results revealed that multi-modality utterances are consistently more likely to lead to a comprehensible response than speech-only utterances, with similar results for dyads 1 and 4 and for dyads 2 and 3.

Social validity

Judges viewed randomly selected baseline and post-training conversational probes and rated the conversations using visual analogue scales on six dimensions. Table 2 displays means and standard deviations for each dimension. Possible differences in baseline versus post-training ratings for each dyad were examined using 2-tailed paired t-tests.

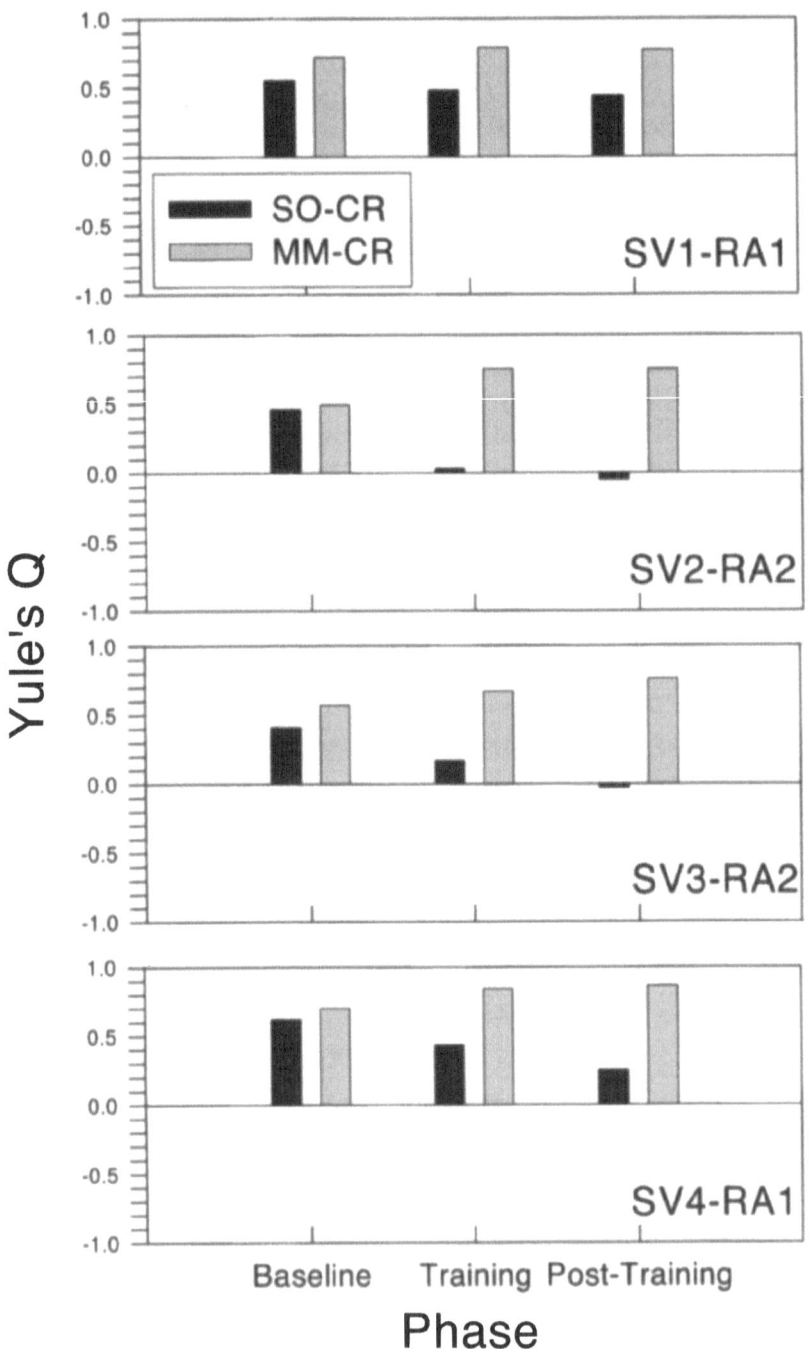

Figure 3. Results of sequential analyses for each dyad. Yule's Q is an index of sequential association between the given and target behaviours. SO-CR = speech-only–comprehensible response sequences. MM-CR = multi-modality–comprehensible response sequences.

TABLE 2
Social validity ratings of unfamiliar judges in samples of baseline and post-training conversations for each dyad

	SV1-RA1	SV2-RA2	SV3-RA2	SV4-RA1
RA comfort				
Baseline	71.2 (17.1)	53.2 (23.4)	50.0 (26.6)	69.6 (21.0)
Post-training	91.2 (9.3)**	75.0 (17.5)**	77.9 (13.1)**	83.6 (21.1)*
SV comfort				
Baseline	74.3 (23.2)	48.6 (24.7)	52.9 (29.5)	70.4 (20.4)
Post-training	95.9 (7.3)**	77.5 (17.8)**	80.7 (13.4)**	85.0 (18.6)**
RA information				
Baseline	40.0 (22.3)	13.9 (10.8)	18.7 (11.9)	50.7 (24.6)
Post-training	70.7 (14.0)**	48.2 (20.1)**	58.6 (16.0)**	69.6 (15.2)**
SV effectiveness				
Baseline	60.0 (27.7)	32.5 (26.4)	36.4 (27.6)	61.7 (26.3)
Post-training	86.9 (11.3)**	75.4 (24.9)**	76.4 (16.5)**	81.8 (16.8)**
Turn-taking				
Baseline	67.9 (26.9)	15.0 (17.9)	20.0 (17.7)	60.7 (25.9)
Post-training	82.2 (14.6)**	50.7 (28.5)**	61.1 (24.8)**	77.1 (16.7)**
Topic maintenance				
Baseline	71.4 (28.6)	25.4 (26.6)	7.5 (27.4)	9.6 (30.2)
Post-training	87.6 (14.3)**	65.0 (24.4)**	65.4 (20.2)**	76.1 (20.2)**

* $p < .05$
** $p < .01$

Post-training conversations were rated significantly higher than the baseline conversations for all dyads on all six dimensions.

DISCUSSION

The results of this study provide preliminary evidence of the effectiveness of a programme to train volunteer conversation partners to use multi-modality communication with persons with aphasia. In baseline, the SVs demonstrated high use of speech-only utterances. After the initial training session, all SVs demonstrated immediate and robust increases in use of multi-modality communication. A change common to all SVs was the use of writing after training began. SV3 and SV4 were the only SVs to use writing during baseline, but this was minimal, and may have been due to the length of baseline.

All four SVs reached criterion in each step of training in one session. Three SVs also reached criterion to withdraw training in five sessions. SV2 needed a sixth session of training to reach criterion in probe conversations. Furthermore, the SVs appeared to have enough training, as they maintained high levels of multi-modality utterances in probe conversations for at least 3 weeks following withdrawal of training.

This evidence for the effectiveness of training volunteer conversation partners of nursing home residents with aphasia contributes to the literature in several important ways. This is the first study to investigate a sample of student volunteers conversing with nursing home residents. All published studies to date include only community-dwelling persons with aphasia. Furthermore, the literature lacks strong scientific evidence for the effectiveness of training volunteer conversation partners. The current study used a multiple baseline experimental design with thorough treatment fidelity procedures to link the changes in the conversation partners' behaviours to the training. In addition, this study examined the sequential association between the trained behaviours of the partner and participation of the person with aphasia, as measured by comprehensible productions. This study also demonstrated the clinical significance of the changes in the quality of the conversations using social validation measures.

Results of sequential analyses revealed that comprehensible responses were always more likely to follow a multi-modality than a speech-only utterance. This effect became stronger after training, and comprehensible responses were less likely to follow a speech-only utterance, and even more likely to follow a multi-modality utterance. The fact that comprehensible responses were always more likely to follow multi-modality utterances than speech-only utterances provides justification for the frequent clinical recommendations to staff and family members to use multi-modality communication with persons with aphasia. This also gives credence to the theory of training partners in order to reveal the "masked competence" of persons with aphasia (Kagan et al., 2001). The RAs' aphasia clearly did not change in this study, yet their ability to reveal communicative competence improved when the SVs used multi-modality communication, and they in turn produced more comprehensible utterances.

The social validity measures revealed increased comfort, more effective communication, and increased turn-taking and topic maintenance between the RAs and SVs. These findings are promising for programmes such as this to reduce social isolation for nursing home residents with aphasia. These increased opportunities to engage in conversation and to be perceived as a competent individual are important for quality of life (Kagan et al., 2001).

The small sample size and homogeneity of the subjects limits the generalisability of the findings of this study. However, this training programme shows promise for the effectiveness of training similar SVs to be conversation partners for nursing home residents with moderate-severe nonfluent aphasia. Future research should be conducted with subjects with a range of aphasia severity and types of language deficits. Volunteers and residents with a variety of demographic characteristics and backgrounds should be studied to examine generalisability of the results. Research should examine the efficacy of this type of training programme with staff, friends, family members, and other residents who interact with residents with aphasia.

Future research should also examine issues related to the training procedures and dependent measures. For example, the specific contributions of each training step should be further explored in order to make the training even more robust or more efficient. Other aspects of the conversations that change as a result of training the conversation partners also need to be determined. For example, unfamiliar judges noted improved topic maintenance after training.

In conclusion, this study provides evidence that training conversation partners of individuals with aphasia is beneficial for both members of the dyad. With concern for social isolation of nursing home residents with aphasia, new service-delivery models are desired. The incorporation of an intergenerational service-learning programme in nursing homes appears to be one viable method to decrease social isolation and to increase opportunities for the residents with aphasia to reveal their communicative competence. Training the SVs to use multi-modality communication was related to increased comprehensibility of the RAs and increased quality of interactions. The changes that occurred in the dyads after just five to six training sessions with the SVs produced effects that could not be expected by directly training the RAs. Nor would training the RAs directly reduce the problem of lack of availability of conversation partners.

REFERENCES

Arkin, S. M. (1998). Volunteers in partnership: An Alzheimer's rehabilitation program delivered by students. *American Journal of Alzheimer's Disease, 11*(1), 12–22.

Bakeman, R., & Gottman, J. (1997). *Observing interaction: An introduction to sequential analysis* (2nd Ed.). Cambridge: Cambridge University Press.

Billingsley, F., White, O. R., & Munson, R. (1980). Procedural reliability: A rationale and an example. *Behavioral Assessment, 2,* 229–241.

Booth, S., & Perkins, L. (1999). The use of conversation analysis to guide individualized advice to carers and evaluate change in aphasia: A case study. *Aphasiology, 13*(4/5), 283–303.

Hersen, M., & Barlow, D. (1976). *Single case experimental designs: Strategies for studying behavioral change.* New York: Pergamon Press.

Hickey, E. M. (2000a). *Effects of training student volunteers to use multi-modality communication in conversations with nursing home residents with aphasia.* Unpublished doctoral dissertation. University of Washington, Seattle, WA, USA.

Hickey, E. M. (2000b). *Training use of multi-modality communication in conversations with persons with aphasia.* Training manual available from E. Hickey, Dalhousie University, Halifax, NS, Canada.

Hickey, E. M., Alarcon, N. B., Rogers, M. A., & Olswang, L. B., (1998). *Social validation measures for Family-based Intervention for Chronic Aphasia (FICA).* Paper presented at the annual Clinical Aphasiology Conference, Asheville, NC, USA.

Hollenbeck, A. R. (1978). Problems of reliability in observational research. In G. P. Sackett (Ed.), *Observing behavior, vol. II, Data collection and analysis methods* (pp. 79–98). Baltimore, MD: University Park Press.

Hopper, T., Holland, A., & Rewega, M. (2002). Conversational coaching: Treatment outcomes and future directions. *Aphasiology, 16*(7), 745–761.

Kagan, A., Black, S. E., Duchan, J. F., Simmons-Mackie, N., & Square, P. (2001). Training volunteers as conversation partners using "Supported Conversation for Adults with Aphasia" (SCA): A controlled trial. *Journal of Speech, Language, and Hearing Research, 44,* 624–634.

Kazdin, A. (1982). *Single case research designs: Methods for clinical and applied settings.* New York: Oxford University Press.

Kertesz, A. (1982). *Western aphasia battery.* Orlando, FL: Grune & Stratton.

Le Dorze, G., & Brassard, C. (1995). A description of the consequences of aphasia on aphasic persons and their relatives and friends, based on the WHO model of chronic diseases. *Aphasiology, 9*(3), 239–255.

Lyon, J. G., Cariski, D., Keisler, L., Rosenbek, J., Levine, R., Kumpula, J. et al. (1997). Communication partners: Enhancing participation in life and communication for adults with aphasia in natural settings. *Aphasiology, 11*(7), 693–708.

McGowan, T. G. (1994). Mentoring-reminiscence: A conceptual and empirical analysis. *International Journal of Aging and Human Development, 39*(4), 321–336.

Miller, J. F., & Chapman, R. S. (1998). *Basic SALT program for Windows, 5.0.* Madison, WI: Waisman Center, Language Analysis Laboratory.

Moncher, F. J., & Prinz, R. J. (1991). Treatment fidelity in outcome studies. *Clinical Psychology Review, 11,* 247–266.

Olswang, L. B., Hickey, E. M., Alarcon, N. B., & Rogers, M. A. (1998). *Treating the disability.* Paper presented at the Symposium on Treatment Efficacy Research in Communication Disorders; Nashville, TN, USA.

Raven, J. C. (1938). *Coloured progressive matrices.* London: H. K. Lewis.

Raven, J. C. (1960). *Guide to the standard progressive matrices.* London: H. K. Lewis.

Simmons, N. M., Kearns, K. P., & Potechin, G. (1987). Treatment of aphasia through family member training. In R. H. Brookshire (Ed.), *Clinical aphasiology, 17,* 106–116. Minneapolis: BRK.

Simmons-Mackie, N., & Kagan, A. (1999). Communication strategies used by 'good' versus 'poor' speaking partners of individuals with aphasia. *Aphasiology, 13*(9–11), 807–820.

Tapp, J. (1996). *MOOSES.* Nashville, TN: Vanderbilt University.

APHASIOLOGY, 2004, *18* (5/6/7), 639–652

Telerehabilitation and its effect on story retelling by adults with neurogenic communication disorders

Amy C. Georgeadis, David M. Brennan, Linsey M. Barker, and Christine R. Baron

National Rehabilitation Hospital, Washington, DC, USA

Background: Telerehabilitation (telerehab) is the method of using technology to provide rehabilitation services at a distance. The concept of delivering remote speech-language pathology (SLP) services using telerehab tools and techniques has been acknowledged for more than 25 years. While research has demonstrated videoconference-based telerehab to be a feasible, effective, and appropriate method for providing SLP services to a broad range of clients, studies have been primarily limited to technical feasibility or demonstration projects with relatively small sample sizes. There is an expressed need in the literature for controlled, randomised studies that track both quantitative outcomes of services delivered via telerehab as well as qualitative measures of satisfaction.

Aims: The purpose of the study was to measure performance of adults with acquired brain injury on a standardised SLP assessment conducted in both face-to-face (FF) and video-conference-based telerehab (T) settings. The objective was to determine if performance on the assessment, or subjective feedback from the participants, differed between settings.

Methods & Procedures: A total of 40 participants with a recent onset of brain injury—12 with traumatic brain injury (TBI), 14 with a left cerebrovascular accident (LCVA), and 14 with a right cerebrovascular accident (RCVA)—were enrolled in the study. Participants were asked to retell stories from the Story Retell Procedure (Doyle, McNeil, Spencer, Goda, Cotrell, & Lustig, 1998) in both FF and T settings. Responses from the stories were scored by the clinician using the percent information unit scoring metric (McNeil, Doyle, Fossett, Park, & Goda, 2001). Additionally, a survey tool was used to probe each participant's level of satisfaction and willingness to use telerehab services in the future.

Outcomes & Results: Across all participants, and within the TBI, LCVA, and RCVA groups, no significant difference in performance between the FF and T settings was found. Feedback from survey data demonstrated a high level of acceptance of the T setting. When compared to participants with LCVA or RCVA, however, participants with TBI were significantly more likely to show a lack of interest in future videoconferencing use.

Conclusions: Story-retelling performance by brain-injured adults was not affected by setting. Additionally, participants expressed a high level of interest in using videoconferencing in the future. These findings offer additional support for telerehab as a viable alternative mode of SLP treatment for survivors of stroke and TBI. Further research is needed to investigate the utility of telerehab for delivering services to clients with attention impairments as well as those with *severe* cognitive-communicative impairment, dysarthria, or aphasia.

Address correspondence to: Amy C. Georgeadis, Speech-Language Pathology Service, National Rehabilitation Hospital, 102 Irving, St., NW, Washington, DC 20010, USA. Email: amy.c.georgeadis@medstar.net

The authors would like to thank Patrick Doyle and Malcolm McNeil of the VA Pittsburgh Healthcare System and the University of Pittsburgh for their consent for and cooperation with use of the story text, accompanying pictures and digital recordings of the SRP stories.

This project was supported by the National Rehabilitation Hospital's Rehabilitation Engineering Research Center on Telerehabilitation funded by the US Department of Education under award number H133E990007.

Telerehabilitation (telerehab) is the method of using technology to provide rehabilitation services at a distance. Telerehab improves access to services in situations where distance and/or immobility are factors and it enables clinicians, clients, family members, educators, and researchers to connect to each other and interact over long distances. Telerehab applications occur through a broad array of techniques and methods ranging from traditional telephone consultations to satellite-based videoconferencing with live audio and video.

The concept of delivering remote speech-language pathology (SLP) services using telerehab tools and techniques has been acknowledged for more than 25 years. Some of the earliest work in this area involved the use of telephone equipment to deliver SLP services for addressing communicative disorders such as articulation impairments, aphasia, and stuttering (Vaughn, 1976). As technology evolved, Wertz et al. (1987, 1992) expanded on the auditory-only technique by using video and computer methods to remotely diagnose neurogenic communication disorders. This approach was demonstrated to be a valid method for appraisal and diagnosis, and viable for improving access and frequency of service to patients living in remote areas.

Videoconferencing is a powerful tool for telerehab applications, as it allows participants to see and hear each other simultaneously across long distances. As videoconferencing technology has evolved and advanced, with improved features and functions, the range of telerehab services that can be delivered has greatly expanded. Videoconferencing has been shown to be an important tool for providing remote therapeutic interventions, as well as for delivering assessment, monitoring, education, and training at a distance. Applications have been demonstrated for the remote delivery of hypnotherapy for pain management (Appel, Bleiberg, & Noiseux, 2002), assessment of cognitive function and depression (Ball & McLaren, 1997; Ball & Puffett, 1998; Menon et al., 2001), vocational rehabilitation (Trepagnier, 2002), assistive technology follow-up (Burns, 1999), nursing management and support for caregivers (Buckley, Tran, & Prandoni, 2002), wound care and assessment (Halstead, Dang, Elrod, Convit, Rosen, & Woods, 2003; Vesmarovich, Walker, Hauber, Temkin, & Burns, 1999), and occupational therapy and physical therapy services (Savard & Borstad, 2002; Savard, Borstad, Tkachuck, Lauderdale, & Conroy, 2003; Tran, Savard, Hayward, & Elliot, 2003; White, 2003).

Research has demonstrated videoconference-based telerehab to be a feasible, effective, and appropriate method for providing SLP services to a broad range of clients. Closed circuit video, computer-controlled video laserdisc, and two-way satellite-based audio-video methods have been described as being valid, reliable, and appropriate approaches for performing SLP diagnostic measures on patients with neurogenic communication disorders in remote locations (Duffy, Werven, & Aronson, 1997; Wertz et al., 1987, 1992). Videoconferencing has also been found to be effective for cognitive assessment of persons with brain injury (Schopp, Johnstone, & Merveille, 2000) and has been used in developing communication skills and promoting parental involvement in the speech therapy of pre-school children with special needs (McCullough, 2001). Results from a study investigating voice therapy at a distance indicated no significant difference in outcomes or satisfaction ratings between telerehab and conventionally treated patients (Mashima, Birkmire-Peters, Holtel, & Syms, 1999).

Videoconferencing is well suited to the primarily verbal/visual interaction between client and clinician typical during SLP diagnosis and treatment (Brennan, Georgeadis, & Baron, 2002; Kully, 2000). While telerehab has been shown to be a viable tool for providing remote SLP services, research has been primarily limited to technical feasibility or demonstration projects with relatively small sample sizes. There is an expressed need for controlled, randomised studies that track both quantitative outcomes of services delivered via telerehab as well as qualitative measures of satisfaction (Hill & Theodoros, 2002).

This study administered a story-retelling task in both face-to-face (FF) and remote telerehab (T) settings to individuals with traumatic brain-injury or stroke. The purpose of this study was to address these questions:

1. Is story retelling performance by participants with neurogenic communication disorders affected by either the FF or T setting?
2. Does feedback from participants with neurogenic communication disorders differ between settings?

METHOD

Study sample

Participants were 40 adults (23 male and 17 female) with a recent history of traumatic brain-injury or stroke who were patients at the National Rehabilitation Hospital. Of these, 12 participants had sustained a traumatic brain injury (TBI), 14 a left-hemisphere cerebrovascular accident (LCVA), and 14 a right-hemisphere cerebrovascular accident (RCVA). Participants ranged in age from 18 to 70 years. All participants were receiving SLP treatment for cognitive-communicative, language and/or speech impairments of varying severity levels. (Detailed information on individual participants' SLP diagnosis is presented in Appendix A.) All participants were less than 14 months post-onset. Participants with uncorrected visual deficits (e.g., visual-spatial neglect, field cuts) or those unable to engage in simple conversation due to inadequate sustained attention or poor intelligibility were excluded from participation. In order to ensure adequate auditory comprehension for the story-retelling task, a score of 8/12 on the Boston Diagnostic Aphasia Examination–Complex Ideational Material (BDAE–CIM) subtest (Goodglass &

TABLE 1
Characteristics of the TBI, LCVA, and RCVA groups

	TBI (n=12)	LCVA (n=14)	RCVA (n=14)
Age (years)			
Mean (SD)	27.9 (11.9)	51.6 (11.2)	51.4 (12.5)
Range	18–51	32–64	31–70
Education (years)			
Mean (SD)	12.7 (2.5)	15.2 (2.7)	14.1 (3.2)
Range	9–18	10–19	9–20
BDAE-CIM score (out of 12)			
Mean (SD)	9.3 (1.4)	9.4 (1.3)	10.3 (0.9)
Range	8–12	8–12	9–12
TPO (days)			
Mean (SD)	90.4 (111.3)	96.9 (104.4)	30.4 (24.1)
Range	20–399	8–336	11–103
Gender			
Male	8	6	9
Female	4	8	5

Kaplan, 1983) was required for participation in the study. A summary description of the study sample is presented in Table 1.

Materials

Stimuli were two randomly selected story sets (each consisting of three stories) from the Story Retell Procedure (SRP) (Brookshire & Nicholas, 1993; Doyle et al., 1998). The SRP measures connected language production by requiring participants to retain the elements of a story and retell them in their own words. For the SRP, the participant listens to a digitised pre-recorded story accompanied by a series of sequenced black and white line drawings illustrating the story. At the conclusion of the story, all of the drawings are displayed together and the participant is asked to retell the story using her/his own words.

A standardised scoring metric, the Percent Information Unit (%IU) (McNeil et al., 2001), was used to evaluate participants' performance on the SRP. For the %IU metric, SRP performance is measured by scoring each participant's responses against a checklist of IUs that have been predetermined for each story. An IU is defined as "an identified word, phrase, or acceptable alternative from the story stimulus that is intelligible and informative and that conveys accurate and relevant information about the story" (McNeil et al., 2001, p. 994). McNeil et al. (2002) used the %IU metric to validate the equivalence of parallel SRP story sets for participants with aphasia. Using the %IU metric with these story sets allows for repeated administration of the SRP for test–retest purposes. Two of the parallel story sets were selected for this study; one story set was used in the FF setting and the other in the T setting.

Procedure

Participants were tested in both FF and T settings. The order in which participants were exposed to the test settings (FF followed by T or T followed by FF) was randomised across participants. The story text, accompanying pictures, and digital recordings of the stories employed for this study (WAVE files in PCM Format [22.050 kHz, 16 bit, Mono] at 43 kb/sec) are those developed and described by Doyle et al. (1998).

The FF setting was structured as a conventional therapy session, with the participant and a speech-language pathologist, certified by the American Speech-Language-Hearing Association, seated together in the testing room. While the stories played, the clinician manually placed the drawings on a bookstand in front of the participant. A noise-cancelling computer microphone was used to digitally record the participant's retelling of the stories.

In the T setting, the participant was located in the testing room in front of a flat panel computer monitor (placed in the same position and orientation as the bookstand used in the FF setting), while the clinician was seated in another room in the hospital. The participant and clinician were able to see and hear each other via computer-based videoconferencing with full-duplex audio and video. As the intent of the study was to test the effects of the intervening telerehab connection at the best available audio and video quality, a high bandwidth (10 Mbps) Local Area Network connection was used. While the stories played, the participant's computer monitor displayed scanned versions of the drawings alongside a video window, approximately $2\frac{1}{2}'' \times 2''$ in size, of the clinician (Figure 1). As in the FF setting, the participant's retellings of the stories were digitally recorded and saved as WAVE files in PCM format (11.025 kHz, 8 bit, Mono) at 10 kb/sec.

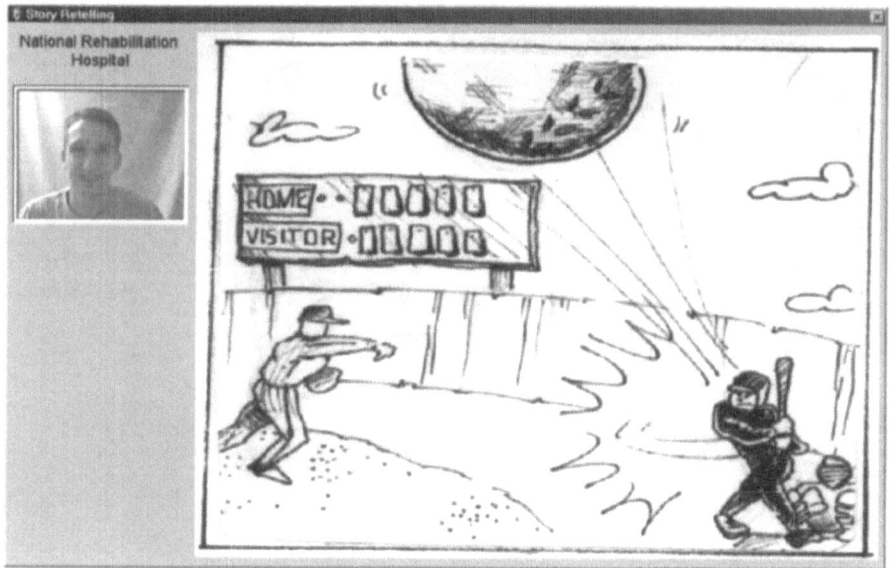

Figure 1.   Image of participant's screen during story playback.

At the conclusion of the testing, the clinician interviewed each participant face-to-face to complete the Participant Exit Survey (see Appendix B). Each participant was asked to self-report her/his own impression of communication in the FF and T settings. In addition, the survey also probed the participant's satisfaction level and willingness to use telerehab services in the future.

Data Analysis

Following completion of the testing session, the participant's responses from the stories in both settings were individually replayed and scored by the clinician using McNeil's %IU scoring metric. For each setting, the %IU scores from the three stories were averaged to determine a final score for the participant's performance in that setting. These scores, FF-Score and T-Score (indicating performance in the FF and T setting, respectively) were then used to analyse and compare performance across all participants and settings.

A second certified speech-language pathologist trained in the %IU scoring metric and blinded to the SRP setting scored a random sample of 12 SRP responses (5% of the total number of SRP responses). Inter-rater agreement between the clinicians for the 12 stories was 92.8% (range = 81.1–100%).

RESULTS

Across all participants, performance in the T setting was slightly better than in the FF setting. The mean T-score, 35.1 (SD = 14.6) and the mean FF-score, 34.5 (SD = 13.2) are illustrated in Figure 2. Results from a two-tailed paired samples t-test indicated no significant difference between performance across settings, $t(39) = 0.69$, $p = .495$. Furthermore, a high correlation between performances in each setting was found ($r = .93$).

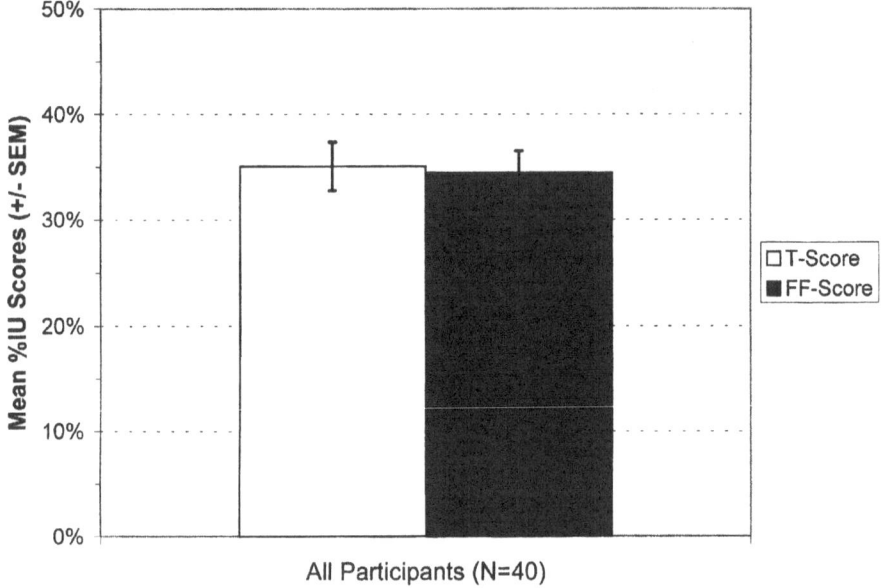

Figure 2. Mean %IU scores across all participants for T and FF settings.

For each group, mean %IU scores are illustrated in Figure 3. The RCVA group performed better in both settings than the LCVA group. The LCVA group performed better in both settings than the TBI group. Results from a series of two-tailed paired samples *t*-tests for each group are presented in Table 2. Performance by the RCVA group indicated a trend towards a significant difference between settings, $t(13) = 2.03, p = .064$. The RCVA group was the only group that scored, on average, higher in the T setting.

In order to further examine the potential variability across groups, difference scores were calculated for each participant by subtracting their FF-score from their T-score. A one-way ANOVA was performed using the $\Delta_{T\text{-}FF}$ scores. A trend towards significance was found for differences in $\Delta_{T\text{-}FF}$, $F(2, 37) = 2.9, p = .069$, among all three groups. Results from post-hoc testing (Table 3) also indicate a trend towards a significant difference between the RCVA and TBI groups.

TABLE 2
Mean %IU scores, paired-samples *t*-test results, and correlations between T and FF settings for each group

	TBI (n=12)	LCVA (n=14)	RCVA (n=14)
T-score (SD)	28.43 (11.02)	31.89 (13.44)	43.96 (14.74)
FF-score (SD)	30.08 (9.82)	31.90 (13.26)	40.83 (13.99)
***t*-test results**	$t(11) = -1.32, p = .213$	$t(13) = -0.01, p = .991$	$t(13) = 2.03, p = .064$
r	.92*	.92*	.92*

* Significant at $p < .001$.

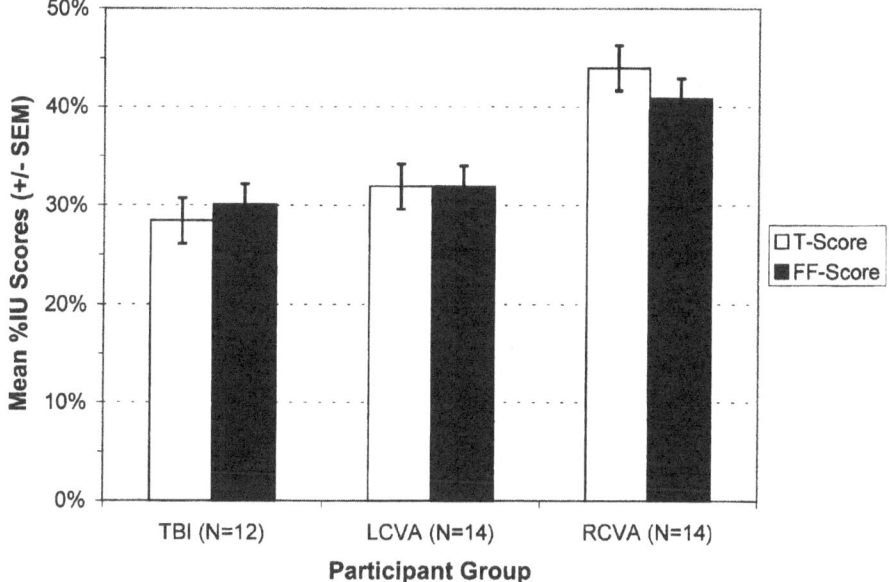

Figure 3.   Mean %IU scores by group for T and FF settings.

TABLE 3
Mean differences and significance levels between
groups for $\Delta_{\text{T-FF}}$ scores

	$\Delta_{T\text{-}FF}$	
Comparison	Mean difference	Sig.
LCVA–RCVA	−3.14	.291
LCVA–TBI	1.63	.729
RCVA–TBI	4.77	.079

Data from the Participant Exit Survey demonstrated a high level of acceptance of the T setting (Figure 4). When asked whether they would use videoconferencing again to talk to a clinician (Figure 4, Q6), participants from the RCVA and LCVA groups all responded favourably. Participants from the TBI group were significantly more likely to respond negatively, $F(2, 37) = 11.2, p < .001$. Specific comments from participants regarding their impressions of the T setting are listed in Appendix C.

DISCUSSION

This study was designed to determine if story retelling by individuals with neurogenic communication impairments differed between FF and T settings. Results demonstrate that participants with TBI, LCVA, and RCVA performed similarly in FF and T settings. Differences between FF and T settings were not significant for any participant group (see Table 2).

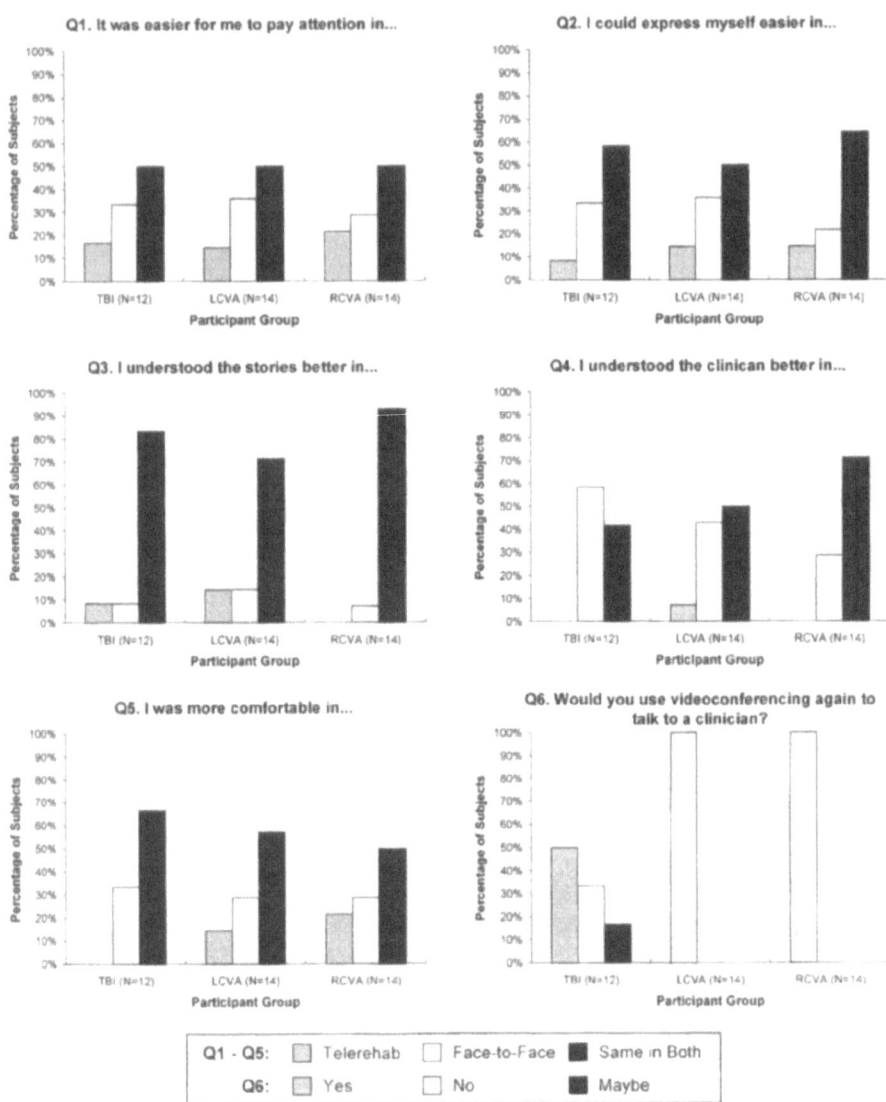

Figure 4. Responses by group to questions on the Participant Exit Survey.

Although differences between settings are not significant for any group, comparing how groups differ between settings (FF versus T) is clinically interesting. The LCVA and RCVA groups performed the same or better in the T setting compared with the FF setting. In contrast, the TBI group performed more poorly in the T setting. It may be that because the SLP was not in the same room for the T setting, the participant needed to demonstrate a greater level of self-initiated attention to interact optimally. Persistent attention deficits following traumatic brain injury are well documented in the literature. Patients complain of poor processing, distractibility, and decreased sustained/divided attention after brain injury (Cicerone, 2002; Mateer & Mapou, 1996). Specific comments provided by participants in the TBI group suggest that impaired attention may have adversely affected their performance in the T setting (e.g., "It was harder to pay attention [in the T setting] ... it was really easy just to look away from the computer and not listen").

This study also examined if feedback provided by participants differed between FF and T settings. Data collected with the Participant Exit Survey indicate that for all parameters examined, the majority of participants reported no difference between settings. However, participants showed a strong preference for the FF setting (17 of 40) when asked to complete the phrase, "I understood the clinician better in ...". This preference may be related to a slight delay and variability in the clarity of the audio transmission during the T setting. As videoconferencing technology has evolved, audio quality has improved through hands-free echo-cancellation microphones and advanced audio compression algorithms. Future research should place a high priority on consistent audio quality to improve user acceptance.

Perhaps the most interesting participant feedback was given to the query regarding use of videoconferencing to talk to a clinician in the future. Overall, a large majority of the participants (34/40) responded "yes" that they would be interested in future videoconferencing use. Of the six "no" or "maybe" responses, all were participants with TBI. When compared to participants with LCVA or RCVA, participants with TBI were significantly more likely to show a lack of interest in future videoconferencing use. Although participants with TBI had not reported increased difficulty in *attending* during the T setting compared with the FF setting (Figure 4), perhaps on some level they were aware that their T *performance* was worse. Awareness of better performance in the FF setting could have led to a preference for that setting. TBI group preference for the FF setting, coupled with better performance in that setting, suggest the need for future research examining the role that attention impairments play during a telerehab session.

Results from this study reported elsewhere (Brennan, Georgeadis, Barker, & Baron, in press) indicate that age, education, technology experience, and gender did not have a significant effect on participant performance in the FF versus T setting. These results, combined with the data presented here, contribute to the support for telerehabilitation as a viable alternative mode of SLP treatment for clients across a range of demographics. Many survivors of stroke and brain injury are unable to receive services due to difficulty in accessing care. This applies not only to those living in rural settings but also in cases where distance and/or mobility are factors. Telerehab has the potential not only to deliver services where they are not currently accessible, but also to provide expanded family education and follow-up services. Additionally, with advancements in technology and the growing role of computers in daily life, telerehab is an increasingly attractive choice for patients who exhibit a preference for technology.

While this study suggests that mild to moderately impaired survivors of stroke and TBI perform similarly on a story-retelling task during FF and T settings, these results may not be applicable to those with *severe* cognitive-communicative impairment, dysarthria, or aphasia. Additionally, this study was conducted in a well-controlled, quiet environment with technical staff on site to provide assistance with and troubleshooting of equipment problems. In future research, it will be essential to examine logistical difficulties that arise when patients receive telerehab services in an uncontrolled setting such as the home (e.g., doorbell ringing, dog barking, computer breaking down, etc.). This team is currently incorporating these considerations into case studies exploring the longitudinal effects of SLP treatment delivered to adult clients with neurogenic communication disorders across a range of SLP diagnoses and severity levels.

REFERENCES

Appel, P. R., Bleiberg, J., & Noiseux, J. (2002). An exploration of behavioral telehealth interventions for pain management and consumer satisfaction. In D. E. Lauderdale (Ed.), *Proceedings of the State of the Science Conference on Telerehabilitation and Applications of Virtual Reality* (pp. 23–30). Washington, DC: NRH Press.

Ball, C., & McLaren, P. (1997). The tele-assessment of cognitive state: A review. *Journal of Telemedicine and Telecare, 3*(3), 126–131.

Ball, C., & Puffett, A. (1998). The assessment of cognitive function in the elderly using videoconferencing. *Journal of Telemedicine and Telecare, 4*(Suppl 1), 36–38.

Brennan, D., Georgeadis, A., Barker, L., & Baron, C. (in press). The effect of videoconference-based telerehab on story retelling performance by brain injured subjects and its implications for remote speech-language therapy. *Telemedicine Journal and e-Health.*

Brennan, D., Georgeadis, A., & Baron, C. (2002). Telerehabilitation tools for the provision of remote speech-language treatment. *Topics in Stroke Rehabilitation, 8*(4), 71–78.

Brookshire, R. H., & Nicholas, L. E. (1993). *Discourse Comprehension Test.* Tucson, AZ: Communication Skill Builders.

Buckley, K. M., Tran, B. Q., & Prandoni, C. (2002). Nursing management and the acceptance/use of telehealth technologies by caregivers of stroke patients in the home setting. In D. E. Lauderdale (Ed.), *Proceedings of the State of the Science Conference on Telerehabilitation and Applications of Virtual Reality* (pp. 35–38). Washington, DC: NRH Press.

Burns, P. (1999). Telehealth or telehype? Some observations and thoughts on the current status and future of telehealth. *Journal of Healthcare Information Management, 13*(4 Suppl), 1–10.

Cicerone, K. D. (2002). Remediation of "working attention" in mild traumatic brain injury. *Brain Injury, 16*(3), 185–195.

Doyle, P., McNeil, M., Spencer, K., Goda, A., Cotrell, K., & Lustig, A. (1998). The effects of concurrent picture presentation on retelling of orally presented stories by adults with aphasia. *Aphasiology, 12*(7/8), 561–574.

Duffy, J. R., Werven, G. W., & Aronson, A. E. (1997). Telemedicine and the diagnosis of speech and language disorders. *Mayo Clinic Proceedings, 72*(12), 1116–1122.

Goodglass, H., & Kaplan, E. (1983). *The assessment of aphasia and related disorders.* Philadelphia: Lea & Febiger.

Halstead, L. S., Dang, T., Elrod, M., Convit, R. J., Rosen, M. J., & Woods, S. (2003). Teleassessment compared with live assessment of pressure ulcers in a wound clinic: A pilot study. *Advances in Skin & Wound Care, 16*(2), 91–96.

Hill, A., & Theodoros, D. (2002). Research into telehealth applications in speech-language pathology. *Journal of Telemedicine and Telecare, 8*(4), 187–196.

Kully, D. (2000). Telehealth in speech pathology: Applications to the treatment of stuttering. *Journal of Telemedicine and Telecare, 6*(Suppl 2), S39–41.

Mashima, P. A., Birkmire-Peters, D. P., Holtel, M. R., & Syms, M. J. (1999). Telehealth applications in speech-language pathology. *Journal of Healthcare Information Management, 13*(4), 71–78.

Mateer, C. A., & Mapou, R. L. (1996). Understanding, evaluating, and managing attention disorders after traumatic brain injury. *Journal of Head Trauma Rehabilitation, 11*(2), 1–16.

McCullough, A. (2001). Viability and effectiveness of teletherapy for pre-school children with special needs. *International Journal of Language and Communication Disorders, 36*(Suppl), 321–326.

McNeil, M., Doyle, P., Fossett, T., Park, G., & Goda, A. (2001). Reliability and concurrent validity of the information unit scoring metric for the story retelling procedure. *Aphasiology, 15*(10/11), 991–1006.

Menon, A. S., Kondapavalru, P., Krishna, P., Chrismer, J. B., Raskin, A., Hebel, J. R. et al. (2001). Evaluation of a portable low cost videophone system in the assessment of depressive symptoms and cognitive function in elderly medically ill veterans. *Journal of Nervous & Mental Disease, 189*(6), 399–401.

Savard, L., & Borstad, A. (2002, February). *Outcomes of specialty consultations using telehealth technologies in physical therapy.* Paper presented at the Combined Sections Meeting of the American Physical Therapy Association, Boston, MA.

Savard, L., Borstad, A., Tkachuck, J., Lauderdale, D., & Conroy, B. (2003). Telerehabilitation consultations for clients with neurologic diagnoses: Cases from rural Minnesota and American Samoa. *NeuroRehabilitation, 18*(2), 93–102.

Schopp, L. H., Johnstone, B. R., & Merveille, O. C. (2000). Multidimensional telecare strategies for rural residents with brain injury. *Journal of Telemedicine and Telecare, 6*(Suppl 1), S146–149.

Tran, B. Q., Savard, L., Hayward, L., & Elliot, J. U. (2003, February). *Use of telehealth in physical therapy: Implications for education and practice.* Paper presented at the Combined Sections Meeting of the American Physical Therapy Association, Tampa, FL.

Trepagnier, C. (2002). Can videotelephones be useful to provision of vocational rehabilitation services? In D. E. Lauderdale (Ed.), *Proceedings of the State of the Science Conference on Telerehabilitation and Applications of Virtual Reality* (pp. 42–44). Washington, DC: NRH Press.

Vaughn, G. R. (1976). Tel-communicology: Health-care delivery system for persons with communicative disorders. *ASHA, 18*, 13–17.

Vesmarovich, S., Walker, T., Hauber, R. P., Temkin, A., & Burns, R. (1999). Use of telerehabilitation to manage pressure ulcers in persons with spinal cord injuries. *Advances in Wound Care, 12*(5), 264–269.

Wertz, R., Dronkers, N., Bernstein-Ellis, E., Shubitowski, Y., Elman, R., Shenaut, G. et al. (1987). Appraisal and diagnosis of neurogenic communication disorders in remote settings. In R. H. Brookshire (Ed.), *Clinical Aphasiology* (Vol. 17, pp. 117–123). Minneapolis: BRK Publishers.

Wertz, R., Dronkers, N., Bernstein-Ellis, E., Sterling, L., Shubitowski, Y., Elman, R. et al. (1992). Potential of telephonic and television technology for appraising and diagnosing neurogenic communication disorders in remote settings. *Aphasiology, 6*(2), 195–202.

White, M. W. (2003, June). *Telerehabilitation: A primer for the OT practitioner.* Paper presented at the Annual Conference of the American Occupational Therapy Association, Washington, DC.

APPENDIX A

SLP Diagnoses of the study sample

Participant	SLP diagnosis[1]
TBI-1	moderate cognitive-communicative impairment
TBI-2	moderate cognitive-communicative impairment and mild non-fluent aphasia
TBI-3	mild cognitive-communicative impairment and moderate dysarthia
TBI-4	mild cognitive-communicative impairment
TBI-5	mild-moderate cognitive-communicative impairment
TBI-6	mild-moderate cognitive-communicative impairment
TBI-7	mild cognitive-communicative impairment
TBI-9	moderate cognitive-communicative impairment
TBI-12	moderate cognitive-communicative impairment
TBI-13	moderate cognitive-communicative impairment
TBI-14	mild-moderate cognitive-communicative impairment
TBI-15	moderate cognitive-communicative impairment
LCVA-2	mild non-fluent aphasia
LCVA-3	moderate dysarthria
LCVA-4	mild-moderate non-fluent aphasia
LCVA-5	mild-moderate fluent aphasia
LCVA-6	moderate non-fluent aphasia moderate apraxia
LCVA-7	mild non-fluent aphasia and mild apraxia
LCVA-8	mild-moderate non-fluent aphasia
LCVA-9	mild-moderate non-fluent aphasia
LCVA-10	moderate non-fluent aphasia
LCVA-11	moderate cognitive-communicative impairment and moderate dysarthria
LCVA-12	moderate dysarthia and mild-mod cognitve-linguistic impairment
LCVA-13	mild-moderate non-fluent aphasia and mild-moderate apraxia
LCVA-14	mild-moderate non-fluent aphasia and mild-mod apraxia
LCVA-15	mild cognitive-communicative impairment
RCVA-1	mild cognitive-communicative impairment
RCVA-2	mild-mod cognitive-communicative impairment
RCVA-3	mild cognitive-communicative impairment and moderate dysarthia
RCVA-4	moderate cognitive-communicative impairment
RCVA-5	mild-moderate dysarthia
RCVA-6	mild cognitive-communicative impairment
RCVA-7	mild-moderate cognitive-communicative impairment
RCVA-8	mild cognitive-communicative impairment and moderate dysarthia
RCVA-9	mild-moderate cognitive-communicative impairment
RCVA-10	mild-moderate cognitive-communicative impairment
RCVA-11	mild-moderate cognitive-communicative impairment
RCVA-12	mild-moderate cognitive-communicative impairment
RCVA-13	functional cognitive-communicative skills
RCVA-14	moderate cognitive-communicative impairment

[1] SLP diagnosis as determined during initial evaluation by each participant's primary speech-language pathologist.

APPENDIX B

Participant Exit Survey

2. I could express myself easier in...
   ☐ Better in Face-to-Face   ☐ Same in Both   ☐ Better in Telerehab

3. I understood the stories better in...
   ☐ Better in Face-to-Face   ☐ Same in Both   ☐ Better in Telerehab

4. I understood the clinician better in...
   ☐ Better in Face-to-Face   ☐ Same in Both   ☐ Better in Telerehab

5. I was more comfortable in...
   ☐ Better in Face-to-Face   ☐ Same in Both   ☐ Better in Telerehab

6. Would you use videoconferencing again to talk to a clinician...
   ☐ No   ☐ No   ☐ No

APPENDIX C

Comments from Participants

Participant	Comments
TBI-1	N/A
TBI-2	The seriousness of the situation needs face to face. You know a lot about people by their expressions ... you can't really see expressions over telerehab.
TBI-3	I liked it.
TBI-4	N/A
TBI-5	It was harder to pay attention. It was really easy just to look away from the computer and not listen. A couple of times I was looking at something else and didn't hear half the story.
TBI-6	I understood the clinician better in face to face, because I was listening closely to you and I wasn't distracted. The computer makes you use your brain and that's good.
TBI-7	It really made a difference—it was really hard to do it over the computer. I saw the pictures and heard the stories, but I did so much better in person.
TBI-9	I'd rather just talk face to face.
TBI-12	I like it better when you are right here ... well it was really okay either way.
TBI-13	It's very hi-tech. It would be real useful for some people. It wouldn't be good for someone who was blind.
TBI-14	N/A
TBI-15	I don't like it. It's not personal.
LCVA-2	I felt more comfortable without the clinician next to me.
LCVA-3	I think it [telerehab] could be an alternative for memory therapy.
LCVA-4	It makes sense that people could get therapy at home. I think people are afraid of technology ... it might intimidate them, but I liked it.
LCVA-5	N/A
LCVA-6	I wasn't doing as well over ... computer. I was getting more mistakes over ... computer. I think I was getting tired during the second setting and maybe that's why it wasn't as good.
LCVA-7	I was more windy in the face-to-face. I seemed to have more ideas or expressions face-to-face. I think it's a good tool.
LCVA-8	You get more feeling with the person right next to you.
LCVA-9	At first I felt apprehensive about the whole computer ordeal, but as I started, either one got my attention. After we got started, I was comfortable either way.
LCVA-10	It is a nice way to do it differently but I felt like I did better when you were right next to me.

(Continued overleaf)

LCVA-11	I am less self-conscious when you were out of the room.
LCVA-12	The last story seemed especially tricky. I didn't get the last one. I thought the pictures were horrible. The woman was grotesque.
LCVA-13	It was good and convenient. I could be at my home and do the teleconference with the speech therapist. I know about teleconferencing and it's okay by me. It's the same to me.
LCVA-14	It was harder over the computer. It's still a good way to get services. It would save people trips to hospital.
LCVA-15	I like the subtleties that you pick up on videoconferencing versus just on phone. You can see the body language.
RCVA-1	It was okay. I have no complaints. I'm just not as comfortable with the technology.
RCVA-2	I was apprehensive before coming, but it turned out okay. "Sound crackling" in telesession made it easier for me to pay attention in face-face.
RCVA-3	I think it's more personal when you are face to face. Modern technology is okay, but nothing beats face to face or personal interaction. It would be nice to not have to deal with transportation.
RCVA-4	N/A
RCVA-5	It could be convenient for some who are not able to get to the therapist.
RCVA-6	It was just as difficult in one setting as it is in the other. I wasn't intimidated by the computer ... and usually I am intimidated by computers.
RCVA-7	I was more shy with face to face interaction.
RCVA-8	I was trying to talk louder in Tele so I did better; I was more comfortable in Tele because I was less distracted because the computer was interesting. I would welcome the opportunity to use videoconferencing again; I think with today's technology anything is possible.
RCVA-9	I am more of a person to person communicator. The image is good and the voice is good. It wasn't because of the system, it's just I prefer face to face.
RCVA-10	I was really focusing on what was going on! I enjoyed it.
RCVA-11	You have high bandwidth—so it works well. It would be hard to do physical therapy this way.
RCVA-12	I paid attention quicker in the face to face. There's nothing wrong with it, I'm just more comfortable face to face. It makes me pay attention more.
RCVA-13	I enjoyed it. It was fun seeing you on the computer.
RCVA-14	I was more nervous with you sitting next to me. I get real nervous around people in general, not just you.

APHASIOLOGY

SUBSCRIPTION INFORMATION

Subscription rates to Volume 18, 2004 (12 issues) are as follows:

To individuals: UK £390.00; Rest of World $644.00

To institutions: UK £925.00; Rest of World $1527.00

A subscription to the print edition includes free access for any number of concurrent users across a local area network to the online edition, ISSN 1464-5041.

Print subscriptions are also available to individual members of the British Aphasiology Society (BAS), on application to the Society.

For a complete and up-to-date guide to Taylor & Francis Group's journals and books publishing programmes, visit the Taylor and Francis website: http://www.tandf.co.uk/

Aphasiology (USPS permit number 001413) is published monthly. The 2004 US Institutional subscription price is $1527.00. Periodicals postage paid at Champlain, NY, by US Mail Agent IMS of New York, 100 Walnut Street, Champlain, NY.

US Postmaster: Please send address changes to pAPH, PO Box 1518, Champlain, NY 12919, USA.

Dollar rates apply to subscribers in all countries except the UK and the Republic of Ireland where the pound sterling price applies. All subscriptions are payable in advance and all rates include postage. Journals are sent by air to the USA, Canada, Mexico, India, Japan and Australasia. Subscriptions are entered on an annual basis, *i.e.* from January to December. Payment may be made by sterling cheque, dollar cheque, international money order, National Giro, or credit card (AMEX, VISA, Mastercard).

Orders originating in the following territories should be sent direct to the local distributor.

India Universal Subscription Agency Pvt. Ltd, 101–102 Community Centre, Malviya Nagar Extn, Post Bag No. 8, Saket, New Delhi 110017.
Japan Kinokuniya Company Ltd, Journal Department, PO Box 55, Chitose, Tokyo 156.
USA, Canada and Mexico Psychology Press, a member of the Taylor & Francis Group, 325 Chestnut St, Philadelphia, PA 19106, USA
UK and other territories Taylor & Francis Ltd, Rankine Road, Basingstoke, Hampshire RG24 8PR.

The print edition of this journal is typeset by DP Photosetting, Aylesbury and printed by Hobbs the Printer, Totton, Hants. The online edition of this journal is hosted by Metapress at journalsonline.tandf.co.uk

Submitting a paper to APHASIOLOGY

Aphasiology is concerned with all aspects of language impairment and related disorders resulting from brain damage. Submissions are encouraged on theoretical, empirical and clinical topics from any disciplinary perspective, and submissions which involve cross disciplinary study are particularly welcome. *Aphasiology* will publish experimental and clinical research papers, reviews, theoretical notes, comments and critiques. Research reports can be group studies, single-case studies or surveys, on psychological, linguistic, medical and social aspects of aphasia. Submissions and ideas for the Review Articles and the Forum are welcome and interdisciplinary peer commentary is encouraged.

Structured Abstracts.

Authors submitting papers should note that from Volume 16 Issue 1 (2002), the journal is introducing Structured Abstracts. There is good evidence that Structured Abstracts are clearer for readers and facilitate better appropriate indexing and citation of papers.

The essential features of the Structured Abstract are given below. Note in particular that any clinical implications should be clearly stated.

Abstract (Between 150-400 words)

Background: Describe the background to the study;

Aims: State the aims and objectives of the study including any clear research questions or hypotheses.

Methods & Procedures: To include outline of the methodology and design of experiments; materials employed and subject/participant numbers with basic relevant demographic information; the nature of the analyses performed.

Outcomes & Results: Outline the important and relevant results of the analyses.

Conclusions: State the basic conclusions and implications of the study. State, clearly and usefully, if there are implications for management, treatment or service delivery.

Review Abstract

Background: Outline the background to the review.

Aims: State the primary objective of the paper; the reasons behind your critical review and analyses of the literature; your approach and methods if relevant.

Main Contribution: The main outcomes of the paper and results of analyses; and any implications for future research and for management, treatment or service delivery.

Conclusions: State your main conclusions.

Papers for consideration should be sent to an Editor. Please send an original and three photocopies. Do not send original MRI scans until accepted for publication.

Papers are accepted for consideration on condition that you will accept and warrant the following conditions:

1. You will transfer copyright to Psychology Press Ltd, should the work be accepted for publication.
2. The work is your original work, and cannot be construed as plagiarising any other published work.
3. You own the copyright in the work.
4. You are empowered by your fellow author(s) to make a submission to this journal, and to make any agreement relating to the work.
5. Your work has not previously been published in the English language.
6. Your work is not under consideration for publication elsewhere, in any form.
7. You have secured the necessary permission in writing from the appropriate authorities for the reproduction in your work of any text, illustration, or other material which is reproduced or derived from a copyrighted source.
8. You have agreed with your fellow author(s) the order of names for publication of the work.
9. You warrant that the work does not include content that is abusive, defamatory, libellous, obscene, fraudulent, or in violation of applicable laws.

If it is found acceptable for publication, you shall retain the right to use the substance of the above work in future works, on condition that you acknowledge its prior publication in the journal, and to the publishers Psychology Press Ltd.

A complimentary copy of the issue in which your article appears will be sent to the principal or sole author of articles; book reviewers will be sent three copies of the issue free of charge. Offprints may be ordered at a special discount price. An order form will accompany the proof.

Submissions and books for, or offers to, review should be sent to an Editor, address on inside front cover.

Style Guides

Please refer to the following website for the journal style guide, and for more information on our other journals and books: http://www.psypress.co.uk

''This publication has been produced with paper manufactured to strict environmental standards and with pulp derived from sustainable forests''.